THE SOCIAL MEDICINE READER

Volume 1, Third Edition

THE SOCIAL MEDICINE READER

VOLUME

1

THIRD EDITION

Ethics and Cultures of Biomedicine

Jonathan Oberlander, Mara Buchbinder, Larry R. Churchill,

Sue E. Estroff, Nancy M. P. King, Barry F. Saunders,

Ronald P. Strauss, and Rebecca L. Walker, eds.

DUKE UNIVERSITY PRESS · DURHAM AND LONDON · 2019

© 2019 Duke University Press
All rights reserved
Printed and bound by CPI Group
(UK) Ltd, Croydon, CR0 4YY
Designed by Matthew Tauch
Typeset in Minion Pro by Westchester
PublishingSer vices

Library of Congress Cataloging-in-Publication Data
Names: Oberlander, Jonathan, editor.
Title: The social medicine reader / Jonathan
Oberlander, Mara Buchbinder, Larry R. Churchill,
Sue E. Estroff, Nancy M. P. King, Barry F. Saunders,
Ronald P. Strauss, Rebecca L. Walker, editors.
Description: Third edition. | Durham : Duke
University Press, 2019– | Includes bibliographical
references and index.
Identifiers: LCCN 2018044276 (print)
LCCN 2019000395 (ebook)
ISBN 9781478004356 (ebook)
ISBN 9781478001737
ISBN 9781478001737 (v. 1 ; hardcover ; alk. paper)
ISBN 9781478002819 (v. 1 ; pbk. ; alk. paper)
Subjects: LCSH: Social medicine.
Classification: LCC RA418 (ebook) | LCC RA418 .S6424
2019 (print) | DDC 362.1—dc23
LC record available at https://lccn.loc.gov/2018044276

Contents

PART III. Health Care Ethics and the Clinician's Role

PART IV. Death, Dying, and Lives at the Margins

PART V. Allocation and Justice

Preface to the Third Edition

The eight editors of this third edition of the *Social Medicine Reader* include six current and two former members of the Department of Social Medicine in the University of North Carolina (UNC) at Chapel Hill School of Medicine. Founded in 1977, the Department of Social Medicine, which includes scholars in medicine, the social sciences, the humanities, and public health, is committed to the promotion and provision of multidisciplinary education, leadership, service, research, and scholarship at the intersection of medicine and society. This includes a focus on the social conditions and characteristics of patients and populations; the social dimensions of illness; the ethical and social contexts of medical care, institutions, and professions; and resource allocation and health care policy.

This two-volume reader reflects the syllabus of a year-long, required interdisciplinary course that has been taught to first-year medical students at UNC since 1978. The goal of the course since its inception has been to demonstrate that medicine and medical practice have a profound influence on—and are influenced by—social, cultural, political, and economic matters. Teaching this perspective requires integrating medical and nonmedical materials and viewpoints. Therefore, this reader incorporates pieces from many fields within medicine, the social sciences, and humanities, representing the most engaging, provocative, and informative materials and issues we have traversed with our students.

Medicine's impact on society is multidimensional. Medicine shapes how we think about the most fundamental, enduring human experiences—conception, birth, maturation, sickness, suffering, healing, aging, and death—as well as the metaphors we use to express our deepest concerns. Medical practices and social responses to them have helped to redefine the meanings of age, race, and gender.

Social forces likewise have a powerful influence on medicine. Medical knowledge and practice, like all knowledge and practice, are shaped by political, cultural, and economic forces. This includes modern science's pursuit of knowledge through ostensibly neutral, objective observation and experimentation. Physicians' ideas about disease—in fact their very definitions of disease—depend on the roles that science and scientists play in particular cultures, as well as on the various cultures of laboratory and clinical science. Despite the power of the biomedical model of disease and the increasing specificity of molecular and genetic knowledge, social factors have always influenced the occurrence and course of most diseases. And once disease has occurred, the power of medicine to alter its course is constrained by the larger social, economic, and political contexts.

While the origin of these volumes lies in teaching medical students, we believe the selections they include will resonate with a broader readership from allied health fields, the medical humanities, bioethics, arts and sciences, and the interested public. The many voices represented in these readings include individual narratives of illness experience, commentaries by physicians, debate about complex medical cases and practices, and conceptually and empirically based scholarly writings. These are readings with the literary and scholarly power to convey the complicated relationships between medicine, health, and society. They do not resolve the most vexing contemporary issues, but they do illuminate their nuances and complexities, inviting discussion and debate.

Repeatedly, the readings throughout these two volumes make clear that much of what we encounter in science, in society, and in everyday and extraordinary lives is indeterminate, ambiguous, complex, and contradictory. And because of this inherent ambiguity, the interwoven selections highlight conflicts about power and authority, autonomy and choice, and security and risk. By critically analyzing these and many other related issues, we can open up possibilities, change what may seem inevitable, and practice professional training and caregiving with an increased capacity for reflection and self-examination. The goal is to ignite and fuel the inner voices of social and moral analysis among health care professionals, and among us all.

Any scholarly anthology is open to challenges about what has been included and what has been left out. This collection is no exception. The study of medicine and society is dynamic, with large and ever-expanding bodies of literature from which to draw. We have omitted some readings widely considered to be "classics" and have included some readings that are exciting and new—that we believe have an indelible impact. We have chosen to include material with literary and scholarly merit and that has worked well in the classroom, provoking discussion and engaging readers' imaginations. These readings invite critical examination, a labor of reading and discussion that is inherently difficult but educationally rewarding.

Volume 1, *Ethics and Cultures of Biomedicine*, examines experiences of illness; the roles and training of health care professionals and their relationships with patients; institutional cultures of bioscience and medicine; health care ethics; death and dying; and resource allocation and justice. Volume 2, *Differences and Inequalities*, explores health and illness, focusing on how difference and disability are defined and experienced in contemporary America, and how social categories commonly used to predict disease outcomes—gender, race/ethnicity, and social class—shape health outcomes and medical care.

We thank our teaching colleagues who helped create and refine all three editions of this reader. These colleagues have come over the years from both within and outside the Department of Social Medicine and the University of North Carolina at Chapel Hill. Equal gratitude goes to our students, whose criticism and enthusiasm over four decades have improved our teaching and have influenced us greatly in making the selections for the reader. We thank the Department's faculty and staff, past and present; students and colleagues from Vanderbilt University School of Medicine and Wake Forest School of Medicine have similarly been instrumental. We especially thank Kathy Crosier, the course coordinator for our first-year class, who assisted with the preparation of the *Reader*. The editors gratefully acknowledge support from the Department of Social Medicine, University of North Carolina at Chapel Hill School of Medicine; the Center for Biomedical Ethics and Society, Vanderbilt University School of Medicine; and the Center for Bioethics, Health, and Society, Wake Forest University.

Introduction

This first of the two volumes that comprise the *Social Medicine Reader* thematically explores the experiences of illness; the roles and training of health care professionals and their relationships with patients alongside the broader cultures of biomedicine; ethics in health care; experiences and decisions regarding death, dying, and struggling to live; and particular manifestations of injustice in the broader health system. The volume's readings, which include narratives, essays, cases studies, fiction, and poetry, have been "road-tested" in social science, ethics, and humanities classes in health professional schools and graduate and undergraduate programs. They have been used to stimulate debate and small-group interactions or exercises, and they have served as launching points for larger class discussions. We do not cover any content area completely; our goal instead is to provide stimulating selected readings from which to engage students in discussion and deeper investigation.

The eight editors of this volume are diverse in their scholarly backgrounds, expertise, and teaching styles. We each teach the same materials differently and have learned much from each other through many years of faculty meetings focused on teaching and pedagogy. Our collaboration exemplifies the adaptability of the volume's readings to a variety of formats, settings, and approaches.

Beginning this volume with experiences of illness helps to ground the nature and meaning of sickness and healing in the familiar yet uniquely experienced state of being a patient. All health care providers have been, and will be again, patients and family members of patients. Vivid narratives about managing illness in daily life help build understanding of the vantage points of patients and family members who participate in illness experiences. Teachers and students unaccustomed to fiction and poetry in the classroom may be surprised at how readily these materials can stimulate rich and nuanced discussion of profoundly significant issues—especially when read aloud. While the first part of the volume is particularly rich in these forms of literature, such selections appear in most other parts of the volume as well.

In the second part of the volume, medical socialization and the doctor-patient relationship are considered. Social scientists have extensively examined the processes that transform medical students into counselors of health and interveners in issues of life and death. Professions, like other social groups, have cultures: they have specialized languages and ways of understanding, norms of behavior, unique customs, rites of passage, and codes of conduct. Students are socialized into the "culture of biomedicine" in a training process that changes the student through direct contact with and knowledge of the most personal aspects of human existence. Many students enter medical school with idealistic views of medicine, its goals, and its basis in evidence. As they learn the ideology and ethics of medicine and uncover the complex evidence base that medicine puts into practice, they may face uncertainty that is too often left unstated in public; they may undergo profound changes in their perspectives and even their identities. These readings promote reflection on the roles of health professional students and practitioners, on the challenges inherent in the physician-patient relationship, and on navigating between professional and personal experiences, values, and truths.

The third part of the volume turns to a more explicit focus on health care ethics. This section includes narratives (fiction and nonfiction) of clinician and patient experiences, as well as theoretical framing and professional guidance. Readings examine moral reasoning and what it means to have a moral life as a clinician in relationships with patients. Fundamental moral precepts in health care practice—truth-telling, informed consent, privacy, autonomy, and beneficence—are addressed in their own right and also presented in cases and stories that pose problems to be unraveled, examined, and debated from a wide range of viewpoints. In this section, complex ethical issues are presented as dynamic: embedded in time, place, society, history, and culture, and entangled in multiple relationships.

The fourth part of this volume employs the prior themes to address decision making, policies, and experiences at the margins of life—including death, dying, and struggling to live. The work of this section includes an effort to clarify concepts; an examination of significant social disagreements and moments in end-of-life decision making; and specific attention to life prolongation, treatment withdrawal, and the ending of life, whether welcome or unwelcome. Questions are raised about the legal, ethical, and practical medical aspects of end-of-life care, the nature and power of medical judgments, and long-standing professional and personal disagreements about the end of life. Poetry, personal narrative, and the voices of patients and their families open the possibility for discussion of morality, meaning, loss, grief, and profound uncertainty in the face of death.

The final section of this volume approaches justice and allocation through a few examples not commonly addressed in texts on distributive justice in health care. Because there are many more comprehensive treatments of health-related justice issues in other volumes, our goal here is to introduce the relevant concepts and illustrate the wide diversity of ways in which injustice is hiding in plain sight in medicine.

The variety of readings in this volume can be addressed productively from different disciplinary perspectives and in many teaching styles and formats. These readings are readily combined with those from volume 2 of the *Social Medicine Reader*, titled *Differences and Inequalities*. Readings from both volumes can be reshuffled and recombined, stand together or alone, or be supplemented by other literature. A key to using these readings successfully is to approach them with flexibility—as helping to shape the right questions rather than giving particular answers. Our hope is that both teachers and students of materials like these will go on asking questions, and finding different and deeper answers, all their lives.

EXPERIENCES OF ILLNESS AND CLINICIAN-PATIENT RELATIONSHIPS

I

Silver Water

Amy Bloom

My sister's voice was like mountain water in a silver pitcher; the clear blue beauty of it cools you and lifts you up beyond your heat, beyond your body. After we went to see *La Traviata*, when she was fourteen and I was twelve, she elbowed me in the parking lot and said, "Check this out." And she opened her mouth unnaturally wide and her voice came out, so crystalline and bright that all the departing operagoers stood frozen by their cars, unable to take out their keys or open their doors until she had finished, and then they cheered like hell.

That's what I like to remember, and that's the story I told to all of her therapists. I wanted them to know her, to know that who they saw was not all there was to see. That before her constant tinkling of commercials and fast-food jingles there had been Puccini and Mozart and hymns so sweet and mighty you expected Jesus to come down off his cross and clap. That before there was a mountain of Thorazined fat, swaying down the halls in nylon maternity tops and sweatpants, there had been the prettiest girl in Arrandale Elementary School, the belle of Landmark Junior High. Maybe there were other pretty girls, but I didn't see them. To me, Rose, my beautiful blond defender, my guide to Tampax and my mother's moods, was perfect.

She had her first psychotic break when she was fifteen. She had been coming home moody and tearful, then quietly beaming, then she stopped coming home. She would go out into the woods behind our house and not come in until my mother went after her at dusk, and stepped gently into the briars and saplings and pulled her out, blank-faced, her pale blue sweater covered with crumbled leaves, her white jeans smeared with dirt. After three weeks of this, my mother, who is a musician and widely regarded as eccentric, said to my father, who is a psychiatrist and a kind, sad man, "She's going off."

"What is that, your professional opinion?" He picked up the newspaper and put it down again, sighing. "I'm sorry, I didn't mean to snap at you. I know something's bothering her. Have you talked to her?"

"What's there to say? David, she's going crazy. She doesn't need a heart-to-heart talk with Mom, she needs a hospital."

They went back and forth, and my father sat down with Rose for a few hours, and she sat there licking the hairs on her forearm, first one way, then the other. My mother stood in the hallway, dry-eyed and pale, watching the two of them. She had already packed, and when three of my father's friends dropped by to offer free consultations and recommendations, my mother and Rose's suitcase were already in the car. My mother hugged me and told me that they would be back that night, but not with Rose. She also said, divining my worst fear, "It won't happen to you, honey. Some people go crazy and some people never do. You never will." She smiled and stroked my hair. "Not even when you want to."

Rose was in hospitals, great and small, for the next ten years. She had lots of terrible therapists and a few good ones. One place had no pictures on the walls, no windows, and the patients all wore slippers with the hospital crest on them. My mother didn't even bother to go to Admissions. She turned Rose around and the two of them marched out, my father walking behind them, apologizing to his colleagues. My mother ignored the psychiatrists, the social workers, and the nurses, and played Handel and Bessie Smith for the patients on whatever was available. At some places, she had a Steinway donated by a grateful, or optimistic, family; at others, she banged out "Gimme a Pigfoot and a Bottle of Beer" on an old, scarred box that hadn't been tuned since there'd been English-speaking physicians on the grounds. My father talked in serious, appreciative tones to the administrators and unit chiefs and tried to be friendly with whoever was managing Rose's case. We all hated the family therapists.

The worst family therapist we ever had sat in a pale green room with us, visibly taking stock of my mother's ethereal beauty and her faded blue T-shirt and girl-sized jeans, my father's rumpled suit and stained tie, and my own unreadable seventeen-year-old fashion statement. Rose was beyond fashion that year, in one of her dancing teddy bear smocks and extra-extra-large Celtics sweatpants. Mr. Walker read Rose's file in front of us and then watched in alarm as Rose began crooning, beautifully, and slowly massaging her breasts. My mother and I laughed, and even my father started to smile. This was Rose's usual opening salvo for new therapists.

Mr. Walker said, "I wonder why it is that everyone is so entertained by Rose behaving inappropriately."

Rose burped and then we all laughed. This was the seventh family therapist we had seen, and none of them had lasted very long. Mr. Walker, unfortunately, was determined to do right by us.

"What do you think of Rose's behavior, Violet?" They did this sometimes. In their manual it must say, If you think the parents are too weird, try talking to the sister.

"I don't know. Maybe she's trying to get you to stop talking about her in the third person."

"Nicely put," my mother said.

"Indeed," my father said.

"Fuckin' A," Rose said.

"Well, this is something that the whole family agrees upon," Mr. Walker said, trying to act as if he understood or even liked us.

"That was not a successful intervention, Ferret Face." Rose tended to function better when she was angry. He did look like a blond ferret, and we all laughed again. Even my father, who tried to give these people a chance, out of some sense of collegiality, had given it up.

After fourteen minutes, Mr. Walker decided that our time was up and walked out, leaving us grinning at each other. Rose was still nuts, but at least we'd all had a little fun.

The day we met our best family therapist started out almost as badly. We scared off a resident and then scared off her supervisor, who sent us Dr. Thorne. Three hundred pounds of Texas chili, cornbread, and Lone Star beer, finished off with big black cowboy boots and a small string tie around the area of his neck.

"O frabjous day, it's Big Nut." Rose was in heaven and stopped massaging her breasts immediately.

"Hey, Little Nut." You have to understand how big a man would have to be to call my sister "little." He christened us all, right away. "And it's the good Doctor Nut, and Madame Hickory Nut, 'cause they are the hardest damn nuts to crack, and over here in the overalls and not much else is No One's Nut"—a name that summed up both my sanity and my loneliness. We all relaxed.

Dr. Thorne was good for us. Rose moved into a halfway house whose director loved Big Nut so much that she kept Rose even when Rose went through a period of having sex with everyone who passed her door. She was in a fever for a while, trying to still the voices by fucking her brains out.

Big Nut said, "Darlin', I can't. I cannot make love to every beautiful woman I meet, and furthermore, I can't do that and be your therapist too. It's a great shame, but I think you might be able to find a really nice guy, someone who treats you just as sweet and kind as I would if I were lucky enough to be your beau. I don't want you to settle for less." And she stopped propositioning the crack addicts and the alcoholics and the guys at the shelter. We loved Dr. Thorne.

My father went back to seeing rich neurotics and helped out one day a week at Dr. Thorne's Walk-In Clinic. My mother finished a recording of Mozart concerti and played at fund-raisers for Rose's halfway house. I went back to college and found a wonderful linebacker from Texas to sleep with. In the dark, I would make him call me "darlin'." Rose took her meds, lost about fifty pounds, and began singing at the A.M.E. Zion Church, down the street from the halfway house.

At first they didn't know what to do with this big blond lady, dressed funny and hovering wistfully in the doorway during their rehearsals, but she gave them a few bars of "Precious Lord" and the choir director felt God's hand and saw that with the help of His sweet child Rose, the Prospect Street Choir was going all the way to the Gospel Olympics.

Amidst a sea of beige, umber, cinnamon, and espresso faces, there was Rose, bigger, blonder, and pinker than any two white women could be. And Rose and the choir's contralto, Addie Robicheaux, laid out their gold and silver voices and wove them together in strands as fine as silk, as strong as steel. And we wept as Rose and Addie, in their billowing garnet robes, swayed together, clasping hands until the last perfect note floated up to God, and then they smiled down at us.

Rose would still go off from time to time and the voices would tell her to do bad things, but Dr. Thorne or Addie or my mother could usually bring her back. After five good years, Big Nut died. Stuffing his face with a chili dog, sitting in his un-air-conditioned office in the middle of July, he had one big, Texas-sized aneurysm and died.

Rose held on tight for seven days; she took her meds, went to choir practice, and rearranged her room about a hundred times. His funeral was like a Lourdes for the mentally ill. If you were psychotic, borderline, bad-off neurotic, or just very hard to get along with, you were there. People shaking so bad from years of heavy meds that they fell out of the pews. People holding hands, crying, moaning, talking to themselves. The crazy people and the not-so-crazy people were all huddled together, like puppies at the pound.

Rose stopped taking her meds, and the halfway house wouldn't keep her after she pitched another patient down the stairs. My father called the insurance company and found out that Rose's new, improved psychiatric coverage wouldn't begin for forty-five days. I put all of her stuff in a garbage bag, and we walked out of the halfway house, Rose winking at the poor drooling boy on the couch.

"This is going to be difficult—not all bad, but difficult—for the whole family, and I thought we should discuss everybody's expectations. I know I have some concerns." My father had convened a family meeting as soon as Rose finished putting each one of her thirty stuffed bears in its own special place.

"No meds," Rose said, her eyes lowered, her stubby fingers, those fingers that had braided my hair and painted tulips on my cheeks, pulling hard on the hem of her dirty smock.

My father looked in despair at my mother.

"Rosie, do you want to drive the new car?" my mother asked.

Rose's face lit up. "I'd love to drive that car. I'd drive to California, I'd go see the bears at the San Diego Zoo. I would take you, Violet, but you always hated the zoo. Remember how she cried at the Bronx Zoo when she found out that the animals didn't get to go home at closing?" Rose put her damp hand on mine and squeezed it sympathetically. "Poor Vi."

"If you take your medication, after a while you'll be able to drive the car. That's the deal. Meds, car." My mother sounded accommodating but unenthusiastic, careful not to heat up Rose's paranoia.

"You got yourself a deal, darlin'."

I was living about an hour away then, teaching English during the day, writing poetry at night. I went home every few days for dinner. I called every night.

My father said, quietly, "It's very hard. We're doing all right, I think. Rose has been walking in the mornings with your mother, and she watches a lot of TV. She won't go to the day hospital, and she won't go back to the choir. Her friend Mrs. Robicheaux came by a couple of times. What a sweet woman. Rose wouldn't even talk to her. She just sat there, staring at the wall and humming. We're not doing all that well, actually, but I guess we're getting by. I'm sorry, sweetheart, I don't mean to depress you."

My mother said, emphatically, "We're doing fine. We've got our routine and we stick to it and we're fine. You don't need to come home so often, you know. Wait 'til Sunday, just come for the day. Lead your life, Vi. She's leading hers."

I stayed away all week, afraid to pick up my phone, grateful to my mother for her harsh calm and her reticence, the qualities that had enraged me throughout my childhood.

I came on Sunday, in the early afternoon, to help my father garden, something we had always enjoyed together. We weeded and staked tomatoes and killed aphids while my mother and Rose were down at the lake. I didn't even go into the house until four, when I needed a glass of water.

Someone had broken the piano bench into five neatly stacked pieces and placed them where the piano bench usually was.

"We were having such a nice time, I couldn't bear to bring it up," my father said, standing in the doorway, carefully keeping his gardening boots out of the kitchen.

"What did Mommy say?"

"She said, 'Better the bench than the piano.' And your sister lay down on the floor and just wept. Then your mother took her down to the lake. This can't go on, Vi. We have twenty-seven days left, your mother gets no sleep because Rose doesn't sleep, and if I could just pay twenty-seven thousand dollars to keep her in the hospital until the insurance takes over, I'd do it."

"All right. Do it. Pay the money and take her back to Hartley-Rees. It was the prettiest place, and she liked the art therapy there."

"I would if I could. The policy states that she must be symptom-free for at least forty-five days before her coverage begins. Symptom-free means no hospitalization."

"Jesus, Daddy, how could you get that kind of policy? She hasn't been symptom-free for forty-five minutes."

"It's the only one I could get for long-term psychiatric." He put his hand over his mouth, to block whatever he was about to say, and went back out to the garden. I couldn't see if he was crying.

He stayed outside and I stayed inside until Rose and my mother came home from the lake. Rose's soggy sweatpants were rolled up to her knees, and she had a bucketful of shells and seaweed, which my mother persuaded her to leave on the back porch. My mother kissed me lightly and told Rose to go up to her room and change out of her wet pants.

Rose's eyes grew very wide. "Never. I will never . . ." She knelt down and began banging her head on the kitchen floor with rhythmic intensity, throwing all her weight behind each attack. My mother put her arms around Rose's waist and tried to hold her back. Rose shook her off, not even looking around to see what was slowing her down. My mother lay up against the refrigerator.

"Violet, please . . ."

I threw myself onto the kitchen floor, becoming the spot that Rose was smacking her head against. She stopped a fraction of an inch short of my stomach.

"Oh, Vi, Mommy, I'm sorry. I'm sorry, don't hate me." She staggered to her feet and ran wailing to her room.

My mother got up and washed her face brusquely, rubbing it dry with a dishcloth. My father heard the wailing and came running in, slipping his long bare feet out of his rubber boots.

"Galen, Galen, let me see." He held her head and looked closely for bruises on her pale, small face. "What happened?" My mother looked at me. "Violet, what happened? Where's Rose?"

"Rose got upset, and when she went running upstairs she pushed Mommy out of the way." I've only told three lies in my life, and that was my second.

"She must feel terrible, pushing you, of all people. It would have to be you, but I know she didn't want it to be." He made my mother a cup of tea, and all the love he had for her, despite her silent rages and her vague stares, came pouring through the teapot, warming her cup, filling her small, long-fingered hands. She rested her head against his hip, and I looked away.

"Let's make dinner, then I'll call her. Or you call her, David, maybe she'd rather see your face first."

Dinner was filled with all of our starts and stops and Rose's desperate efforts to control herself. She could barely eat and hummed the McDonald's theme song over and over again, pausing only to spill her juice down the front of her smock and begin weeping. My father looked at my mother and handed Rose his napkin. She dabbed at herself listlessly, but the tears stopped.

"I want to go to bed. I want to go to bed and be in my head. I want to go to bed and be in my bed and in my head and just wear red. For red is the color that my baby wore and once more, it's true, yes, it is, it's true. Please don't wear red tonight, oh, oh, please don't wear red tonight, for red is the color—"

"Okay, okay, Rose. It's okay. I'll go upstairs with you and you can get ready for bed. Then Mommy will come up and say good night too. It's okay, Rose." My father reached out his hand and Rose grasped it, and they walked out of the dining room together, his long arm around her middle.

My mother sat at the table for a moment, her face in her hands, and then she began clearing the plates. We cleared without talking, my mother humming Schubert's "Schlummerlied," a lullaby about the woods and the river calling to the child to go to sleep. She sang it to us every night when we were small.

My father came into the kitchen and signaled to my mother. They went upstairs and came back down together a few minutes later.

"She's asleep," they said, and we went to sit on the porch and listen to the crickets. I don't remember the rest of the evening, but I remember it as quietly sad, and I remember the rare sight of my parents holding hands, sitting on the picnic table, watching the sunset.

I woke up at three o'clock in the morning, feeling the cool night air through my sheet. I went down the hall for a blanket and looked into Rose's room, for no reason. She wasn't there. I put on my jeans and a sweater and went downstairs. I could feel her absence. I went outside and saw her wide, draggy footprints darkening the wet grass into the woods.

"Rosie," I called, too softly, not wanting to wake my parents, not wanting to startle Rose. "Rosie, it's me. Are you here? Are you all right?"

I almost fell over her. Huge and white in the moonlight, her flowered smock bleached in the light and shadow, her sweatpants now completely wet. Her head was flung back, her white, white neck exposed like a lost Greek column.

"Rosie, Rosie—" Her breathing was very slow, and her lips were not as pink as they usually were. Her eyelids fluttered.

"Closing time," she whispered. I believe that's what she said.

I sat with her, uncovering the bottle of white pills by her hand, and watched the stars fade.

When the stars were invisible and the sun was warming the air, I went back to the house. My mother was standing on the porch, wrapped in a blanket, watching me. Every step I took overwhelmed me; I could picture my mother slapping me, shooting me for letting her favorite die.

"Warrior queens," she said, wrapping her thin strong arms around me. "I raised warrior queens." She kissed me fiercely and went into the woods by herself.

Later in the morning she woke my father, who could not go into the woods, and still later she called the police and the funeral parlor. She hung up the phone, lay down, and didn't get back out of bed until the day of the funeral. My father fed us both and called the people who needed to be called and picked out Rose's coffin by himself.

My mother played the piano and Addie sang her pure gold notes and I closed my eyes and saw my sister, fourteen years old, lion's mane thrown back and eyes tightly closed against the glare of the parking lot lights. That sweet sound held us tight, flowing around us, eddying through our hearts, rising, still rising.

"Is *She* Experiencing Any Pain?"

Disability and the Physician-Patient Relationship

S. K. Toombs

As a person who lives with chronic progressive neurological disease (multiple sclerosis) and significant disability, I have an intimate knowledge of the physician-patient relationship from the perspective of the patient. Over the years, I have become aware that chronic disability poses unique challenges in the clinical context—challenges that, if unrecognized, can unwittingly undermine even the most well-intentioned efforts to provide optimal care.

In reflecting on these challenges, I want to begin by stressing that chronic disability means much more to the patient than simply a mechanical dysfunction or discrete disease process. Living with permanent incapacity represents a distinct way of being-in-the-world, a way of being that affects one's sense of self, one's relationships with others, one's ability to interact in (and with) the surrounding world, one's family and professional life, one's ability to exercise control and to be autonomous, and one's relationship with one's body.[1] Given the chronic nature of such bodily disorder, it is not possible to restore the patient to a former state of health characterized by the absence of bodily malfunction. Consequently, the clinical goal must be broadened to encompass not only the cure of disease but, as importantly, the project of assisting patients to live well in the face of ongoing bodily limitation. An important way to conceive this project is to focus on personal (and not simply bodily) well-being. By functioning well at the personal level, I have in mind such things as being able to engage in activities that are meaningful, sustaining important relationships, and retaining a sense of personal integrity.

S. K. Toombs, "'Is *She* Experiencing Any Pain?': Disability and the Physician-Patient Relationship," from *Internal Medicine Journal* 34, no. 11 (2004): 645–647. Reprinted by permission of John Wiley and Sons.

In stressing personal, as opposed to bodily, well-being, it is important to make a sharp distinction between the functioning of the body and the functioning of the person. The prevailing biomedical model of illness and the overriding focus on physical pathology gives priority to the well functioning of the physical organism—with the assumption that if the body functions well so does the person. In the case of chronic disability, this assumption is deeply problematic. For example, quantitative measurements of disability, in and of themselves, do not convey whether a patient can function well at the personal level. In my own case, functioning well at the personal level does not depend on whether I can walk, although it does relate to my ability to manage my illness in such a way that I can pursue those projects that are meaningful to me.

Focusing primarily on assessments of physical functioning as the most accurate measure of wellness can paradoxically disrupt the task of functioning well at the personal level. Patients and medical professionals alike might be tempted to pursue medical interventions that are extremely disruptive of the patient's life and that result in minimal improvement in bodily function. I learned this lesson personally when undergoing a course of chemotherapy in an attempt to slow down the progression of my disease. The treatment was worse than the illness. Monthly infusions of Cytoxan (cyclophosphamide; Bristol-Myers Squibbs, New York, NY) caused nausea, vomiting and prostrating weakness for three of every four weeks. After four months, I chose to discontinue the treatment on the grounds that it totally disrupted my life. Although my neurologist supported my decision, he voiced disappointment and pointed out that tests indicated a slight improvement in my ability to lift my right leg. However, for me, this minimal gain in physical function was not worth the erosion in my quality of life.

Weighing the harms and benefits of treatment is more difficult for those living with chronic disability. If one has an acute disease, one knows that the disruption of treatment will be short lived, with an end result of cure. Consequently, the certainty of future benefit enables one to "put up with" temporary discomfort, even if it is extreme. However, when future benefit is uncertain and disruption is ongoing, patients and physicians must take seriously the impact of therapy on the patient's quality of life. Even noninvasive tests can be particularly difficult for people with disabilities. As an example, for someone like myself with compromised bladder and bowel control, tests that involve drinking large amounts of fluids (or cleansing the gastrointestinal tract) can be especially burdensome.

Physical barriers also make testing difficult for people with disabilities. A survey in the United States showed that women with severe disabilities are less likely to receive annual pelvic exams than able-bodied women, and 23 percent of women with spinal cord injuries reported that it was impossible to have a mammogram, either because the equipment could not be positioned for them or because there was no accessible room for mammograms.[2] Indeed, very few doctors' offices have accessible examining tables, which makes even a routine physical examination problematic for someone who uses a wheelchair.

One of the most debilitating aspects of chronic disability is the loss of bodily control. An important task for clinicians is that of assisting patients to develop concrete strategies to compensate for bodily limitation. It is vitally important that patients recognize there is always some level of control that one can exercise, even in the face of increasingly disruptive symptoms. This task is not limited to instituting medical treatment. Rather, it involves exploring with the individual patient the specific manner in which bodily malfunction disrupts his or her life at the personal level. In this connection, it is helpful not simply to ask patients specific questions, such as "Are you experiencing increased spasticity?," but to include more global inquiries, such as "What is the most difficult thing for you to deal with in your daily life?" Sometimes even simple strategies, such as controlling intake of fluids to minimize the risk of incontinence in social situations, learning to adjust daily schedules to compensate for fatigue, or acquiring mobility aids to counteract weakening muscles, can significantly improve a patient's quality of life. For example, if a patient is greatly fatigued by the effort of walking, using a wheelchair might conserve energy and permit increased social interaction, resulting in a much fuller personal and social life. In this respect, choosing to use a wheelchair is not to be equated with "giving in" to the disease. Rather, "giving up" in one area might well free the patient to embrace other important areas of life.

Of course, it is vital that physicians recognize the extent to which negative cultural attitudes make it extraordinarily difficult for people with disabilities to retain a sense of personal well-being in the face of permanent physical incapacity. We live in a culture that places inordinate value on independence, beauty, health, and physical fitness. People with disabilities are far from the ideal. In the eyes of the able-bodied, there is a widespread assumption that disability is incompatible with living a meaningful life. When others observe I am in a wheelchair, they make the immediate judgement that my situation is an essentially negative one, that I am unable to engage in professional activities, and that I am wholly dependent on others. On many occasions strangers have said to me "Aren't you *lucky* to have your husband?" This is not so much a comment about my husband's character as it is a perception that my relationship with him is purely one of burdensome dependence. In observing my physical incapacities, people assume that my intellect is likewise affected. Strangers invariably address questions to my companion and refer to me in the third person: "Where would *she* like to sit?," "Would *she* like us to move this chair?" Such negative responses from others are demeaning and reinforce the sense that disability reduces personal and social worth. Unfortunately, such attitudes also exist in the clinical context. In a national survey, women with severe disabilities reported that if they were accompanied by another person, more often than not the doctor addressed questions to their companion rather than speaking to them directly (Nosek *et al.* unpubl. data 1992, 1995): "Is *she* experiencing any pain?"

An important way for physicians to promote personal well-being is to consciously reject such stereotypical attitudes about persons with disabilities. Indeed, patients with chronic disabilities have an especially important role to play in the physician-patient relationship. Those of us who live with permanent bodily disorder have an intimate knowledge of our bodies as we must constantly pay attention to them. Thus, we are often aware of even minute changes in function and sensation (changes that might not be readily apparent to the physician). Although physicians have the expert medical knowledge to comprehend and assess the disease process, patients with chronic disabilities have an equally expert knowledge of what is "normal" and "abnormal" with respect to their own bodily experience. Both types of knowledge are essential to the task of assessing and dealing with bodily disorder. People with disabilities are also experts at knowing how best to work with their recalcitrant bodies—a knowledge that is too often disregarded by medical professionals. As an example, Robillard (a quadriplegic) describes his frustration when trying to tell X-ray crews how to position his body to avoid muscle and coughing spasms, only to be ignored and informed erroneously that (as professionals) they "knew what they were doing."[3]

In conclusion, I would like to stress that, although chronic disability poses specific challenges, it also provides a significant opportunity in the doctor-patient relationship. The shift in focus from bodily to personal well-being (a shift that involves exploring with patients the multiplicity of ways in which ongoing disability impacts on their daily lives) and the necessity of including the patient as an active participant in the long-term management of a chronic condition provide an exceptional occasion for clinicians to forge close and rewarding partnerships with patients.

1   Toombs SK. Reflections on bodily change: the lived experience of disability. In: Toombs
    SK, ed. *Handbook of Phenomenology and Medicine*. Dordrecht, The Netherlands: Klu-
    wer Academic Publications; 2001:247–261.

2   Nosek MA, Howland CA. Breast and cervical cancer screening among women with
    physical disabilities. *Arch Phys Med Rehabil*. 1997;78(Suppl 5):S39–44.

3   Robillard AB. *The Meaning of Disability: The Lived Experience of Paralysis*. Philadel-
    phia: Temple University Press; 1999.

The Cost of Appearances

Arthur Frank

Society praises ill persons with words such as "courageous," "optimistic," and "cheerful." Family and friends speak approvingly of the patient who jokes or just smiles, making them, the visitors, feel good. Everyone around the ill person becomes committed to the idea that recovery is the only outcome worth thinking about. No matter what the actual odds, an attitude of "You're going to be fine" dominates the sickroom. Everyone works to sustain it. But how much work does the ill person have to do to make others feel good?

Two kinds of emotional work are involved in being ill. One kind I have written about takes place when the ill person, alone or with true caregivers, works with the emotions of fear, frustration, and loss and tries to find some coherence about what it means to be ill. The other kind is the work the ill person does to keep up an appearance. This appearance is the expectation that a society of healthy friends, coworkers, medical staff, and others places on an ill person.

The appearance most praised is "I'd hardly have known she was sick." At home the ill person must appear to be engaged in normal family routines; in the hospital she should appear to be just resting. When the ill person can no longer conceal the effects of illness, she is expected to convince others that being ill isn't that bad. The minimal acceptable behavior is praised, faintly, as "stoical." But the ill person may not feel like acting good-humored and positive; much of the time it takes hard work to hold this appearance in place.

I have never heard an ill person praised for how well she expressed fear or grief or was openly sad. On the contrary, ill persons feel a need to apologize if they show any emotions other than laughter. Occasional tears may be passed off as the ill person's need to "let go"; the tears are categorized as temporary outbursts instead of understood as part of an ongoing emotion. Sustained "negative" emotions are out of place. If a patient shows too much sadness, he must be depressed, and "depression" is a treatable medical disease.

Too few people, whether medical staff, family, or friends, seem willing to accept the possibility that depression may be the ill person's most appropriate response to the situation. I am not recommending depression but I do want to suggest that at some moments even fairly deep depression must be accepted as part of the experience of illness.

A couple of days before my mother-in-law died, she shared a room with a woman who was also being treated for cancer. My mother-in-law was this woman's second dying roommate, and the woman was seriously ill herself. I have no doubt that her diagnosis of clinical depression was accurate. The issue is how the medical staff responded to her depression. Instead of trying to understand it as a reasonable response to her situation, her doctors treated her with antidepressant drugs. When a hospital psychologist came to visit her, his questions were designed only to evaluate her "mental status." What day is it? Where are you and what floor are you on? Who is prime minister? and so forth. His sole interest was whether the dosage of antidepressant drug was too high, upsetting her "cognitive orientation." The hospital needed her to be mentally competent so she would remain a "good patient" requiring little extra care; it did not need her emotions. No one attempted to explore her fears with her. No one asked what it was like to have two roommates die within a couple of days of each other, and how this affected her own fear of death. No one was willing to witness her experience.

What makes me saddest is seeing the work ill persons do to sustain this "cheerful patient" image. A close friend of ours, dying of cancer, seriously wondered how her condition could be getting worse, since she had brought homemade cookies to the treatment center whenever she had chemotherapy. She believed there had to be a causal connection between attitude and physical improvement. From early childhood on we are taught that attitude and effort count. "Good citizenship" is supposed to bring us extra points. The nurses all said what a wonderful woman our friend was. She was the perfectly brave, positive, cheerful cancer patient. To me she was most wonderful at the end, when she grieved her illness openly, dropped her act, and clearly demonstrated her anger. She lived her illness as she chose, and by the time she was acting on her anger and sadness, she was too sick for me to ask her if she wished she had expressed more of those emotions earlier. I can only wonder what it had cost her to sustain her happy image for so long.

When I tried to sustain a cheerful and tidy image, it cost me energy, which was scarce. It also cost me opportunities to express what *was* happening in my life with cancer and to understand that life. Finally, my attempts at a positive image diminished my relationships with others by preventing them from sharing my experience. But this image is all that many of those around an ill person are willing to see.

The other side of sustaining a "positive" image is denying that illness can end in death. Medical staff argue that patients who need to deny dying should be allowed to do so. The sad end of this process comes when the person is dying but has become too sick to express what he might now want to say to his loved ones, about his life and theirs. Then that person and his family are denied a final experience together; not all will choose this moment, but all have a right to it.

The medical staff do not have to be part of the tragedy of living with what was left unsaid. For them a patient who denies is one who is cheerful, makes few demands, and asks fewer questions. Some ill persons may need to deny, for reasons we cannot know. But it is too convenient for treatment providers to assume that the denial comes entirely from the patient, because this allows them not to recognize that they are cueing the patient. Labeling the ill person's behavior as denial describes it as a need of the patient, instead of understanding it as the patient's *response* to his situation. That situation, made up of the cues given by treatment providers and caregivers, is what shapes the ill person's behavior.

To be ill is to be dependent on medical staff, family, and friends. Since all these people value cheerfulness, the ill must summon up their energies to be cheerful. Denial may not be what they want or need, but it is what they perceive those around them wanting and needing. This is not the ill person's own denial, but rather his accommodation to the denial of others. When others around you are denying what is happening to you, denying it yourself can seem like your best deal.

To live among others is to make deals. We have to decide what support we need and what we must give others to get that support. Then we make our "best deal" of behavior to get what we need. This process is rarely a conscious one. It develops over a long time in so many experiences that it becomes the way we are, or what we call our personality. But behind much of what we call personality, deals are being made. In a crisis such as illness the terms of the deal rise to the surface and can be seen more clearly.

One incident can stand for all the deals I made during treatment. During my chemotherapy I had to spend three-day periods as an inpatient, receiving continuous drugs. In the three weeks or so between treatments I was examined weekly in the day-care part of the cancer center. Day care is a large room filled with easy chairs where patients sit while they are given briefer intravenous chemotherapy than mine. There are also beds, closely spaced with curtains between. Everyone can see everyone else and hear most of what is being said. Hospitals, however, depend on a myth of privacy. As soon as a curtain is pulled, that space is defined as private, and the patient is expected to answer all questions, no matter how intimate. The first time we went to day care, a young nurse interviewed Cathie and me to assess our "psychosocial" needs. In the middle of this medical bus station she began asking some reasonable questions. Were we experiencing difficulties at work because of my illness? Were we having any problems with our families? Were we getting support from them? These questions were precisely what a caregiver should ask. The problem was where they were being asked.

Our response to most of these questions was to lie. Without even looking at each other, we both understood that whatever problems we were having, we were not going to talk about them there. Why? To figure out our best deal, we had to assess the kind of support we thought we could get in that setting from that nurse. Nothing she did convinced us that what she could offer was equal to what we would risk by telling her the truth.

Admitting that you have problems makes you vulnerable, but it is also the only way to get help. Throughout my illness Cathie and I constantly weighed our need for help against the risk involved in making ourselves vulnerable. If we did not feel that support was forthcoming, we suppressed our need for expression. If we had expressed our problems and emotions in that very public setting, we would have been extremely vulnerable. If we had then received anything less than total support, it would have been devastating. The nurse showed no awareness or appreciation of how much her questions required us to risk, so we gave only a cheerful "no problems" response. That was all the setting seemed able to support.

Maybe we were wrong. Maybe the staff would have supported us if we had opened up about our problems with others' responses to my illness, our stress trying to keep our jobs going, and our fears and doubts about treatment. We certainly were aware that our responses cut off that support. It was double or nothing; we chose safety. Ill persons face such choices constantly. We still believe we were right to keep quiet. If the staff had had real support to offer, they would have offered it in a setting that encouraged our response. When we were alone with nurses in an inpatient room, the questions they asked were those on medical history forms. In the privacy of that room the nurses were vulnerable to the emotions we might have expressed, so they asked no "psychosocial" questions.

It was a lot of work for us to answer the day-care nurse's questions with a smile. Giving her the impression that we felt all right was draining, and illness and its care had drained us both already. But expending our energies this way seemed our best deal.

Anybody who wants to be a caregiver, particularly a professional, must not only have real support to offer but must also learn to convince the ill person that this support is there. My defenses have never been stronger than they were when I was ill. I have never watched others more closely or been more guarded around them. I needed others more than I ever have, and I was also most vulnerable to them. The behavior I worked to let others see was my most conservative estimate of what I thought they would support.

Again I can give no formula, only questions. To the ill person: How much is this best deal costing you in terms of emotional work? What are you compromising of your own expression of illness in order to present those around you with the cheerful appearance they want? What do you fear will happen if you act otherwise? And to those around the ill person: What cues are you giving the ill person that tell her how you want her to act? In what way is her behavior a response to your own? Whose denial, whose needs?

Fear and depression are a part of life. In illness there are no "negative emotions," only experiences that have to be lived through. What is needed in these moments is not denial but recognition. The ill person's suffering should be affirmed, whether or not it can be treated. What I wanted when I was most ill was the response, "Yes, we see your pain; we accept your fear." I needed others to recognize not only that I was suffering, but also that we had this suffering in common. I can accept that doctors and nurses sometimes fail to provide the correct treatment. But I cannot accept it when medical staff, family, and friends fail to recognize that they are equal participants in the process of illness. Their actions shape the behavior of the ill person, and their bodies share the potential of illness.

Those who make cheerfulness and bravery the price they require for support deny their own humanity. They deny that to be human is to be mortal, to become ill, and die. Ill persons need others to share in recognizing with them the frailty of the human body. When others join the ill person in this recognition, courage and cheer may be the result, not as an appearance to be worked at, but as a spontaneous expression of a common emotion.

The Ship Pounding

Donald Hall

Each morning I made my way
among gangways, elevators,
and nurses' pods to Jane's room
to interrogate grave helpers
who had tended her all night
like the ship's massive engines
that kept its propellers turning.
Week after week, I sat by her bed
with black coffee and the *Globe.*
The passengers on this voyage
wore masks or cannulae
or dangled devices that dripped
chemicals into their wrists,
but I believed that the ship
traveled to a harbor of breakfast,
work, and love.
I wrote: "When the infusions
are infused entirely, bone
marrow restored and lymphoblasts
remitted, I will take my wife,
as bald as Michael Jordan,
home to our dog and day."
Months later these words turn up
among papers on my desk at home,
as I listen to hear Jane call
for help, or speak in delirium,

Donald Hall, "The Ship Pounding," from *White Apples and the Taste of Stone: Selected Poems, 1946–2006,* by Donald Hall. © 2006 by Donald Hall. Reprinted by permission of Houghton Mifflin Harcourt Publishing Company. All rights reserved.

waiting to make the agitated
drive to Emergency again,
for re-admission to the huge
vessel that heaves water month
after month, without leaving
port, without moving a knot,
without arrival or destination,
its great engines pounding.

God at the Bedside

Jerome Groopman

Not long ago, in the oncology clinic where I work, my patient Anna Angelo asked me to pray to God. At the time, prayer was far from the forefront of my mind. Anna (her name has been changed to maintain confidentiality) is a 71-year-old woman from Boston's North End with longstanding cardiac and hepatobiliary disease. Six years ago, breast cancer developed. The tumor was incurable from the time of diagnosis, since it had already spread to bone. The cancer cells tested positive for estrogen and progesterone receptors, and Anna was treated with a series of hormonal agents, which, over the ensuing years, largely controlled the disease. A devout Catholic, she regularly attended Mass and counted her priest among her closest friends. "God has been good to me," Anna said at the end of each visit.

Over the previous two months, Anna had been complaining to her internist about loss of appetite and fatigue. He ordered blood tests and then a CAT scan. The cancer had metastasized to her liver. A biopsy showed that the hepatic metastases no longer expressed hormone receptors. When Anna arrived for her appointment with me, she had already been informed of her biopsy results. The first thing she said was that she wanted to live as long as possible but was concerned about the toll of chemotherapy.

I explained that the choice of a treatment plan would not be simple, given her complicating medical problems. Many of the drugs could have serious side effects on her heart and would be metabolized by her liver. So, before recommending a regimen, I would consult with her internist, cardiologist, and gastroenterologist. Anna took in my words and then said, "Doctor, I'm frightened. I pray every day. I want you to pray for me."

Anna looked squarely at me. It was clear she wanted a response. For a long while, I did not know what to say. A doctor's words have great power

Jerome Groopman, "God at the Bedside," from the *New England Journal of Medicine* 350 (2004): 1176–1178. © 2004 by Massachusetts Medical Society. Reprinted by permission of Massachusetts Medical Society.

for a patient; they can help to heal, and they can do great harm. The specialty of oncology routinely involves treating people who are in dire circumstances and find themselves facing their own mortality. Many of my patients seek strength and solace in their faith.

None of the training I received in medical school, residency, fellowship, or practice had taught me how to reply to Anna. And although I am religious, I consider my beliefs and prayers a private matter. Should I sidestep Anna's request, in effect distancing myself from her at a moment of great need? Or should I cross the boundary from the purely professional to the personal and join her in prayer?

Dilemmas like this one have become points of sharp contention in the medical world. How should doctors examine and engage religion in the lives of their patients and in their own lives as clinicians? Is there any place for God at the bedside during rounds?

The United States is a deeply religious country, and several surveys show both that a large majority of patients want physicians to be engaged in their spiritual lives and that the sick believe in miraculous healing when medicine can offer no proven cure. But religious beliefs are not always positive or beneficial. One of my most instructive experiences of the effects of religious belief occurred some three decades ago, when I was a third-year medical student. An Orthodox Jewish woman in her 20s was admitted to the surgical service with a large breast mass. She seemed intelligent and animated, and it made no sense to me that she would have ignored a growth in her breast that was the size of a walnut. In my naïveté, I thought that our shared heritage positioned me to communicate with her in a particularly effective way, and I encouraged her to confide in me the reason why she had let the mass grow so large before seeking a surgeon. It turned out that she had had an affair with her employer, and she saw her tumor as God's punishment for her sin. There was no hope for her, no reason to continue living, because her death was God's will.

I was in over my head. I had brashly treaded into theological territory without a clinical compass. Was her confession meant as a call for absolution or a confirmation of her transgression? It was not my place to afford either, and with a mix of confusion and shame, I retreated from her. Later she shared her secret with the attending surgeon. I never knew what he had said to her that convinced her to be treated. Nor, during my subsequent medical training, was I ever taught how to speak to patients about matters of faith.

Centuries ago, when healers came primarily from the ranks of monks, rabbis, and imams, and when nurses were nuns or members of religious orders, there was no clear divide between biology and acts of God in the genesis of an illness or between the physical and spiritual components of its treatment. In the modern era, religion and science are understood to be sharply divided, the two occupying very different domains. Religion explores the nature of God and offers rituals for implementing God's will, whereas science eschews any such metaphysics and through experimentation unveils the workings of the material world.

But in the minds of many of our patients, there is no such schism. Religion, perhaps more than any other single force, can sculpt the experience of illness. In America today, religious influence can go beyond concepts embodied in the three Abrahamic faiths. Some patients and their doctors have turned to Eastern philosophies, seeking to integrate Buddhist, Taoist, and Ayurvedic ideas and practices into clinical care.

Different faiths dictate different forms of behavior, social interactions, and views about how to live and how to die. For this reason, some medical educators have argued that religion is a clinical variable to be considered in every case and that a "spiritual history" should become a regular part of the patient interview. Indeed, such a history may yield key diagnostic clues or guide recommendations about disease prevention and suggest strategies to ensure compliance with treatment. But if this kind of history taking becomes common practice, when, by whom, and how should it be done? At the first visit, or only after a close bond has been formed between patient and doctor? By the medical student, resident, or attending physician? And how would doctors manage the theological fallout?

Many doctors, understandably, are leery of moving outside the strictly clinical and venturing into the spiritual realm. As was clear in the case of the Orthodox woman I met as a student, theologies can sometimes be toxic. Religion can be a wellspring of great strength and comfort or a pool of guilt and pain. If we begin taking a spiritual history, then we risk becoming clinical judges of what we hear. But although doctors should not presume to take on the mantle of the clergy, I believe that they cannot always avoid evaluating whether the personal religious beliefs of their patients are salubrious. Unfortunately, this type of evaluation requires deeper knowledge of different religions and their clinically beneficial and harmful conceptions than most of us possess. Venturing into the spiritual domain also means confronting a patient's expectations about the outcome of an illness, particularly what it means not to be cured despite faith and prayer. If a patient prays for a medical miracle and it doesn't occur, does that mean that God doesn't love her or that she is unworthy because her will and character were too weak to exert the "power of prayer"? Popular culture makes much of the ability of will and faith to miraculously overcome dreaded diseases for which modern medicine has no proven remedies. Rigorous documentation of such widely touted spontaneous remissions is scant, and even in those rare true cases, cause and effect are obscure.

A doctor's practice can also be influenced, consciously or subconsciously, by his own religious beliefs. Moreover, his own faith, like that of his patients, may be tested by the trauma and travail that he witnesses. I came from a home where faith was strong but not fundamentalist, where belief coexisted with doubt. After spending six weeks on a pediatric oncology ward at a time when most children with cancer died terrible deaths, I was on the verge of losing my faith. Theodicy, the question of why a benevolent God would permit such suffering in the universe, can be brought into sharp focus in the hospital. The intimacy of the physician-patient dialogue could cause this question to emerge. What if Anna had asked me why God had chosen her to suffer? Should a doctor participate in such a dialogue?

Even as we ponder whether or how we should step inside the religious worlds of our patients, we should also ask whether members of the clergy should enter more deeply into our clinical sphere. There is a great imbalance of power between patient and doctor. Often, I have been insensitive to this imbalance and have taken a patient's silence to represent tacit assent to my recommendations. A member of the clergy can speak to a doctor at eye level and act as an advocate for a patient who may be intimidated by a physician and reluctant to question or oppose his or her advice. A priest, a rabbi, or an imam can help patients to determine which clinical options are in concert with their religious imperatives and can give the physician the language with which to address the patient's spiritual needs.

Facing Anna, I searched for a response. I reminded myself that whenever I wear that white coat I am a physician and that whatever I say or do should be for the clinical benefit of my patient. I briefly pondered the question of whether prayer was "good for health." This issue had captured the public's imagination, but published research on the subject was often preliminary and inconclusive. It was a legitimate and intriguing subject of scientific inquiry, but somehow, at the moment, it seemed remote from what Anna was asking for—a heartfelt answer.

And so, unsure of where to fix the boundary between the professional and the personal, unsure what words were appropriate, I drew on the Talmudic custom of my ancestors and the pedagogical practice of my mentors and answered her question with a question.

"What is the prayer you want?"

"Pray for God to give my doctors wisdom," Anna said.

To that, I silently echoed, "Amen."

The Use of Force

William Carlos Williams

They were new patients to me, all I had was the name, Olson. Please come down as soon as you can, my daughter is very sick.

When I arrived I was met by the mother, a big startled looking woman, very clean and apologetic who merely said, Is this the doctor? and let me in. In the back, she added. You must excuse us, doctor, we have her in the kitchen where it is warm. It is very damp here sometimes.

The child was fully dressed and sitting on her father's lap near the kitchen table. He tried to get up, but I motioned for him not to bother, took off my overcoat and started to look things over. I could see that they were all very nervous, eyeing me up and down distrustfully. As often, in such cases, they weren't telling me more than they had to, it was up to me to tell them; that's why they were spending three dollars on me.

The child was fairly eating me up with her cold, steady eyes, and no expression to her face whatever. She did not move and seemed, inwardly, quiet; an unusually attractive little thing, and as strong as a heifer in appearance. But her face was flushed, she was breathing rapidly, and I realized that she had a high fever. She had magnificent blonde hair, in profusion. One of those picture children often reproduced in advertising leaflets and the photogravure sections of the Sunday papers.

She's had a fever for three days, began the father and we don't know what it comes from. My wife has given her things, you know, like people do, but it don't do no good. And there's been a lot of sickness around. So we tho't you'd better look her over and tell us what is the matter.

As doctors often do I took a trial shot at it as a point of departure. Has she had a sore throat?

Both parents answered me together, No . . . No, she says her throat don't hurt her.

Does your throat hurt you? added the mother to the child. But the little girl's expression didn't change nor did she move her eyes from my face.

Have you looked?

I tried to, said the mother, but I couldn't see.

As it happens we had been having a number of cases of diphtheria in the school to which this child went during that month and we were all, quite apparently, thinking of that, though no one had as yet spoken of the thing.

Well, I said, suppose we take a look at the throat first. I smiled in my best professional manner and asking for the child's first name I said, come on, Mathilda, open your mouth and let's take a look at your throat.

Nothing doing.

Aw, come on, I coaxed, just open your mouth wide and let me take a look. Look, I said opening both hands wide, I haven't anything in my hands. Just open up and let me see.

Such a nice man, put in the mother. Look how kind he is to you. Come on, do what he tells you to. He won't hurt you.

At that I ground my teeth in disgust. If only they wouldn't use the word "hurt" I might be able to get somewhere. But I did not allow myself to be hurried or disturbed but speaking quietly and slowly I approached the child again.

As I moved my chair a little nearer suddenly with one catlike movement both her hands clawed instinctively for my eyes and she almost reached them too. In fact she knocked my glasses flying and they fell, though unbroken, several feet away from me on the kitchen floor.

Both the mother and father almost turned themselves inside out in embarrassment and apology. You bad girl, said the mother, taking her and shaking her by one arm. Look what you've done. The nice man . . .

For heaven's sake, I broke in. Don't call me a nice man to her. I'm here to look at her throat on the chance that she might have diphtheria and possibly die of it. But that's nothing to her. Look here, I said to the child, we're going to look at your throat. You're old enough to understand what I'm saying. Will you open it now by yourself or shall we have to open it for you?

Not a move. Even her expression hadn't changed. Her breaths however were coming faster and faster. Then the battle began. I had to do it. I had to have a throat culture for her own protection. But first I told the parents that it was entirely up to them. I explained the danger but said that I would not insist on a throat examination so long as they would take the responsibility.

If you don't do what the doctor says you'll have to go to the hospital, the mother admonished her severely.

Oh yeah? I had to smile to myself. After all, I had already fallen in love with the savage brat, the parents were contemptible to me. In the ensuing struggle they grew more and more abject, crushed, exhausted while she surely rose to magnificent heights of insane fury of effort bred of her terror of me.

The father tried his best, and he was a big man but the fact that she was his daughter, his shame at her behavior and his dread of hurting her made him release her just at the critical moment several times when I had almost achieved success, till I wanted to kill him. But his dread also that she might have diphtheria made him tell me to go on, go on though he himself was almost fainting, while the mother moved back and forth behind us raising and lowering her hands in an agony of apprehension.

Put her in front of you on your lap, I ordered, and hold both her wrists.

But as soon as he did the child let out a scream. Don't, you're hurting me. Let go of my hands. Let them go I tell you. Then she shrieked terrifyingly, hysterically. Stop it! Stop it! You're killing me!

Do you think she can stand it, doctor! said the mother.

You get out, said the husband to his wife. Do you want her to die of diphtheria?

Come on now, hold her, I said.

Then I grasped the child's head with my left hand and tried to get the wooden tongue depressor between her teeth. She fought, with clenched teeth, desperately! But now I also had grown furious—at a child. I tried to hold myself down but I couldn't. I know how to expose a throat for inspection. And I did my best. When finally I got the wooden spatula behind the last teeth and just the point of it into the mouth cavity, she opened up for an instant but before I could see anything she came down again and gripping the wooden blade between her molars she reduced it to splinters before I could get it out again.

Aren't you ashamed, the mother yelled at her. Aren't you ashamed to act like that in front of the doctor?

Get me a smooth-handled spoon of some sort, I told the mother. We're going through with this. The child's mouth was already bleeding. Her tongue was cut and she was screaming in wild hysterical shrieks. Perhaps I should have desisted and come back in an hour or more. No doubt it would have been better. But I have seen at least two children lying dead in bed of neglect in such cases, and feeling that I must get a diagnosis now or never I went at it again. But the worst of it was that I too had got beyond reason. I could have torn the child apart in my own fury and enjoyed it. It was a pleasure to attack her. My face was burning with it.

The damned little brat must be protected against her own idiocy, one says to one's self at such times. Others must be protected against her. It is social necessity. And all these things are true. But a blind fury, a feeling of adult shame, bred of a longing for muscular release are the operatives. One goes on to the end.

In a final unreasoning assault I overpowered the child's neck and jaws. I forced the heavy silver spoon back of her teeth and down her throat till she gagged. And there it was—both tonsils covered with membrane. She had fought valiantly to keep me from knowing her secret. She had been hiding that sore throat for three days at least and lying to her parents in order to escape just such an outcome as this.

Now truly she *was* furious. She had been on the defensive before but now she attacked. Tried to get off her father's lap and fly at me while tears of defeat blinded her eyes.

Sunday Dialogue

Conversations between Doctor and Patient

Rebecca Dresser

The Letter

TO THE EDITOR:

The old days of medical paternalism are gone. Today we have shared decision making, in which doctors describe treatment options and patients choose the one they prefer.

It sounds simple, but it's not. I learned this when I had to decide whether to have a feeding tube during cancer treatment. Doctors explained the tube's benefits and risks, then left it to me to decide. I said no. I had my reasons—I didn't want a foreign object in my body or an overnight stay in the hospital. I wanted to prove that I was tough enough to get through treatment without extra help.

But this was a bad decision. As time passed, I became too weak to continue daily radiation sessions. People kept trying to get me to change my mind, and finally a nurse succeeded. Consenting to the tube was the right thing to do, but it took a lot of persuasion for me to accept that.

Argument is a legitimate part of shared decision making, but not everyone understands this. Some clinicians think that respect for autonomy means they should never disagree with a patient. Some think that it would be cruel to question what a seriously ill person says she wants. Some don't want to devote time to the hard conversations that produce good decisions.

Patients avoid arguments, too. Many are too intimidated to take issue with anything a doctor says. But doctors aren't always right, and patients who are

Rebecca Dresser, "Sunday Dialogue: Conversations between Doctor and Patient" (Letter to the Editor), from *New York Times*, August 25, 2012. Reprinted by permission of the author.

afraid to argue can pay the price. A friend had his cancer properly diagnosed only after he challenged his doctors' opinions about what was wrong.

In everyday life, arguments with family and friends help us think through the consequences of our choices and sometimes change our minds. Patients and doctors should do the same for one another.

Rebecca Dresser

ST. LOUIS, AUG. 21, 2012

The writer is a professor of law and medical humanities at Washington University and the editor of *Malignant: Medical Ethicists Confront Cancer*.

Readers React

Ms. Dresser advocates having patients take a more active role in questioning and arguing with physicians to help the patients think through the consequences of their choices.

An alternative but more attractive approach would be to shift more responsibility back on the physician, who is better equipped to manage medical decision making than distraught and less knowledgeable patients. This can be done without paternalism.

Society accepts expert opinion. We allow our lawyers, accountants, decorators, and plumbers to tell us what to do based on expertise that they have, and that we do not. Why shouldn't this be true for physicians?

On controversial issues, such as treatments for breast or prostate cancer, the physician should inform the patient of the various options and provide patient-specific expert opinion. Complete neutrality doesn't work, as patients will wind up asking doctors what they would do if their relative had the condition.

When the choice is not clear because of conflicting medical evidence or a lack of it, the doctor can be helpful by providing the patient with well-written, easily understandable discussions of the issue, leaving the choice up to the patient.

Edward R. Burns

EXECUTIVE DEAN

ALBERT EINSTEIN COLLEGE OF MEDICINE

BRONX, AUG. 22, 2012

I am a second-year medical student and a Crohn's disease patient. Before starting medical school I always just assumed that my doctors knew what was best for me. I've come to realize that the medical profession is fallible.

Crohn's in a pathology textbook is not the same as the Crohn's I've seen in clinic offices, and it's also not the same as what I've experienced myself. While we're taught to recognize that every patient is unique, what we learn is largely based on studies of large populations and data from the laboratory.

To be empowered as a patient, you really need to express what your specific needs are. Doctors can give their informed opinion and might be legally and ethically held responsible for your standard of care, but ultimately it is your own health and well-being.

R. Jacobowitz

VALHALLA, NY, AUG. 22, 2012

I differ with both the diagnosis and the cure. The days of medical paternalism are far from over, and argument works only when both sides are equally equipped. But in the world of medicine, patients are amateurs who must negotiate a scary foreign terrain.

So it's no wonder that we latch onto parental figures, follow blindly whatever they say, and then learn, too late, that there were a lot of questions we should have asked.

As a malpractice attorney, I often meet patients who wish that they had asked more questions and engaged in a deeper conversation before agreeing to the proposed treatment. Argument, though, is the wrong approach. An adult conversation is needed.

Just for starters: On the provider side: "Here are the key facts: the pros, the cons, the options, the unknowns (always plentiful), my own biases." On the patient side: "Here's what scares me, and here's what my body is telling me that I'm not sure you've appreciated."

Patrick Malone

WASHINGTON, AUG. 22, 2012

The writer is the author of *The Life You Save: Nine Steps to Finding the Best Medical Care—and Avoiding the Worst.*

One of the most difficult challenges that physicians face is allowing patients to make what appear to be unwise decisions—even decisions that may lead to increased suffering or premature death. The reason we do this is because we recognize that the patient is ultimately the best judge of her own personal values and goals.

That does not mean that doctors should refuse to offer recommendations or personal perspectives to patients. If asked, I always tell my patients what I would do if I found myself standing in their shoes or if they were my own relative.

At the same time, it is extremely important to keep in mind the highly unequal power dynamic that exists between physicians and their patients. Many patients are easily influenced by the expertise of doctors and fear that rejecting their physician's advice will lead to lower-quality care.

So while gentle persuasion may at times be appropriate, the role of the clinician must be principally to inform rather than to influence. There is a world of difference between helping the patient figure out what she wants to do and persuading the patient to do what you want her to do.

Jacob M. Appel
NEW YORK, AUG. 22, 2012

The writer is a psychiatrist and medical ethicist at Mount Sinai Hospital.

The doctor-patient dialogue is the key to success. Arguments over best medical practices may not be as simple as Ms. Dresser describes, primarily because only one party in the argument (the doctor) has at least a decade of medical education. But the other party (the patient) can level the playing field by better articulating the goals of treatment.

"Will this make me feel better?" is an important question, but "Will this allow me to again be the person I want to be?" is a better question when facing a treatment decision. The dialogue that will ensue, about lifestyle, hobbies, interests, and the reasons for needing to get healthier, will yield better health outcomes, happier patients and more successful doctors.

Seth Ginsberg
UPPER NYACK, NY, AUG. 22, 2012

The writer is president of the Global Healthy Living Foundation, a patient advocacy organization.

The status of the physician has shifted from revered expert to hired consultant. Physicians are no longer looked upon as the final word in medical decisions. The reasons for this change are twofold.

First, patients have easily available information from the Internet, and consequently they are much better informed about their health than they were 30 years ago. Second, medicine has become a commodity subject to being priced and regulated like any other commodity. The patient, as the consumer of health care, acts like the consumer of any product and chooses based on availability, price, insurance coverage, recommendations, and reputation.

Whether this shift proves advantageous for the health of our patients, only time will tell.

Paul W. Adams
Christina Frohock
OXFORD, FL, AUG. 22, 2012

Dr. Adams is a radiation oncologist. Ms. Frohock is a lecturer at the University of Miami School of Law.

Yes, medical paternalism has been replaced by shared decision-making, and patients are usually asked to choose among options presented by their physicians. And yes, some clinicians are so influenced by the concept of patient autonomy that they hesitate to press their own judgment and will allow patients to determine every decision without challenge.

Too often, however, the reverse is true. Notwithstanding the decline of medical paternalism, some patients still tend to defer to medical opinion and accept treatments that they would prefer to avoid. In such instances, it may be helpful to use the analogy of civilian authority over the military. Once the generals have proposed their strategic plans, it is civilian government that must weigh the final objectives and decide on the ultimate strategy (think Douglas MacArthur and Harry S. Truman).

In medical decision making, the patient should see herself as the ultimate authority—paying close attention to professional advice but having the self-confidence to exercise her authority and say yes or no. Such a concept will make it easier for patients to enter into a constructive dialogue with their physicians.

Peter Rogatz
PORT WASHINGTON, NY, AUG. 22, 2012

The writer, a doctor, is vice president of Compassion and Choices of New York, which offers counseling on end-of-life choices.

The Writer Responds

When patients and doctors discuss treatment alternatives, each has something to learn from the other. Doctors know medicine, and experienced doctors know how previous patients responded to different treatment approaches. Patients know their bodies, their histories, and what is most important to them as individuals. Experienced patients like Ms. Jacobowitz also know what strategies are more or less likely to work for them.

It takes time, in-depth conversation and—sometimes—argument for the necessary learning to occur. By argument, I mean the expression of different views. Argument involves giving reasons for one's position and then hearing what others think about those reasons.

As Dr. Appel points out, patients have the freedom to make unwise decisions. But before putting those decisions into effect, doctors should ask patients to explain their choices.

As I learned, unwise decisions sometimes rest on misunderstanding or shortsightedness. I wouldn't have learned this if my doctors, nurses, and family hadn't openly and persistently questioned my treatment refusal.

There are also times when patients should challenge doctors. I wish I had challenged the doctor who dismissed my symptoms and delayed my cancer diagnosis. As several letter writers observe, relatively few patients are confident enough to do this. But what Mr. Ginsberg calls "doctor-patient dialogue" and what Mr. Malone calls "adult conversation" often involve the give-and-take that characterizes constructive argument.

None of this is easy. Patients are facing some of the most difficult decisions they will ever make. Doctors are facing frightened people who need lots of support, but also control over their medical care. Active engagement, not passivity, is the best way to proceed in these unwelcome, unsettling circumstances.

Rebecca Dresser
ST. LOUIS, AUG. 23, 2012

What the Doctor Said

Raymond Carver

He said it doesn't look good
he said it looks bad in fact real bad
he said I counted thirty-two of them on one lung before
I quit counting them
I said I'm glad I wouldn't want to know
about any more being there than that
he said are you a religious man do you kneel down
in forest groves and let yourself ask for help
when you come to a waterfall
mist blowing against your face and arms
do you stop and ask for understanding at those moments
I said not yet but I intend to start today
he said I'm real sorry he said
I wish I had some other kind of news to give you
I said Amen and he said something else
I didn't catch and not knowing what else to do
and not wanting him to have to repeat it
and me to have to fully digest it
I just looked at him
for a minute and he looked back it was then
I jumped up and shook hands with this man who'd just given me
something no one else on earth had ever given me
I may even have thanked him habit being so strong

PROFESSIONALISM AND THE
CULTURE OF MEDICINE

II

The Learning Curve

Atul Gawande

The patient needed a central line. "Here's your chance," S., the chief resident, said. I had never done one before. "Get set up and then page me when you're ready to start."

It was my fourth week in surgical training. The pockets of my short white coat bulged with patient printouts, laminated cards with instructions for doing CPR and reading EKGs and using the dictation system, two surgical handbooks, a stethoscope, wound-dressing supplies, meal tickets, a penlight, scissors, and about a dollar in loose change. As I headed up the stairs to the patient's floor, I rattled.

This will be good, I tried to tell myself: my first real procedure. The patient—fiftyish, stout, taciturn—was recovering from abdominal surgery he'd had about a week earlier. His bowel function hadn't yet returned, and he was unable to eat. I explained to him that he needed intravenous nutrition and that this required a "special line" that would go into his chest. I said that I would put the line in him while he was in his bed, and that it would involve my numbing a spot on his chest with a local anesthetic, and then threading the line in. I did not say that the line was eight inches long and would go into his vena cava, the main blood vessel to his heart. Nor did I say how tricky the procedure could be. There were "slight risks" involved, I said, such as bleeding and lung collapse; in experienced hands, complications of this sort occur in fewer than one case in a hundred.

But, of course, mine were not experienced hands. And the disasters I knew about weighed on my mind: the woman who had died within minutes from massive bleeding when a resident lacerated her vena cava; the man whose chest had to be opened because a resident lost hold of a wire inside the line, which then floated down to the patient's heart; the man who had a cardiac arrest when the procedure put him into ventricular fibrillation. I said

---

nothing of such things, naturally, when I asked the patient's permission to do his line. He said, "OK."

I had seen S. do two central lines; one was the day before, and I'd attended to every step. I watched how she set out her instruments and laid her patient down and put a rolled towel between his shoulder blades to make his chest arch out. I watched how she swabbed his chest with antiseptic, injected lidocaine, which is a local anesthetic, and then, in full sterile garb, punctured his chest near his clavicle with a fat three-inch needle on a syringe. The patient hadn't even flinched. She told me how to avoid hitting the lung ("Go in at a steep angle," she'd said. "Stay *right* under the clavicle"), and how to find the subclavian vein, a branch to the vena cava lying atop the lung near its apex ("Go in at a steep angle. Stay *right* under the clavicle"). She pushed the needle in almost all the way. She drew back on the syringe. And she was in. You knew because the syringe filled with maroon blood. ("If it's bright red, you've hit an artery," she said. "That's not good.") Once you have the tip of this needle poking in the vein, you somehow have to widen the hole in the vein wall, fit the catheter in, and snake it in the right direction—down to the heart, rather than up to the brain—all without tearing through vessels, lung, or anything else.

To do this, S. explained, you start by getting a guide wire in place. She pulled the syringe off, leaving the needle in. Blood flowed out. She picked up a two-foot-long twenty-gauge wire that looked like the steel D string of an electric guitar, and passed nearly its full length through the needle's bore, into the vein, and onward toward the vena cava. "Never force it in," she warned, "and never, ever let go of it." A string of rapid heartbeats fired off on the cardiac monitor, and she quickly pulled the wire back an inch. It had poked into the heart, causing momentary fibrillation. "Guess we're in the right place," she said to me quietly. Then to the patient: "You're doing great. Only a few minutes now." She pulled the needle out over the wire and replaced it with a bullet of thick, stiff plastic, which she pushed in tight to widen the vein opening. She then removed this dilator and threaded the central line—a spaghetti-thick, flexible yellow plastic tube—over the wire until it was all the way in. Now she could remove the wire. She flushed the line with a heparin solution and sutured it to the patient's chest. And that was it.

Today, it was my turn to try. First, I had to gather supplies—a central-line kit, gloves, gown, cap, mask, lidocaine—which took me forever. When I finally had the stuff together, I stopped for a minute outside the patient's door, trying to recall the steps. They remained frustratingly hazy. But I couldn't put it off any longer. I had a page-long list of other things to get done:

Mrs. A needed to be discharged; Mr. B needed an abdominal ultrasound arranged; Mrs. C needed her skin staples removed. And every fifteen minutes or so I was getting paged with more tasks: Mr. X was nauseated and needed to be seen; Miss Y's family was here and needed "someone" to talk to them; Mr. Z needed a laxative. I took a deep breath, put on my best don't-worry-I-know-what-I'm-doing look, and went in.

I placed the supplies on a bedside table, untied the patient's gown, and laid him down flat on the mattress, with his chest bare and his arms at his sides. I flipped on a fluorescent overhead light and raised his bed to my height. I paged S. I put on my gown and gloves and, on a sterile tray, laid out the central line, the guide wire, and other materials from the kit. I drew up five cc's of lidocaine in a syringe, soaked two sponge sticks in the yellow-brown Betadine, and opened up the suture packaging.

S. arrived. "What's his platelet count?"

My stomach knotted. I hadn't checked. That was bad: too low and he could have a serious bleed from the procedure. She went to check a computer. The count was acceptable.

Chastened, I started swabbing his chest with the sponge sticks. "Got the shoulder roll underneath him?" S. asked. Well, no, I had forgotten that, too. The patient gave me a look. S., saying nothing, got a towel, rolled it up, and slipped it under his back for me. I finished applying the antiseptic and then draped him so that only his right upper chest was exposed. He squirmed a bit beneath the drapes. S. now inspected my tray. I girded myself.

"Where's the extra syringe for flushing the line when it's in?" Damn. She went out and got it.

I felt for my landmarks. *Here*? I asked with my eyes, not wanting to undermine the patient's confidence any further. She nodded. I numbed the spot with lidocaine. ("You'll feel a stick and a burn now, sir.") Next, I took the three-inch needle in hand and poked it through the skin. I advanced it slowly and uncertainly, a few millimetres at a time. This is a big goddam needle, I kept thinking. I couldn't believe I was sticking it into someone's chest. I concentrated on maintaining a steep angle of entry, but kept spearing his clavicle instead of slipping beneath it.

"Ow!" he shouted.

"Sorry," I said. S. signalled with a kind of surfing hand gesture to go underneath the clavicle. This time, it went in. I drew back on the syringe. Nothing. She pointed deeper. I went in deeper. Nothing. I withdrew the needle, flushed out some bits of tissue clogging it, and tried again.

"Ow!"

Too steep again. I found my way underneath the clavicle once more. I drew the syringe back. Still nothing. He's too obese, I thought. S. slipped on gloves and a gown. "How about I have a look?" she said. I handed her the needle and stepped aside. She plunged the needle in, drew back on the syringe, and, just like that, she was in. "We'll be done shortly," she told the patient.

She let me continue with the next steps, which I bumbled through. I didn't realize how long and floppy the guide wire was until I pulled the coil out of its plastic sleeve, and, putting one end of it into the patient, I very nearly contaminated the other. I forgot about the dilating step until she reminded me. Then, when I put in the dilator, I didn't push quite hard enough, and it was really S. who pushed it all the way in. Finally, we got the line in, flushed it, and sutured it in place.

Outside the room, S. said that I could be less tentative the next time, but that I shouldn't worry too much about how things had gone. "You'll get it," she said. "It just takes practice." I wasn't so sure. The procedure remained wholly mysterious to me. And I could not get over the idea of jabbing a needle into someone's chest so deeply and so blindly. I awaited the X-ray afterward with trepidation. But it came back fine: I had not injured the lung and the line was in the right place.

Not everyone appreciates the attractions of surgery. When you are a medical student in the operating room for the first time, and you see the surgeon press the scalpel to someone's body and open it like a piece of fruit, you either shudder in horror or gape in awe. I gaped. It was not just the blood and guts that enthralled me. It was also the idea that a person, a mere mortal, would have the confidence to wield that scalpel in the first place.

There is a saying about surgeons: "Sometimes wrong; never in doubt." This is meant as a reproof, but to me it seemed their strength. Every day, surgeons are faced with uncertainties. Information is inadequate; the science is ambiguous; one's knowledge and abilities are never perfect. Even with the simplest operation, it cannot be taken for granted that a patient will come through better off—or even alive. Standing at the operating table, I wondered how the surgeon knew that all the steps would go as planned, that bleeding would be controlled and infection would not set in and organs would not be injured. He didn't, of course. But he cut anyway.

Later, while still a student, I was allowed to make an incision myself. The surgeon drew a six-inch dotted line with a marking pen across an anesthetized patient's abdomen and then, to my surprise, had the nurse hand me the knife. It was still warm from the autoclave. The surgeon had me stretch the skin taut with the thumb and forefinger of my free hand. He told me to make one smooth slice down to the fat. I put the belly of the blade to the skin and cut. The experience was odd and addictive, mixing exhilaration from the calculated violence of the act, anxiety about getting it right, and a righteous faith that it was somehow for the person's good. There was also the slightly nauseating feeling of finding that it took more force than I'd realized. (Skin is thick and springy, and on my first pass I did not go nearly deep enough; I had to cut twice to get through.) The moment made me want to be a surgeon—not an amateur handed the knife for a brief moment but someone with the confidence and ability to proceed as if it were routine.

A resident begins, however, with none of this air of mastery—only an overpowering instinct against doing anything like pressing a knife against flesh or jabbing a needle into someone's chest. On my first day as a surgical resident, I was assigned to the emergency room. Among my first patients was a skinny, dark-haired woman in her late twenties who hobbled in, teeth gritted, with a two-foot-long wooden chair leg somehow nailed to the bottom of her foot. She explained that a kitchen chair had collapsed under her and, as she leaped up to keep from falling, her bare foot had stomped down on a three-inch screw sticking out of one of the chair legs. I tried very hard to look like someone who had not got his medical diploma just the week before. Instead, I was determined to be nonchalant, the kind of guy who had seen this sort of thing a hundred times before. I inspected her foot, and could see that the screw was embedded in the bone at the base of her big toe. There was no bleeding and, as far as I could feel, no fracture.

"Wow, that must hurt," I blurted out, idiotically.

The obvious thing to do was give her a tetanus shot and pull out the screw. I ordered the tetanus shot, but I began to have doubts about pulling out the screw. Suppose she bled? Or suppose I fractured her foot? Or something worse? I excused myself and tracked down Dr. W., the senior surgeon on duty. I found him tending to a car-crash victim. The patient was a mess, and the floor was covered with blood. People were shouting. It was not a good time to ask questions.

I ordered an X-ray. I figured it would buy time and let me check my amateur impression that she didn't have a fracture. Sure enough, getting the X-ray took about an hour, and it showed no fracture—just a common screw embedded, the radiologist said, "in the head of the first metatarsal." I showed the patient the X-ray. "You see, the screw's embedded in the head of the first metatarsal," I said. And the plan? she wanted to know. Ah, yes, the plan.

I went to find Dr. W. He was still busy with the crash victim, but I was able to interrupt to show him the X-ray. He chuckled at the sight of it and asked me what I wanted to do. "Pull the screw out?" I ventured. "Yes," he said, by which he meant "Duh." He made sure I'd given the patient a tetanus shot and then shooed me away.

Back in the examining room, I told her that I would pull the screw out, prepared for her to say something like "You?" Instead she said, "OK, Doctor." At first, I had her sitting on the exam table, dangling her leg off the side. But that didn't look as if it would work. Eventually, I had her lie with her foot jutting off the table end, the board poking out into the air. With every move, her pain increased. I injected a local anesthetic where the screw had gone in and that helped a little. Now I grabbed her foot in one hand, the board in the other, and for a moment I froze. Could I really do this? Who was I to presume?

Finally, I gave her a one-two-three and pulled, gingerly at first and then hard. She groaned. The screw wasn't budging. I twisted, and abruptly it came free. There was no bleeding. I washed the wound out, and she found she could walk. I warned her of the risks of infection and the signs to look for. Her gratitude was immense and flattering, like the lion's for the mouse—and that night I went home elated.

In surgery, as in anything else, skill, judgment, and confidence are learned through experience, haltingly and humiliatingly. Like the tennis player and the oboist and the guy who fixes hard drives, we need practice to get good at what we do. There is one difference in medicine, though: we practice on people.

My second try at placing a central line went no better than the first. The patient was in intensive care, mortally ill, on a ventilator, and needed the line so that powerful cardiac drugs could be delivered directly to her heart. She was also heavily sedated, and for this I was grateful. She'd be oblivious of my fumbling.

My preparation was better this time. I got the towel roll in place and the syringes of heparin on the tray. I checked her lab results, which were fine. I also made a point of draping more widely, so that if I flopped the guide wire around by mistake again, it wouldn't hit anything unsterile.

For all that, the procedure was a bust. I stabbed the needle in too shallow and then too deep. Frustration overcame tentativeness and I tried one angle after another. Nothing worked. Then, for one brief moment, I got a flash of blood in the syringe, indicating that I was in the vein. I anchored the needle with one hand and went to pull the syringe off with the other. But the syringe was jammed on too tightly, so that when I pulled it free I dislodged the needle from the vein. The patient began bleeding into her chest wall. I held pressure the best I could for a solid five minutes, but her chest turned black and blue around the site. The hematoma made it impossible to put a line through there anymore. I wanted to give up. But she needed a line and the resident supervising me—a second-year this time—was determined that I succeed. After an X-ray showed that I had not injured her lung, he had me try on the other side, with a whole new kit. I missed again, and he took over. It took him several minutes and two or three sticks to find the vein himself and that made me feel better. Maybe she was an unusually tough case.

When I failed with a third patient a few days later, though, the doubts really set in. Again, it was stick, stick, stick, and nothing. I stepped aside. The resident watching me got it on the next try.

Surgeons, as a group, adhere to a curious egalitarianism. They believe in practice, not talent. People often assume that you have to have great hands to become a surgeon, but it's not true. When I interviewed to get into surgery programs, no one made me sew or take a dexterity test or checked to see if my hands were steady. You do not even need all ten fingers to be accepted. To be sure, talent helps. Professors say that every two or three years they'll see someone truly gifted come through a program—someone who picks up complex manual skills unusually quickly, sees tissue planes before others do, anticipates trouble before it happens. Nonetheless, attending surgeons say that what's most important to them is finding people who are conscientious, industrious, and boneheaded enough to keep at practicing this one difficult thing day and night for years on end. As a former residency director put it to me, given a choice between a Ph.D. who had cloned a gene and a sculptor, he'd pick the Ph.D. every time. Sure, he said, he'd bet on the sculptor's being more physically talented; but he'd bet on the Ph.D.'s being less "flaky." And in the end that matters more. Skill, surgeons believe, can be taught; tenacity cannot. It's an odd approach to recruitment, but it continues all the way up the ranks, even in top surgery departments. They start with minions with no experience in surgery, spend years training them, and then take more of their faculty from these same homegrown ranks.

And it works. There have now been many studies of élite performers—concert violinists, chess grand masters, professional ice-skaters, mathematicians, and so forth—and the biggest difference researchers find between them and lesser performers is the amount of deliberate practice they've accumulated. Indeed, the most important talent may be the talent for practice itself. K. Anders Ericsson, a cognitive psychologist and an expert on performance, notes that the most important role that innate factors play may be in a person's *willingness* to engage in sustained training. He has found, for example, that top performers dislike practicing just as much as others do. (That's why, for example, athletes and musicians usually quit practicing when they retire.) But, more than others, they have the will to keep at it anyway.

I wasn't sure I did. What good was it, I wondered, to keep doing central lines when I wasn't coming close to hitting them? If I had a clear idea of what I was doing wrong, then maybe I'd have something to focus on. But I didn't. Everyone, of course, had suggestions. Go in with the bevel of the needle up. No, go in with the bevel down. Put a bend in the middle of the needle. No, curve the needle. For a while, I tried to avoid doing another line. Soon enough, however, a new case arose.

The circumstances were miserable. It was late in the day, and I'd had to work through the previous night. The patient weighed more than 300 pounds. He couldn't tolerate lying flat because the weight of his chest and abdomen made it hard for him to breathe. Yet he had a badly infected wound, needed intravenous antibiotics, and no one could find veins in his arms for a peripheral IV. I had little hope of succeeding. But a resident does what he is told, and I was told to try the line.

I went to his room. He looked scared and said he didn't think he'd last more than a minute on his back. But he said he understood the situation and was willing to make his best effort. He and I decided that he'd be left sitting propped up in bed until the last possible minute. We'd see how far we got after that.

I went through my preparations: checking his blood counts from the lab, putting out the kit, placing the towel roll, and so on. I swabbed and draped his chest while he was still sitting up. S., the chief resident, was watching me this time, and when everything was ready I had her tip him back, an oxygen mask on his face. His flesh rolled up his chest like a wave. I couldn't find his clavicle with my fingertips to line up the right point of entry. And already he was looking short of breath, his face red. I gave S. a "Do you want to take over?" look. Keep going, she signalled. I made a rough guess about where the right spot was, numbed it with lidocaine, and pushed the big needle in. For a second, I thought it wouldn't be long enough to reach through, but then I felt the tip slip underneath his clavicle. I pushed a little deeper and drew back on the syringe. Unbelievably, it filled with blood. I was in. I concentrated on anchoring the needle firmly in place, not moving it a millimetre as I pulled the syringe off and threaded the guide wire in. The wire fed in smoothly. The patient was struggling hard for air now. We sat him up and let him catch his breath. And then, laying him down one more time, I got the entry dilated and slid the central line in. "Nice job" was all S. said, and then she left.

I still have no idea what I did differently that day. But from then on my lines went in. That's the funny thing about practice. For days and days, you make out only the fragments of what to do. And then one day you've got the thing whole. Conscious learning becomes unconscious knowledge, and you cannot say precisely how.

I have now put in more than a hundred central lines. I am by no means infallible. Certainly, I have had my fair share of complications. I punctured a patient's lung, for example—the right lung of a chief of surgery from another hospital, no less—and, given the odds, I'm sure such things will happen again. I still have the occasional case that should go easily but doesn't, no matter what I do. (We have a term for this. "How'd it go?" a colleague asks. "It was a total flog," I reply. I don't have to say anything more.)

But other times everything unfolds effortlessly. You take the needle. You stick the chest. You feel the needle travel—a distinct glide through the fat, a slight catch in the dense muscle, then the subtle pop through the vein wall—and you're in. At such moments, it is more than easy; it is beautiful.

Surgical training is the recapitulation of this process—floundering followed by fragments followed by knowledge and, occasionally, a moment of elegance—over and over again, for ever harder tasks with ever greater risks. At first, you work on the basics: how to glove and gown, how to drape patients, how to hold the knife, how to tie a square knot in a length of silk suture (not to mention how to dictate, work the computers, order drugs). But then the tasks become more daunting: how to cut through skin, handle the electrocautery, open the breast, tie off a bleeder, excise a tumor, close up a wound. At the end of six months, I had done lines, lumpectomies, appendectomies, skin grafts, hernia repairs, and mastectomies. At the end of a year, I was doing limb amputations, hemorrhoidectomies, and laparoscopic gallbladder operations. At the end of two years, I was beginning to do tracheotomies, small-bowel operations, and leg artery bypasses.

I am in my seventh year of training, of which three years have been spent doing research. Only now has a simple slice through skin begun to seem like the mere start of a case. These days, I'm trying to learn how to fix an abdominal aortic aneurysm, remove a pancreatic cancer, open blocked carotid arteries. I am, I have found, neither gifted nor maladroit. With practice and more practice, I get the hang of it.

Doctors find it hard to talk about this with patients. The moral burden of practicing on people is always with us, but for the most part it is unspoken. Before each operation, I go over to the holding area in my scrubs and introduce myself to the patient. I do it the same way every time "Hello, I'm

Dr. Gawande. I'm one of the surgical residents, and I'll be assisting your surgeon." That is pretty much all I say on the subject. I extend my hand and smile. I ask the patient if everything is going OK so far. We chat. I answer questions. Very occasionally, patients are taken aback. "No resident is doing my surgery," they say. I try to be reassuring. "Not to worry—I just assist," I say. "The attending surgeon is always in charge."

None of this is exactly a lie. The attending *is* in charge, and a resident knows better than to forget that. Consider the operation I did recently to remove a seventy-five-year-old woman's colon cancer. The attending stood across from me from the start. And it was he, not I, who decided where to cut, how to position the opened abdomen, how to isolate the cancer, and how much colon to take.

Yet I'm the one who held the knife. I'm the one who stood on the operator's side of the table, and it was raised to my six-foot-plus height. I was there to help, yes, but I was there to practice, too. This was clear when it came time to reconnect the colon. There are two ways of putting the ends together—handsewing and stapling. Stapling is swifter and easier, but the attending suggested I handsew the ends—not because it was better for the patient but because I had had much less experience doing it. When it's performed correctly, the results are similar, but he needed to watch me like a hawk. My stitching was slow and imprecise. At one point, he caught me putting the stitches too far apart and made me go back and put extras in between so the connection would not leak. At another point, he found I wasn't taking deep enough bites of tissue with the needle to insure a strong closure. "Turn your wrist more," he told me. "Like this?" I asked. "Uh, sort of," he said.

In medicine, there has long been a conflict between the imperative to give patients the best possible care and the need to provide novices with experience. Residencies attempt to mitigate potential harm through supervision and graduated responsibility. And there is reason to think that patients actually benefit from teaching. Studies commonly find that teaching hospitals have better outcomes than nonteaching hospitals. Residents may be amateurs, but having them around checking on patients, asking questions, and keeping faculty on their toes seems to help. But there is still no avoiding those first few unsteady times a young physician tries to put in a central line, remove a breast cancer, or sew together two segments of colon. No matter how many protections are in place, on average these cases go less well with the novice than with someone experienced.

Doctors have no illusions about this. When an attending physician brings a sick family member in for surgery, people at the hospital think twice about letting trainees participate. Even when the attending insists that they participate as usual, the residents scrubbing in know that it will be far from a teaching case. And if a central line must be put in, a first-timer is certainly not going to do it. Conversely, the ward services and clinics where residents have the most responsibility are populated by the poor, the uninsured, the drunk, and the demented. Residents have few opportunities nowadays to operate independently, without the attending docs scrubbed in, but when we do—as we must before graduating and going out to operate on our own—it is generally with these, the humblest of patients.

And this is the uncomfortable truth about teaching. By traditional ethics and public insistence (not to mention court rulings), a patient's right to the best care possible must trump the objective of training novices. We want perfection without practice. Yet everyone is harmed if no one is trained for the future. So learning is hidden, behind drapes and anesthesia and the elisions of language. And the dilemma doesn't apply just to residents, physicians in training. The process of learning goes on longer than most people know.

I grew up in the small Appalachian town of Athens, Ohio, where my parents are both doctors. My mother is a pediatrician and my father is a urologist. Long ago, my mother chose to practice part time, which she could afford to do because my father's practice became so busy and successful. He has now been at it for more than twenty-five years, and his office is cluttered with the evidence of this. There is an overflowing wall of medical files, gifts from patients displayed everywhere (books, ceramics with Biblical sayings, hand-painted paperweights, blown glass, carved boxes, a figurine of a boy who, when you pull down his pants, pees on you), and, in an acrylic case behind his oak desk, a few dozen of the thousands of kidney stones he has removed.

Only now, as I get glimpses of the end of my training, have I begun to think hard about my father's success. For most of my residency, I thought of surgery as a more or less fixed body of knowledge and skill which is acquired in training and perfected in practice. There was, I thought, a smooth, upward-sloping arc of proficiency at some rarefied set of tasks (for me, taking out gallbladders, colon cancers, bullets, and appendixes; for him, taking out kidney stones, testicular cancers, and swollen prostates). The arc would peak at, say, ten or fifteen years, plateau for a long time, and perhaps tail off a little in the final five years before retirement. The reality, however, turns out to be far messier. You do get good at certain things, my father tells me, but no sooner do you master something than you find that what you know is outmoded. New technologies and operations emerge to supplant the old, and the learning curve starts all over again. "Three-quarters of what I do today I never learned in residency," he says. On his own, fifty miles from his nearest colleague—let alone a doctor who could tell him anything like "You need to turn your wrist more"—he has had to learn to put in penile prostheses, to perform microsurgery, to reverse vasectomies, to do nerve-sparing prostatectomies, to implant artificial urinary sphincters. He's had to learn to use shock-wave lithotripters, electrohydraulic lithotripters, and laser lithotripters (all instruments for breaking up kidney stones); to deploy Double J ureteral stents and Silicone Figure Four Coil stents and Retro-Inject Multi-Length stents (don't even ask); and to maneuver fiber-optic ureteroscopes. All these technologies and techniques were introduced after he finished training. Some of the procedures built on skills he already had. Many did not.

This is the experience that all surgeons have. The pace of medical innovation has been unceasing, and surgeons have no choice but to give the new thing a try. To fail to adopt new techniques would mean denying patients meaningful medical advances. Yet the perils of the learning curve are inescapable—no less in practice than in residency.

For the established surgeon, inevitably, the opportunities for learning are far less structured than for a resident. When an important new device or procedure comes along, as happens every year, surgeons start by taking a course about it—typically a day or two of lectures by some surgical grandees with a few film clips and step-by-step handouts. You take home a video to watch. Perhaps you pay a visit to observe a colleague perform the operation—my father often goes up to the Cleveland Clinic for this. But there's not much by way of hands-on training. Unlike a resident, a visitor cannot scrub in on cases, and opportunities to practice on animals or cadavers are few and far between. (Britain, being Britain, actually bans surgeons from practicing on animals.) When the pulse-dye laser came out, the manufacturer set up a lab in Columbus where urologists from the area could gain experience. But when my father went there the main experience provided was destroying kidney stones in test tubes filled with a urinelike liquid and trying to penetrate the shell of an egg without hitting the membrane underneath. My surgery department recently bought a robotic surgery device—a staggeringly sophisticated $980,000 robot with three arms, two wrists, and a camera, all millimetres in diameter, which, controlled from a console, allows a surgeon to do almost any operation with no hand tremor and with only tiny incisions. A team of two surgeons and two nurses flew out to the manufacturer's headquarters, in Mountain View, California, for a full day of training on the machine. And they did get to practice on a pig and on a human cadaver.

(The company apparently buys the cadavers from the city of San Francisco.) But even this was hardly thorough training. They learned enough to grasp the principles of using the robot, to start getting a feel for using it, and to understand how to plan an operation. That was about it. Sooner or later, you just have to go home and give the thing a try on someone.

Patients do eventually benefit—often enormously—but the first few patients may not, and may even be harmed. Consider the experience reported by the pediatric cardiac-surgery unit of the renowned Great Ormond Street Hospital, in London, as detailed in the *British Medical Journal* last April. The doctors described their results from 325 consecutive operations between 1978 and 1998 on babies with a severe heart defect known as transposition of the great arteries. Such children are born with their heart's outflow vessels transposed: the aorta emerges from the right side of the heart instead of the left and the artery to the lungs emerges from the left instead of the right. As a result, blood coming in is pumped right back out to the body instead of first to the lungs, where it can be oxygenated. The babies died blue, fatigued, never knowing what it was to get enough breath. For years, it wasn't technically feasible to switch the vessels to their proper positions. Instead, surgeons did something known as the Senning procedure: they created a passage inside the heart to let blood from the lungs cross backward to the right heart. The Senning procedure allowed children to live into adulthood. The weaker right heart, however, cannot sustain the body's entire blood flow as long as the left. Eventually, these patients' hearts failed, and although most survived to adulthood, few lived to old age.

By the 1980s, a series of technological advances made it possible to do a switch operation safely, and this became the favored procedure. In 1986, the Great Ormond Street surgeons made the changeover themselves, and their report shows that it was unquestionably an improvement. The annual death rate after a successful switch procedure was less than a quarter that of the Senning, resulting in a life expectancy of 63 years instead of 47. But the price of learning to do it was appalling. In their first 70 switch operations, the doctors had a 25 percent surgical death rate, compared with just 6 percent with the Senning procedure. Eighteen babies died, more than twice the number during the entire Senning era. Only with time did they master it: in their next 100 switch operations, five babies died.

As patients, we want both expertise and progress; we don't want to acknowledge that these are contradictory desires. In the words of one British public report, "There should be no learning curve as far as patient safety is concerned." But this is entirely wishful thinking.

Recently, a group of Harvard Business School researchers who have made a specialty of studying learning curves in industry decided to examine learning curves among surgeons instead of in semiconductor manufacture or airplane construction, or any of the usual fields their colleagues examine. They followed eighteen cardiac surgeons and their teams as they took on the new technique of minimally invasive cardiac surgery. This study, I was surprised to discover, is the first of its kind. Learning is ubiquitous in medicine, and yet no one had ever compared how well different teams actually do it.

The new heart operation—in which new technologies allow a surgeon to operate through a small incision between ribs instead of splitting the chest open down the middle—proved substantially more difficult than the conventional one. Because the incision is too small to admit the usual tubes and clamps for rerouting blood to the heart-bypass machine, surgeons had to learn a trickier method, which involved balloons and catheters placed through groin vessels. And the nurses, anesthesiologists, and perfusionists all had new roles to master. As you'd expect, everyone experienced a substantial learning curve. Whereas a fully proficient team takes three to six hours for such an operation, these teams took on average three times as long for their early cases. The researchers could not track complication rates in detail, but it would be foolish to imagine that they were not affected.

What's more, the researchers found striking disparities in the speed with which different teams learned. All teams came from highly respected institutions with experience in adopting innovations and received the same three-day training session. Yet, in the course of 50 cases, some teams managed to halve their operating time while others improved hardly at all. Practice, it turned out, did not necessarily make perfect. The crucial variable was *how* the surgeons and their teams practiced.

Richard Bohmer, the only physician among the Harvard researchers, made several visits to observe one of the quickest-learning teams and one of the slowest, and he was startled by the contrast. The surgeon on the fast-learning team was actually quite inexperienced compared with the one on the slow-learning team. But he made sure to pick team members with whom he had worked well before and to keep them together through the first 15 cases before allowing any new members. He had the team go through a dry run before the first case, then deliberately scheduled six operations in the first week, so little would be forgotten in between. He convened the team before each case to discuss it in detail and afterward to debrief. He made sure results were tracked carefully. And Bohmer noticed that the surgeon was not the stereotypical Napoleon with a knife. Unbidden, he told Bohmer,

"The surgeon needs to be willing to allow himself to become a partner [with the rest of the team] so he can accept input." At the other hospital, by contrast, the surgeon chose his operating team almost randomly and did not keep it together. In the first seven cases, the team had different members every time, which is to say that it was no team at all. And the surgeon had no pre-briefings, no debriefings, no tracking of ongoing results.

The Harvard Business School study offered some hopeful news. We can do things that have a dramatic effect on our rate of improvement—like being more deliberate about how we train, and about tracking progress, whether with students and residents or with senior surgeons and nurses. But the study's other implications are less reassuring. No matter how accomplished, surgeons trying something new got worse before they got better, and the learning curve proved longer, and was affected by a far more complicated range of factors, than anyone had realized.

This, I suspect, is the reason for the physician's dodge: the "I just assist" rap; the "We have a new procedure for this that you are perfect for" speech; the "You need a central line" without the "I am still learning how to do this." Sometimes we do feel obliged to admit when we're doing something for the first time, but even then we tend to quote the published complication rates of experienced surgeons. Do we ever tell patients that, because we are still new at something, their risks will inevitably be higher, and that they'd likely do better with doctors who are more experienced? Do we ever say that we need them to agree to it anyway? I've never seen it. Given the stakes, who in his right mind would agree to be practiced upon?

Many dispute this presumption: "Look, most people understand what it is to be a doctor," a health policy expert insisted, when I visited him in his office not long ago. "We have to stop lying to our patients. Can people take on choices for societal benefit?" He paused and then answered his question. "Yes," he said firmly.

It would certainly be a graceful and happy solution. We'd ask patients—honestly, openly—and they'd say yes. Hard to imagine, though. I noticed on the expert's desk a picture of his child, born just a few months before, and a completely unfair question popped into my mind. "So did you let the resident deliver?" I asked.

There was silence for a moment. "No," he admitted. "We didn't even allow residents in the room."

One reason I doubt whether we could sustain a system of medical training that depended on people saying "Yes, you can practice on me" is that I myself have said no. When my eldest child, Walker, was 11 days old, he suddenly went into congestive heart failure from what proved to be a severe cardiac defect. His aorta was not transposed, but a long segment of it had failed to grow at all. My wife and I were beside ourselves with fear—his kidneys and liver began failing, too—but he made it to surgery, the repair was a success, and although his recovery was erratic, after two and a half weeks he was ready to come home.

We were by no means in the clear, however. He was born a healthy six pounds plus but now, a month old, he weighed only five, and would need strict monitoring to insure that he gained weight. He was on two cardiac medications from which he would have to be weaned. And in the longer term, the doctors warned us, his repair would prove inadequate. As Walker grew, his aorta would require either dilation with a balloon or replacement by surgery. They could not say precisely when and how many such procedures would be necessary over the years. A pediatric cardiologist would have to follow him closely and decide.

Walker was about to be discharged, and we had not indicated who that cardiologist would be. In the hospital, he had been cared for by a full team of cardiologists, ranging from fellows in specialty training to attendings who had practiced for decades. The day before we took Walker home, one of the young fellows approached me, offering his card and suggesting a time to bring Walker to see him. Of those on the team, he had put in the most time caring for Walker. He saw Walker when we brought him in inexplicably short of breath, made the diagnosis, got Walker the drugs that stabilized him, coordinated with the surgeons, and came to see us twice a day to answer our questions. Moreover, I knew, this was how fellows always got their patients. Most families don't know the subtle gradations among players, and after a team has saved their child's life they take whatever appointment they're handed.

But I knew the differences. "I'm afraid we're thinking of seeing Dr. Newburger," I said. She was the hospital's associate cardiologist-in-chief, and a published expert on conditions like Walker's. The young physician looked crestfallen. It was nothing against him, I said. She just had more experience, that was all.

"You know, there is always an attending backing me up," he said. I shook my head.

I know this was not fair. My son had an unusual problem. The fellow needed the experience. As a resident, I of all people should have understood this. But I was not torn about the decision. This was my child. Given a choice, I will always choose the best care I can for him. How can anybody be expected to do otherwise? Certainly, the future of medicine should not rely on it.

In a sense, then, the physician's dodge is inevitable. Learning must be stolen, taken as a kind of bodily eminent domain. And it was, during Walker's stay—on many occasions, now that I think back on it. A resident intubated him. A surgical trainee scrubbed in for his operation. The cardiology fellow put in one of his central lines. If I had the option to have someone more experienced, I would have taken it. But this was simply how the system worked—no such choices were offered—and so I went along.

The advantage of this coldhearted machinery is not merely that it gets the learning done. If learning is necessary but causes harm, then above all it ought to apply to everyone alike. Given a choice, people wriggle out, and such choices are not offered equally. They belong to the connected and the knowledgeable, to insiders over outsiders, to the doctor's child but not the truck driver's. If everyone cannot have a choice, maybe it is better if no one can.

It is 2 P.M. I am in the intensive-care unit. A nurse tells me Mr. G.'s central line has clotted off. Mr. G. has been in the hospital for more than a month now. He is in his late sixties, from South Boston, emaciated, exhausted, holding on by a thread—or a line, to be precise. He has several holes in his small bowel, and the bilious contents leak out onto his skin through two small reddened openings in the concavity of his abdomen. His only chance is to be fed by vein and wait for these fistulae to heal. He needs a new central line.

I could do it, I suppose. I am the experienced one now. But experience brings a new role: I am expected to teach the procedure instead. "See one, do one, teach one," the saying goes, and it is only half in jest.

There is a junior resident on the service. She has done only one or two lines before. I tell her about Mr. G. I ask her if she is free to do a new line. She misinterprets this as a question. She says she still has patients to see and a case coming up later. Could I do the line? I tell her no. She is unable to hide a grimace. She is burdened, as I was burdened, and perhaps frightened, as I was frightened.

She begins to focus when I make her talk through the steps—a kind of dry run, I figure. She hits nearly all the steps, but forgets about checking the labs and about Mr. G.'s nasty allergy to heparin, which is in the flush for the line. I make sure she registers this, then tell her to get set up and page me.

I am still adjusting to this role. It is painful enough taking responsibility for one's own failures. Being handmaiden to another's is something else entirely. It occurs to me that I could have broken open a kit and had her do an actual dry run. Then again maybe I can't. The kits must cost a couple of hundred dollars each. I'll have to find out for the next time.

Half an hour later, I get the page. The patient is draped. The resident is in her gown and gloves. She tells me that she has saline to flush the line with and that his labs are fine.

"Have you got the towel roll?" I ask.

She forgot the towel roll. I roll up a towel and slip it beneath Mr. G.'s back. I ask him if he's all right. He nods. After all he's been through, there is only resignation in his eyes.

The junior resident picks out a spot for the stick. The patient is hauntingly thin. I see every rib and fear that the resident will puncture his lung. She injects the numbing medication. Then she puts the big needle in, and the angle looks all wrong. I motion for her to reposition. This only makes her more uncertain. She pushes in deeper and I know she does not have it. She draws back on the syringe: no blood. She takes out the needle and tries again. And again the angle looks wrong. This time, Mr. G. feels the jab and jerks up in pain. I hold his arm. She gives him more numbing medication. It is all I can do not to take over. But she cannot learn without doing, I tell myself. I decide to let her have one more try.

The Perfect Code

Terrence Holt

A faint click opens the air. A disembodied voice calls out, "Adult Code 100, Adult Code 100, 5 East. Adult Code 100, 5 East." Or it might be "Code Blue, Code Blue 3C, Code Blue 3C." From place to place the wording varies, but the message thinly hidden in the code is always the same: somewhere in the hospital, someone is dying.

The nature of the emergency varies as well. Hearts stop. Vital signs droop. We give up the ghost. But whatever the nature of the emergency, the response is the same: from all over the hospital the code team comes running, and the attempt at resuscitation begins.

The team is an invention of the 1960s, when evidence began to suggest that people suffering cardiopulmonary arrest had a much better chance of surviving if organized help reached them within two minutes. The "code" part was a response to public relations concerns that the laity might be upset by announcements of "Cardiac arrest on 4 North." Hence the "Code"—100, blue, pick your meaningless term. Thanks to television, I doubt anyone is taken in by it these days. But it adds another element of insider status to a culture that values that sort of thing.

Despite being no secret to anyone, the code still holds its mysteries. I'm not sure, still, just what I have learned by running to so many codes. But the experience haunts me, long after the fact. As if, somewhere in the tangle of tubes and wires, knotted sheets, Betadine, and blood, I lost track of something important. Listen.

In the hospital where I work, codes go something like this. A nurse finds a patient slumped over in bed. The nurse calls her name. No answer. The nurse shakes her. No answer. Harder. Still no answer. The nurse steps to the door and calls, in tones that rise at each syllable, "I need some help here." The rest of the nurses on the floor converge. Within a minute, every bystander within hearing is gathered at the door.

In the basement of the hospital, a hospital operator listens intently to her headset. She flips a switch, and a faint click opens the hospital to the microphone on her console. "Adult Code 100, 6 South. Adult Code 100, 6 South." The message goes out on the hospital PA system, her bodiless voice filling the hallways. It also goes out to a system of antique voice pagers, from which the operator's measured words emerge as inarticulate squealing. The pagers are largely backup, in case some member of the team is, say, in the bathroom, or otherwise out of reach of the PA system.

The team consists of eight or nine people: respiratory techs, anesthesiologists, pharmacists, and the residents on call for the cardiac ICU. On hearing the summons, the residents drop whatever they are doing and sprint. People running full-tilt in a hospital is unavoidably a spectacle. In their voluminous white coats, from whose pockets fall stethoscopes, penlights, reflex hammers, EKG calipers, tuning forks, ballpoint pens (these clatter across the floors, to be scooped up by the medical student who follows behind), the medical team's passing is a curious combination of high drama and burlesque.

The medical team arrives on a scene of Bedlam. The room is so crowded with nurses, CNAs, janitors, and miscellaneous onlookers that it can be physically impossible to enter. Shouldering your way through the mob at the door, you are stopped by a crowd around the bed; the crash cart, a rolling red metal Sears Roebuck toolchest, is also in the way, its open drawers a menace to knees and elbows. There are wires draped from the crash cart, and tubing everywhere.

At the center of all this lies the patient, the only one in the room who isn't shouting. She doesn't move at all. This time it is an elderly woman, frail to the point of wasting; her ribs arch above her hollow belly. Her eyes are half open, her jaw is slack, pink tongue protruding slightly. Her gown and the bedding are tangled in a mass at the foot of the bed; at a glance you take in the old mastectomy scar, the scaphoid abdomen, the gray tuft between her legs. At the head of the bed, a nurse is pressing a mask over her face, squeezing oxygen through a large bag; the woman's cheeks puff out with each squeeze, which isn't right. Another nurse is compressing the chest, not hard enough. You shoulder her aside and press two fingers under the angle of the jaw. Nothing. A quick listen at her chest: only the hubbub in the room, dulled by silent flesh. Pile the heels of both hands over her breastbone and start to push: the bed rolls away. Falling half onto the patient, you holler above the commotion, "Somebody please lock the bed." Alternate this with, "Does anyone have the chart?"

A nurse near the door hoists a thick brown binder, passing it over the heads jamming the room. "Code status," you bawl out. "Full code," the nurse bawls back. You reposition your hands and push down on her breastbone. "Why's she here?" There is a palpable crunch as her ribs separate from her sternum. "Metastatic breast cancer," the nurse calls, flipping pages in the chart. "Admitted for pain control." You lighten up the pressure and continue to push, rhythmically, fast. You look around, trying to pick out from the mass of excited bystanders the people who belong; the background is a weird frieze of faces and limbs reaching, pointing, gesticulating, mouths open. The noise is immense. On the opposite side of the bed you see one of the respiratory techs has arrived. "Airway," you shout, and the tech nods: she has already seen the puffing cheeks. She takes the mask and bag from the nurse and adjusts the patient's neck. The patient's chest starts to rise and fall beneath your hands.

"What's she getting for pain?"

"Morphine PCA."

"What rate?"

The question sets off a flurry of activity among some nurses, one of whom stoops to examine the IV pump at the patient's bedside. "Two per hour, one q fifteen on the lockout."

"Narcan," you order.

By this time the pharmacist has arrived, which is fortunate because you can't remember the dose of opiate-blocker. You doubt this is overdose here, but it's the first thing to try. Out of the corner of your eye you see the pharmacist load a clear ampule into a syringe and pass it to a nurse.

Meanwhile, on your left, the other resident and the intern are plunging large needles into both groins, probing for the femoral vein. The intern strikes blood first, removes the syringe, throws it onto the sheets. "Send that off for labs," you shout. Blood dribbles from the needle's hub as the intern threads a long, coiled wire through it into the vein. The other resident stops jabbing and watches the intern's progress. With a free hand she feels for the femoral pulse, but the bed is bouncing. You stop compressing. The resident focuses, shakes her head. Start compressing again.

A nurse reaches around you on the right, trying to fit a pair of metallic adhesive pads onto the patient's chest. You shake your head. "Paddles," you shout. "Get me the paddles." Then, into the general roar, "Somebody take that syringe and send it off for labs." A hand grabs the syringe and whisks it off. "You," you shout at the med student, who is hanging by the resident's elbow. "Get a gas." The resident throws a package from the crash cart, then steps back to give the student access to the patient's groin. The student fits the needle—it's a sixteen-gauge, two inches long—to the blood gas syringe, feels for the pulse your compressions are making in the groin, and stabs it home: blood, dark purple, fills the barrel. The student looks worried; he may have missed the artery. It doesn't matter. The student passes it around the foot of the bed to another hand and it vanishes.

The nurse at your elbow is still there, holding the defibrillator paddles. She stands as though she has been holding these out to you for some time. Clap the paddles on the patient's chest. Over your shoulder on the tiny screen of the defibrillator a wavy line of green light scrawls horizontally onward. You look back at the other resident. "Anything?" you both say at once, and both of you shake your heads. The intern has finished with the femoral catheter, very fast. He holds up one of the access ports. "Amp of epi," you say, but there's no response. Louder: "I need an amp of epi." Finally someone shoves a big blunt-nosed syringe into your hand. Without stopping to verify that it's what you asked for, you lean over and fit it to the port and push the plunger. Another look at the screen. Still nothing. "Atropine," you call out, and this time a nurse has it ready. "Push it," you say, and she does. Stop compressions, check the screen.

Suddenly the wavery tracing leaps into life, a jagged irregular line, teeth of a painful saw. "V fib," the other resident calls out, annoying you for a moment. You clamp the paddles down on the patient's ribs. "Everyone clear?" Everyone has moved back two feet from the bed. You check your own legs, arch your back: "Clear?" You push the button. The patient spasms, then lies limp again. The pattern on the screen is unchanged. The other resident shakes her head. You call over your shoulder, "Three hundred," and shock again. The body twitches again. An unpleasant smell rises from the bed.

The pattern on the screen subsides, back to the long lazy wave. Still no pulse. You start compressing again. "Epi," you call out. "Atropine." There is another flutter of activity on the screen, but before you can shock, it goes flat again, almost flat, perhaps there is a suggestion of a ragged rhythm there, fine sawteeth. "Clear," you call again, and everybody draws back. "Three-sixty," you remember to say over your shoulder, and when the answering call comes back you shock again, knowing this is futile. But the patient is dead and there is no harm in trying. As the body slumps again, there is a palpable slackening of the noise level in the room, and even though you go on another ten minutes, pushing on the chest until your shoulders are burning and your breath is short, and a total of ten milligrams of epinephrine have gone in, there is nothing more on the monitor that looks remotely shockable.

Finally, you straighten up, and find the clock on the wall. "I'm calling it," you say. Against the wall, a nurse with a clipboard makes a note. "Time?" she says. You tell her.

There is more. Picking up, writing notes, a phone call or two. There is a family member in the hallway, sitting stricken on a bench beside a nurse or volunteer holding a hand. You need to speak to her, but before you do you have to find out the patient's name. Or you don't. And then you go back to whatever you were doing before the code went out over the PA.

———

What I'm thinking, usually, as we trickle out at the end, is this: What a mess.

There is a great deal of mess in hospital medicine, literal and figurative, and the code bunches it all up into a dense mass that on some days seems to represent everything wrong with the world. The haste, the turmoil, the anonymity, the smell, the futility: all of it brought to bear on a single body, the body inert at the center of the mess, as if at the center of all wrong it remains somehow inviolate, beyond help or harm; as if to point to a moral I would understand better if I only had time to stop and contemplate it. Which I don't, not that day. We're admitting and there are three patients, two on the floor and one down in the ER, waiting to be seen. There is no time to read the fine print on anything, least of all the mortal contract just executed on the anonymous woman lying back in that room. I can barely make out the large block letters at the top: Our Patients Die. And very often they do so in the middle of a scene with all the dignity of a food fight in a high school cafeteria. We can't cure everybody, but I think most of us treasure as a small consolation that at least we can afford people some kind of dignity at the end, something quiet and solemn in which whatever meaning resides in all of this may be—if we watch and listen carefully—perceptible.

Which may be why one particular code persists in my memory, long after the event, as the perfect code.

———

David Gillet was the name I got from the medicine admitting officer. I wasn't sure what to make of the MAO's story, but I knew I didn't like it.

The story was an eighty-two-year-old guy with a broken neck. He had apparently fallen in his bathroom that morning, cracking his first and second vertebrae. I had a vague memory from medical school that this wasn't a good thing—the expression "hangman's fracture" kept bobbing up from the well of facts I do not use—but I had a much more distinct impression that this was not a case for cardiology.

"And Ortho isn't taking him because?" I said wearily.

"Because he's got internal organs, dude."

I sighed. "So why me?"

"Because they got an EKG."

The MAO was clearly enjoying himself. I remembered he had recently been accepted to a cardiology fellowship. I braced myself for the punch line.

"And?"

"And there's ectopy on it. *Ectopy.*" He then made a noise intended to suggest a ghost haunting something.

"Ectopy," meaning literally "out of place," refers to a heartbeat generated anywhere in the heart but the little knob in the upper right-hand corner where heartbeats are supposed to start. Such beats appear with an unusual shape and timing on the EKG. They can be caused by any number of things, from too much caffeine to fatigue to an impending heart attack, but in the absence of other warning signs ectopy is not something we generally get excited about. And it sounded to me as though a man with a broken neck had enough reasons for ectopy without sending him to the Cardiology service.

"So?" I said, trying not to sound indignant.

"So he's also got a history. Angioplasty about ten years ago, no definite history of MI. You can't really read his EKG because he's got a left bundle, no old strips so I don't know if it's new."

We were down to business.

"So I rule him out."

"You rule him out. Ortho says they'll follow with you."

"Lovely. And once I rule him out?"

"Ortho says they'll follow with you."

I said something unpleasant.

The MAO understood. "Sucks, I know, but there you are."

And there I was, down in the ER on a Sunday afternoon, turning over the stack of papers that David Gillet had generated over his six hours in the ED. There was a sheaf of EKGs covered with bizarre ectopic beats, through which occasionally emerged a stretch of normal sinus rhythm, enough to see that there was, indeed, a left bundle branch block, and not much else. The heart has several bundles, cables in its internal wiring. When some disease process disrupts a bundle, the result is an EKG too distorted to answer the question we usually ask it: Is this patient having a heart attack? Of course, the bundle itself is not a reassuring sign, and if new it merits an investigation, but plenty of people in their eighties have them and it's pretty much a so-what. But the ectopy on today's strips was impressive—if you didn't know what you were looking at you might think he was suffering some catastrophic event. I read between the lines of the consult note the orthopedic surgeons had left, and it was clear they regarded David Gillet as a time bomb and didn't want him on their service.

Which I couldn't help noting was exactly how I felt about having a patient with a broken neck on my service. But I didn't get to make decisions like that. Instead I wadded the stack of papers back in their cubby and took a brief glance through the curtains of Bay 12. From my somewhat distorted perspective, most of what I saw of the patient was his feet, which were large, bare, and protruding from the lower end of his ER blankets in a way that suggested he would be tall if I could stand him up. At his side sat a small, iron-haired woman who at that moment was speaking to him, leaning close while she spoke. She wore a faint, affectionate smile on a face that looked otherwise tired. I watched her for a moment, her profile held precisely per-pendicular to my line of sight as though posed. For a moment her face took on an almost luminous clarity, the single real object in the pallid blur of the ED, a study in patience, in care—and then it wavered, receding into a small tired woman with gray hair beside a gurney in Bay 12. The patient's face was obscured by the pink plastic horse collar that immobilized his neck. I watched the woman for a minute. Her expression, the calm progress of their conversation, suggested that nothing too drastic was going on. I took a walk to the radiology reading room to get a look at the neck films.

There were many of these, too. They showed the vulture-neck silhou-ette all C-spine films share. There were several unusual views, including one that I decided must have been shot straight down the patient's open mouth: it showed, framed by teeth palisaded with spiky metal, the pale ring of the first vertebra, the massive bone called the atlas, and clear (even to me) on both sides of it were two jagged dark lines angling in on the empty center where the spinal cord had failed to register on film. The break in the second vertebra was harder to make out, but I took the surgeons at their word: *C1/2 fx. Will need immobilization pending installation of halo. Will follow w/you.*

———————

I was not in the best of moods as I made my way back to the ER, grabbed a clipboard, and parted the curtains to Bay 12. I still managed an adequate smile as I introduced myself. "David Gillet?" I said tentatively.

The woman at his shoulder blinked up at me, wearing that same weary smile, brushing an iron-colored lock of hair from her face.

"It's '*Zhee-ay*,'" she said, with an odd combination of self-deprecation and something else—perhaps it was warmth?—that made me like her. "It's French," she explained. Her smile widened, one of those dazzling white things older people sometimes possess (dentures, I believe), and she welcomed me into Bay 12, which I had been inside of more times than I cared to count, with a curious air of apology, as if concerned about the quality of her housekeeping. I was charmed. This was still relatively early in the day and I was capable of being charmed. I shook myself a little, straightened my back (her posture was perfect), trying to escape some of the lethargy that had been piling on me over the day.

Her husband made a less distinct impression. The cervical stabilization collar tends to have a dampening effect on most people, as would the eight milligrams of morphine he'd absorbed over the past six hours, so it was a bleary and not very articulate history I got from him. His wife filled in the relevant bits. No prior MI. Occasional chest pain, hard to pin down (arthritis in the picture as well, of course). Otherwise a generally healthy, alert, and active man. On the one really critical point—what had caused the fall—Mr. Gillet insisted on giving account. He had *not* fainted. He had not been dizzy or breathless or experienced palpitations or anything of that sort. He had tripped. He had caught his toes on the damned bath mat, and gone down like a stupid ox. As he said the last he shook his head vehemently within the confines of his collar, and I caught my breath: you're not supposed to do that with a broken neck.

Even so I was partially reassured. The history didn't suggest a cardiac cause to his fall, and he denied any of the other symptoms that go along with impending doom. The physical exam was similarly reassuring, although hampered by the cervical collar and my dread of doing anything that might disturb his neck. He was a tall, bony man, with a nasty-looking cut across the scalp above his right eye, and dried blood crusted in his bushy eyebrows. The cut had been sutured already, and the blood made it look much worse than it was. Aside from the cut and a large bruise on his right ribs (none broken), he seemed fine. Except for the neck, of course. I stayed another few minutes, making idle chat with the wife, and then excused myself to write my orders.

He ruled out with the four A.M. blood draw the next morning, which I announced on rounds a few hours later with less pleasure than I would have ordinarily. I knew what was coming.

"So now what?" the attending asked.

"I guess I call Ortho."

Everybody—from attending to fellow to the other resident on the team and the intern, even the two medical students—started to smile. Then laugh.

"Well, I can call them, can't I?"

"Go ahead," the attending said.

There are attendings who will actually fight to make a transfer happen. They will call the attending on the other service and make the case, at least. Usually, when it comes to this, the transfer goes through. Which might be why most attendings are loath to let things get that far. If the patient's welfare requires it, they'll make the call (except for those dreadful individuals—and we know who they are—who believe themselves capable of caring for cases far outside their subspecialization). Or if they're dealing with some critical shortage of space. But if it's simply a matter of one patient more or less on their census, most attendings will let things be. And this attending was one of the more notoriously laissez-faire, happy enough to let the house staff run the show.

I made the call, and after three or four hours the Ortho resident returned the page. I knew by that time that I was already defeated, but I went ahead and asked the obligatory question, and received the inevitable answer (the Ortho resident having anticipated as well) that the Ortho attending did not feel comfortable taking the case—"and besides, it's not that bad a break. We'll follow."

"How long?" I asked.

"What do you mean?"

"How long does he need to be in the hospital?"

Puzzled. "When will you be done with him?"

"We've been done since eight this morning."

"You mean you'd send him home?"

"Except for the neck thing, yeah."

"Oh." This he hadn't anticipated.

"So what does he need from you?"

"He needs a halo."

I knew what a halo was. They're those excruciating-looking devices you may have seen somebody wearing in the mall: a ring of shiny metal that encircles the head (hence the name), supported by a cage that rests on a harness braced on the shoulders. Four large bolts run through the halo and into the patient's skull, gripping the head rigidly in place like a Christmas tree in its stand. A little crust of blood where the bolts penetrate the skin completes the picture. They look terrible, but patients tell me that after the first day or so they don't really hurt. Getting one put on, however: that hurts.

"So when does he get it?" I asked. Again, I knew the answer. It was already past noon. I was pretty sure it was Monday.

"Well," the Ortho resident replied, "it's already past noon."

"And you're in surgery."

"Yeah."

"And tomorrow?"

"Clinic. All-day clinic."

I didn't say anything. I waited a long time, biting my tongue.

"I guess we could do it tonight."

"That'd be nice."

"Unless there's an emergency, of course."

"Of course."

Of course there was. And clinic ran overtime the next day, or so I was told. Their notes on the chart (they came by each morning at five forty-five) ran to five scribbled lines, ending each time with *Plan halo. Will follow*, and a signature and pager number I couldn't quite decipher. This left me, of course, holding the bag. Not only had I one more unnecessary patient crowding my census, one more patient to see in the morning, round on, and write notes about (this during the month our team set the record for admissions to cardiology), but I also had the unpleasant responsibility of walking into Mr. Gillet's room on Tuesday and Wednesday morning to find him unhaloed, and making apologies for it.

It would have been unpleasant, at least, but for Mrs. Gillet. Her quiet grace put me in mind of faces I'd seen in old oil paintings, looking off to one side at something beyond the frame, eyes lit by what she saw there, the rest of the scene lost in dark chiaroscuro. All of which only made the situation even more intolerable, driving me to want to *do* something—and the only thing I had to offer lay in the gift of the inaccessible Ortho resident.

Wednesday I was on call again, and had pledged myself, in the brief moments between admissions, to track down the Ortho team and make them come up and put that halo on. Unfortunately, this was the day we admitted fifteen patients, as the failure clinic opened its floodgates and the Cath Lab pumped out case after case. Nobody was any too sick—the ER was blessedly free of chest pain—but the sheer volume of histories to take, physicals to perform, notes and orders to compose was overwhelming. The phone call—with its necessary sequel of waiting for the paged resident to call back—never happened.

Sometime in the late afternoon, however, I looked up from the counter where I had been leaning, trying to absorb the salient features of yet another failure patient's complex history, and saw through the open door of Mr. Gillet's room a strange tableau: two tall men in green scrubs wielding socket wrenches around the patient's head, a tangle of chrome, and the patient's hands quivering in the air, fingers spread as if calling on the seas to part. Some time later I looked up again and the green scrubs were gone: Mr. Gillet lay propped up in his bed, his head in a halo. From the side, his nose was a hawk's beak, the rest of his face sunk in drugged sleep, but his mouth still snarled as if it remembered recent pain. I remembered him in the ER, the flash of injured pride he had been able to conjure even through the morphine. That was gone now. He looked like a strange, sad bird in a very small cage.

Still later—time on that service being marked by missed meals and sleep, I can say only that I was hungry, but not yet punchy—a nurse stopped me.

"Fourteen," she said.

She meant Mr. Gillet. "How's he doing?" I was harboring some vague hope that he was awake and asking to go home.

"He's complaining of chest pain. Ten out of ten."

"Crap," I said. The nurse looked at me. "Get an EKG."

My vague hope vanished entirely ten minutes later as I watched the red graph paper emerge from the side of the box. The squiggle on it looked better than the initial set from the ER, but that was only because the ectopy was gone. What was there instead—Mr. Gillet's souvenir of the activities of the afternoon—were T-wave inversions marching across his precordium. This is not good. T-wave inversions generally signify heart muscle that isn't getting oxygen. What I was seeing here suggested that his LAD—a major artery supplying blood to the heart's strongest muscle—was about to choke off. I looked up at the nurse. She had been reading the strip as well—upside down, as cardiology nurses can.

"You gonna move him?" she asked.

"Yeah."

"Write me some orders."

"I'll write you orders. Just get him to the Unit. Quickly," I added, with a backward glance through the door of fourteen. Gillet's beaked face lay still in its silver cage. I scratched out a set of orders and turned to the next disaster.

———————

I didn't give Gillet much thought the rest of the evening, beyond seeing him settled in the CCU, and getting him scheduled as an add-on for the Cath Lab the next day. Around two in the morning the three of us—my partner Sasha, the intern Jeff, and I—were gathered at one end of the long counter, pushing stacks of paper around and trying to count up the score. We were on admission twelve for the day, we decided, but couldn't remember who was up next. I was digging in my pockets for a coin to flip when my pager went off. I swore as I tugged it from my belt, expecting to find yet again the number for the ER. I found instead the number for the CCU, followed by "911." At that moment the overhead paging system called a code in the CCU. The three of us ran.

It was perhaps thirty yards to the CCU, but by the time we got there three of the six nurses on shift were in Gillet's room, one at the head squeezing oxygen through a bag-valve mask, another compressing his chest, a third readying the crash cart. I had a moment's awareness that something was unusual—the whole thing looked too emptily staged, some kind of diorama in the Museum of Human Misery—but the scene only appeared that way for an instant and then we were in it and perspective fell apart in a surge of activity that picked us all up on its back and hurried us on.

Sasha and I had never made any formal arrangement about who did what in a code. I was the first one on the far side of the bed and started feeling the groin for a pulse. It was faint, driven solely by the nurse's compressions, but clear enough. I grabbed a finder syringe from the tray a nurse held out to me and plunged it in. Nothing. Pull back, change angle, feel for the pulse again and drive. Needle ground against bone. Again, and on this pass I saw the flash in the syringe, flung it aside and put a thumb over the welling blood while reaching for the wire. The nurse had it out already, handle turned toward me. It threaded the vein without resistance.

I had the catheter in place a minute or two later, met at each step in the process by the right item held out at the right time. No one spoke a word.

On the other side of the bed, Sasha stood with her arms folded across her chest, nodding at two nurses in turn as they pushed drugs, placed pads on the chest, and warmed up the defibrillator. Her eyes were on the monitor overhead, where green light drew lazy lines across the screen. At some point in the proceedings Anesthesia had shown up and slipped an endotracheal tube down Gillet's throat; respiratory therapy was wheeling a ventilator to the head of the bed, looping tubing through the bars of the halo and cursing at it.

"Hold compressions," Sasha said. The nurse stopped pushing on the chest. I saw for the first time that the halo was supported by a broad sheet of plastic backed with sheepskin that covered the upper half of the chest: the nurse had to get her hands underneath it to press; with each compression Gillet's head bobbed up and down, up and down. He was out, his eyes blank at the ceiling. The nurse at my elbow was hooking up the ports of my catheter, pushing one of the blunt syringes of epinephrine. We were all staring at the monitor above the bed, the long horizontal drift of asystole. As the second amp of atropine ran in, the lines all leapt to life, frantic peaks filling the screen.

"V-fib," a nurse said quietly.

"Paddles," Sasha replied in the same voice, taking the offered handgrips of the defibrillator from the nurse as she spoke.

"Clear," she said quietly, and thumbed the button.

David Gillet's body rose from the mattress, hung for a moment, collapsed. On the screen we saw scrambled green light settle for a moment, a rhythm emerge. Then the peaked lines consolidated into a high picket fence.

"V-tach," said the nurse, and turned up the power on the defibrillator.

"Clear," said Sasha. The body arched and fell again.

It went on for twelve more minutes (we knew this later, as we reviewed the printed strips of telemetry paper, trying to reconstruct what had gone on), Gillet's heart flying through one arrhythmia after another. Each time we responded it would settle briefly into sinus rhythm before flinging out again into some lethal variation, until finally, after two grams of magnesium sulfate and another round of shocks, it found a rhythm and held it through another flurry of activity when his systolics dropped to the sixties, then rallied on a minimal infusion of dopamine. And through all of this, as the atmosphere in the room maintained its eerie calm, the nurses kept up their surreal economy of gesture, and Sasha intoned the ritual of the ACLS algorithm, I felt my own adrenaline surging through the night's fatigue in an approach to exultation. It was almost beautiful.

This, I thought as we left the room, the lines on the monitor dancing their steady dance, the ventilator measuring breath and time to its own slower rhythm, this is what a code should be. A clean thing. A beautiful thing. The patient hadn't died.

––––––––––

The rest of the night was anticlimax, of course. There was a note to write (there is always a note to write), for which we had to puzzle some time over the strips churned out by the telemetry system, the notes scribbled on a paper towel recording what drugs had been given when, the values called over the phone from Core Lab and written in black marker on the leg of a nurse's scrubs. There was the call to the wife: I had to temper my enthusiasm as I searched for words to use when calling from the CCU at 2:35 in the morning. She took the news well enough, asked if I thought she needed to come now. I assured her he was stable. I assured her everything was under control; I had anticipated the code, I realized, when I moved him to the CCU. He was in the safest possible place. "In the morning, then," she said softly.

"In the morning," I agreed, and turned to the call room at last, where I spent perhaps forty-five minutes on my back, replaying the code against the springs of the empty bunk above me, until my pager went off again and this time it was the ER. And then around five another code on 4 West, where we found a man bleeding from a ruptured arterial graft and I had to threaten him with death if he did not hold still while I put yet another catheter in yet another groin, and this time there were fourteen nurses in the room, all shouting at once, so that I had to bellow over them to be heard as I requested, repeatedly, the proper catheter kit, something big enough to pour in fluid as fast as he was losing it. The patient was alive when I saw him last, a scared and tousled surgery intern kneeling right on top of him to hold pressure as the entire ungainly assemblage—patient, intern, and tree of IV bags—wheeled out the door to the OR. Back to normal life, I said to Sasha as we trudged back to the cardiology ward. Whether she knew what I was talking about I couldn't say, and didn't really care. I was still warmed by a vague sense of something right having happened. Mr. Gillet had coded, coded beautifully, and he had survived. We had done everything right.

––––––––––

The next morning on rounds, we were congratulated for our management of Mr. Gillet's arrest, although there was an ominous pH value from a blood gas obtained early on in the event that occasioned some shaking of heads. He had not responded since the code, being content to lie there unconscious in his halo, his chest rising and falling in response to the ventilator's efforts.

But his vital signs were stable, his labs from the four A.M. draw were looking good, and I had my hopes. No longer for an early discharge, but I was hopeful, all the same.

I shared these hopes with Mrs. Gillet when she arrived at seven. She stood at the bedside looking down, and her eyes were wet, her mouth unstably mobile. She reached out almost to touch the bars supporting the halo, down one of the threaded rods that pierced her husband's skin above the temple, almost touched there, then withdrew. "Is this the . . . thing? What do they call it?"

I was silent a moment.

"A halo," I said finally. "They call it a halo."

"Ah," she said.

I left her at the bedside, Mrs. Gillet with one hand through the chrome that cradled her husband's head.

David Gillet died five days later, having never regained consciousness. As each day passed and he gave no sign of mental activity, eventually it became clear that not all of him had survived the code. Mrs. Gillet decided, once pneumonia set in, to withdraw support. I had to agree. Even though I had anticipated the pneumonia, and was pretty sure I could get him through it, I had to agree it was for the best. Much as I wanted to keep him around.

He had become something unreal for me—something beautiful, like a work of art, but unreal. Amid all the mess and squalor of the hospital, with its blind random unraveling of lives, in their patient dignity and kindness he and his wife stood apart. In his case, for a little while at least, everything had gone exactly as it should have. The perfect code. And it hadn't made any difference. No difference at all. I pulled his tube early in the afternoon, after a bedside service, and took my place at the wall while the usual drama worked to its conclusion.

She sent me a card that Christmas, Mrs. Gillet. I kept it for a while, until it vanished in the clutter on my desk. She had written a text inside, something from the New Testament I had admired at the bedside service, but soon forgot. I do remember vividly the picture on the card. It was like her: sober, attractive. It showed a medieval nativity scene, all saints and angels with their burnished golden ovals overhead. Their faces were sorrowful in profile, as if anticipating what will crown that rosy newborn, perfection laid in straw, with pain in time to come.

Coeur d'Alene

Richard B. Weinberg

Despite the fact that Colossus, our new electronic health record program, had a confusing interface of unintuitive icons, dead-end click paths, and unwanted functions that could only have been designed by a cabal of computer geeks and business administrators, I did my best to adapt it to the needs of my practice. But I immediately noted a distressing problem: using Colossus to enter even the simplest note required more of my time—a lot more. Soon I was spending as much time tending to my charts as I was talking to my patients. And Colossus was monitoring my every click, the amount of time a chart stayed open, my billing codes. Every day, I was greeted by a Doctor's Dashboard that rated my (subpar) performance and urged me to be faster. I did not need to be reminded that these data would be used to determine my compensation.

It intrigued me that these issues did not seem to bother our trainees. Born into the information age, familiar with computers and the Internet since infancy, they treated the installation of Colossus like the appearance of just another smartphone app and blithely clicked their way through their patient encounters with impressive speed. But it troubled me that their efficiency did not necessarily equate with delivering good medical care. Dr. Manning, the resident assigned to my clinic one Friday morning, was no different. Our first patient was a 54-year-old man referred for chronic diarrhea. Dr. Manning exited the examination room after a scant 10 minutes but was able to present a reasonable, if not generic, differential diagnosis and care plan. Upon visiting the patient, I concurred. "Let's go see the next patient," I said. "You can finish the encounter note later."

"Oh, I've already finished the note."

"How did you do that?"

Richard B. Weinberg, "Coeur d'Alene," from *Annals of Internal Medicine* 165, no. 11 (2016): 822–823. DOI:10.7326/M16-0258. Reprinted by permission of American College of Physicians.

"I used a disease-specific macro template that I programmed to auto-populate with patient data just before the visit, then I clicked in the history as I was talking to the patient, entered my orders, and closed out the note before I left the room."

I looked over at my computer screen and saw that, indeed, his encounter note had already been forwarded to my inbox for authentication and signature—which, I reflected sadly, would probably take me more time than it took him to write it. I also noted that all of the meaningful use boxes had been checked and the patient information sheets and after-visit summary had been printed out. I reviewed his note; it read as follows:

CC: diarrhea

HPI: loose stools ×6 mo; 4–6×/day; (+) postprandial, (±) nocturnal; (−) heme, fever

PMH, FH: on chart

ROS: all other systems (−)

PEX: {normal template}

DDX: Diarrhea, infectious v osmotic v secretory

Plan: stool for GI pathogens, C. diff, lactoferrin, osm, lytes; CBC, CMP, celiac serology panel; colonoscopy w/Bx; trial of Cipro; diarrhea info sheet

It was concise, efficient—and soulless.

"Where's the social history?" I inquired.

"The nurses already asked him about tobacco and alcohol use."

"There's a bit more to the social history than that. Where was he born?"

He looked at me as if I had asked how many folds were in his patient's cerebellum.

"I don't know," he replied in bewilderment.

"Is he married? Does he have any children?"

"That's probably in the chart somewhere," he offered lamely.

"What does he do for a living?"

"I'm sorry. I didn't ask."

"So, you don't really know who this person is at all, do you?"

Dr. Manning looked down in dismay. Why was I asking such strange questions?

"Let me tell you the advice that my physical diagnosis teacher gave me over 40 years ago. Right off, ask every patient four questions: Where were you born? Are you married, and do you have children? Where did you go to school? What kind of work do you do? If you do this, it will be a rare patient with whom you don't find some point of connection."

He seemed very dubious but soldiered off to see our next patient, a 78-year-old woman referred for bloating and abdominal pain. After more than an hour he still had not emerged from the examination room. Perhaps he was trapped by a loquacious patient who had commandeered the interview, I mused. Just as I was about to go rescue him, he reappeared in the doctor's workroom, his face beaming with excitement.

"I asked the four questions," he announced proudly. "My patient was born in Coeur d'Alene, Idaho!"

"Really? Not many Idahoans here in North Carolina."

"Yes, but I'm one of them. I was born in Coeur d'Alene, too! And Dr. Weinberg—you're not going to believe this—her sister was my first-grade teacher! We started talking about all the people we knew back home, and I almost forgot to ask about her problem. But then I asked if she was married, and she told me that her husband died suddenly last year from a stroke. Her brother lives in Charlotte—that's why she moved here. She and her husband used to eat dinner together every single night for 60 years. She can't bear to eat alone at home now, so she eats most of her meals at a K&W Cafeteria."

A narrative story! In prose!

"I think I know what's wrong," he continued. "She's been eating a lot of Southern food—biscuits, cream gravy, mashed potatoes, custard pies. There's a lot of milk in those foods the way they make them here. I think she has lactose intolerance, and it's her new diet that's causing her bloating and cramps! All she needs is some lactase pills!"

We returned to the examination room, and I introduced myself to the white-haired lady who sat next to the consultation desk. "I hear it's been old home week in here," I joked.

"Yes. I think this fine young doctor has me figured out," she replied. She reached out and took his hand. "Now, I know you're an expert, Dr. Weinberg, and I mean no disrespect, but I would like Dr. Manning to be my doctor from now on. He knows where I'm from."

Dr. Manning looked up at me sheepishly; I nodded back.

"I agree completely, Mrs. Sorenson. You're in very good hands."

Back in the doctor's workroom, I praised my resident. "Excellent job! Please keep me informed how she's doing. Now, did you write all this down in your progress note?"

"No, not yet. I was too busy talking. I'll finish the note later today. Uh—is that okay?"

"Yes, it most certainly is."

"Thank you, Dr. Weinberg. No one has ever taught me something like this before."

"You're welcome. And thank you for showing me that autotext trick. Very cool."

Dr. Manning departed for his noon conference, and I went to see my last two patients. By now, I was more than an hour behind schedule. The Dashboard was not going to be kind to me, but I didn't care. I don't need a computer to tell me how to be a doctor.

The "Worthy" Patient

Rethinking the "Hidden Curriculum" in Medical Education

Robin T. Higashi, Allison Tillack, Michael A. Steinman,
C. Bree Johnston, and G. Michael Harper

During clinical training, medical students and residents in major U.S. medical schools learn to provide daily care for numerous patients in a limited amount of time. Providing the "best care possible" becomes a highly qualified, subjective endeavor, and strategies for accomplishing this are learned "on the job" during clinical rotations. How do physicians decide how much time to devote to each patient in order to provide care? How is this determination made, and how is this process taught to physicians-in-training? It is argued in this paper that these decisions are dictated by a moral economy rather than a knowledge economy in which values, behavioral norms, and ethical assumptions guide transactions as much, if not more, than knowledge and skill. Drawing from research at two major American metropolitan teaching hospitals, this paper illuminates how this process of evaluation occurs.

Background

The "Hidden Curriculum"

The ritual behaviors, assumptions, and commonly held beliefs of teaching physicians constitute what has been termed the "hidden curriculum" (Jackson 1968; Hafferty and Franks 1994; Wear 1998).[1] As opposed to the formal

Robin T. Higashi, Allison Tillack, Michael A. Steinman, C. Bree Johnston, and G. Michael Harper, "The 'Worthy' Patient: Rethinking the 'Hidden Curriculum' in Medical Education," from *Anthropology and Medicine* 20, no. 1 (2013): 13–23. Reprinted by permission of Taylor and Francis Ltd.

curriculum, which involves knowledge communicated via such mechanisms as lectures, planned small group activities, texts, and online learning modules, the basic premise of the hidden curriculum is that medical education is a cultural process through which students learn what is and what should be valued and how to discriminate between "good" and "bad" clinical practices. In doing so, physicians-in-training learn to subjectively define patients in ways that guide their interactions and influence decisions about the patient's medical care (Fineman 1991).

While the formal curriculum is implicitly directed at helping students resist making value judgments of patients, the hidden curriculum encourages students to cultivate an index of value judgments that enable them to act within a moral economy of care. Perceptions of patient worthiness are one aspect of the hidden curriculum, and participant narratives show how the moral economy is taught to physicians-in-training via the hidden curriculum. However, physicians-in-training are not simply passive recipients of the hidden curriculum but instead are active agents, "pushing back against and transforming the structure, even as they operate within its constraints" (Davenport 2000, 324).

A Moral Economy of Care

The concept of moral economy is a derivative of political economy, a theoretical approach to understanding the structural relationship between political institutions and economic power. Kohli (1987, 125) defines the moral economy as "the collectively shared moral assumptions underlying norms of reciprocity in which a market economy is grounded." In other words, a moral economy perspective seeks to understand the ethics and dispositions that influence economic exchanges, and vice versa. For example, the concept has often been used in the context of health care to understand how managed care policies are influenced by culturally defined notions of basic medical needs (Sprinkle 2001). In turn, ideas about what constitutes basic medical needs are reified or contradicted by insurance policies that define which services are covered.

Physicians' own cultural beliefs, rooted in biomedicine as shared social values, include moralizing assumptions about patients and their illnesses. Physicians-in-training learn to use these cultural beliefs and values to make assessments about patient worthiness, and these determinations guide decisions about the quality and quantity of care provided to each patient. Instead of money or material goods, time is the currency that is spent and saved by physicians. As exchange for this capital, physicians may expect to receive, among other things, a sense of competence and purpose, measurable improvement in the patient's health status, and perhaps positive feedback from their superiors or from patients. From a moral economy perspective, a patient whose health will improve little despite medical intervention has less capital than a patient who stands to make a full recovery given the same amount of time spent. In arguing a moral economy of clinical practice, it is not posited that the interactions between physician and patient are reduced to a simple economic equation. Instead, it is argued that moralizing assumptions and values are inherent in physician training, and however subtly they may be communicated, judgments about varying degrees of patient worthiness influence patient care.

Methods

The data for this paper were gathered through ethnographic field research over a period of four months in 2005. Research was conducted at two tertiary care teaching hospitals, both located in a large city in Northern California. While both hospitals served ethnically diverse patients, one hospital primarily cared for low-income patients while the other had a more economically varied patient population. Ethnographic research involved following a total of ten medical teams, each for a period of one week.[2] A team typically consisted of one attending (clinical faculty member), one resident (second-year resident), one intern (first-year resident), one fourth-year medical student, and one third-year medical student. All members of the team except for the attending were defined as "physicians-in-training" and were potential study participants.

Data were gathered using in-depth interviews and direct observation, allowing for the comparison of behaviors and opinions expressed in both more and less formal environments.

Observations focused on activities in which physicians-in-training interacted with other members of the medical team, namely during morning rounds. In the afternoons, participants were observed in unstructured, less formal interactions, usually in and around the staff work area, but also in call rooms, the cafeteria, hallways, and stairwells. A total of 21 interviews were conducted, digitally recorded, and transcribed. Qualitative data analysis consists of iterative readings of all transcriptions and observation notes to distill emerging themes, patterns, and areas of interest (Schensul, Schensul, and LeCompte 1999). Information obtained through interviews was related to observational data, and recurring ideas were assigned code names (e.g., "frustration," "money," "team dynamic"), which were used to organize, categorize, and rank key themes in an ongoing process. This paper reflects on one of the key themes that emerged through this analysis: patient worthiness.

Who Are the "Less Worthy" Patients?

The "Frequent Flyer"

Participants felt most negatively toward patients who were known to cycle in and out of the hospital. Such patients, who were often homeless and/or drug users or had chronic conditions, were often described as especially "frustrating." Some participants openly called them by the pejorative "frequent flyers" (for making frequent trips to the hospital). If a patient was admitted on multiple occasions, or if the patient had previously left the hospital against medical advice (AMA), this information was included during the presentation. As one fourth-year medical student said, "Patients who are very well-known to the doctors, they've come in many times, and they sign out AMA. And you know even if you put a ton of money into them they're going to leave." Similarly, an intern stated,

> It's frustrating because you know it's a patient that you're just sort of tuning up and they're going to go home and they're going to come back in three days and there's nothing you can really do about it . . . you have so many patients on your team and you have this patient that has the same issues every time. And if you know that probably no matter what you do they're going to end up going home and coming back, then you may not try as hard as possible to get them into a good situation because you think probably you're going to spend hours and hours and hours and the result is going to be the same. . . .

Some participants reflected on the fact that not all "frequent flyers" were purposely taking advantage of the system, but in fact had few alternatives to receive treatment by any other means. Thus, while they didn't feel that these patients were less worthy of care, per se, they felt frustrated by the fact that significant health care dollars were "drained" on such patients. Reflecting on this situation, an intern commented, "We spend a lot of money on care for patients in the hospitals, but we really devote none to what happens when they leave the hospital."

Drug Addicts

In response to questions about whether he has received negative messages about certain patients, one intern said, "If I had to target a group that was spoken poorly of and who people rolled their eyes to . . . it would be drug users and drug seekers." Many participants felt such patients exploited the system because they seemed less interested in receiving medical care than they were in securing food and housing, and because they were unlikely to make any changes in the behaviors that caused their medical problems. Another intern commented,

> The prototype patient who wouldn't be worthy of care would be the crack addict who comes in with chest pain, and this is his fifth time that he's come in recently, and wants a lunch bag, and isn't interested in medical care.

Ideas about distributive justice governed many determinations of patient worthiness. Several participants expressed strong feelings about which patients they felt were more deserving of health care dollars, and which, in actuality, received those resources. One second-year resident felt embittered by a particular patient, a homeless man with a history of poly-substance abuse who had been admitted several times for the same underlying issues. He asserted, frankly, "There's probably not a lot of reason to keep using medical resources on these people and rediscovering the same things that you already knew." This participant recalled learning this lesson early on as a medical student. "It's not explicitly said that they deserve less care, but it *is* explicitly said that you don't need to reinvent the wheel. In other words, they've had a full, significant workup over the course of multiple hospitalizations" (emphasis in original).

The Nonadherent Patient

Almost universally, participants felt at a loss to understand why patients would refuse to follow through with various treatment regimens when doing so would result in an improvement in their condition. Nonadherent patients were deemed less worthy of care because, in the participants' views, the team's efforts were futile in resolving the underlying medical problem. One fourth-year student indicated, "You kind of start catering your care to what you know they will do to take care of themselves." If patients didn't invest the time and energy required to improve their medical condition, then participants felt justified in investing less in them as well.

Sometimes nonadherence centered on a patient's refusal to refrain from engaging in certain self-harm behaviors. One second-year resident stated that the message that patients who "don't take care of themselves, don't take their meds, and instead use illicit stuff that's harmful to their health, and they're seen in the hospital over and over again" are less worthy is one that is communicated early and often. "I've definitely had attendings who feel quite strongly on that," she added. The frustration in these cases seemed to focus less on the fact that the patients engaged in self-harm behaviors, but more on the fact that they received expensive treatments that would likely be undone by the patient's continued self-harming. From a moral economy perspective, health care dollars should provide the greatest good for the greatest number of people. Participants felt strongly that the amount of resources spent on one patient—especially if that patient had actively caused his own medical problems—would be better spent on preventive care for thousands of other patients, who presumably did not engage in self-harm.

The Defiant Patient

Regardless of their medical condition, patients who behaved rudely toward staff were almost universally perceived as being less worthy of time and attention. Several participants recalled experiences with patients whose behavior ranged from moderately unpleasant to physically and verbally abusive. Participants admitted that they deliberately spent minimal time with such patients. For example, during the week in which the researcher observed his team, an intern reported that one of his patients was throwing his dirty diapers at the nurses and urinating on the floor (instead of in a diaper) because he was unhappy that the nurses had not responded quickly enough to his request for help getting to the bathroom. Following this incident, the intern overheard staff saying they would do the absolute minimum for this patient and try to have him discharged or transferred out of their unit as soon as possible.

Similarly, a third-year medical student recalled her very first patient in the department:

> For three weeks he was very abusive to everyone, he would swear at people and would refuse to do things and would call people various ethnic slurs and horrible things. So people would treat him very badly a lot of times in return. . . . [The intern] was spending very little time with him and some days not even do a physical exam on him because he was

so unpleasant. . . . It was a perfect example of "treat others the way you want to be treated," and he was getting bad care because he was treating people so badly.

While her tone reflected a certain level of discomfort with the way the situation was handled and she seemed to recognize that the team's behavior was morally questionable, this student also clearly stated that the team's behavior with this patient was "justified in a lot of ways, but it was difficult to see." By saying "treat others the way you want to be treated," this physician-in-training indicates that she learned from her team and from her very first patient that reciprocity is valued and practiced in the moral economy of clinical care.

The Elderly

An opinion commonly voiced was that older patients were more "needy" in a way that made interactions slow and frustrating. Several participants felt that interactions with older patients took more time and felt less productive. Participants said that they often had to repeat themselves and speak more slowly, and that older patients took longer to "get the words out," wanted to talk a long time about unrelated things, and sometimes complained about things that participants felt were petty or irrelevant. One intern commented,

A lot of older patients are what we could traditionally call "poor historians." So someone who's 85 comes in . . . and can't recall his symptoms or when things started or the precise characteristics of what's going on, and for a physician that can be really frustrating. And I think there's a certain amount of discrimination going on that those patients may not get as good care as someone that comes in with a similar problem who's 10 to 15 years younger and can describe the problem well and establish a better rapport with the physician.

Other participants' comments revealed that their frustration stemmed less from the patients themselves than it did from the recognition that patients with progressive or chronic illnesses, especially as they were older, simply did not have a lot of alternatives for more comprehensive care within the medical system. For example, an intern expressed that it was common for older patients not to have enough social and economic support, which left him helpless to set up better, more continuous care outside the hospital. Older patients were perceived as frustrating and less worthy of some participants' attention primarily because they were assumed to have multiple chronic illnesses that were ultimately incurable and required intervention and support beyond the hospital, and because treating them required a lot of time in spite of the interventions being relatively minor or unexciting (e.g., rehydration, basic antibiotics, etc.).

Unfortunately, the net effect of these negative experiences was an overall frustration displaced on all homeless, drug addicted, and "difficult" patients, including new admits who had not yet been assessed but who were known to have certain unfavorable characteristics. In other words, messages about a given patient's worthiness had rippling effects beyond that single patient. They predisposed other patients in similar circumstances to be labeled less worthy as well.

Who Are the "More Worthy" Patients?

Participants spoke more often of "less worthy" than of "more worthy" patients, but some recalled experiences in which their superiors clearly communicated the message that certain patients should receive preferential treatment. Participants typically identified wealthy patients and colleagues in the medical profession as chief among these. One resident recalled, "Either they're benefactors of the hospital or in certain circumstances they've been wives of important attending physicians." A fourth-year student commented, "People who are wealthier get their own room, and they get treated better by the attending. And if the attending babys them, you have to baby them." When asked by the researcher what she meant by "babys them," she added, "The attending a lot of times wants to know as soon as they come in, versus other people they don't need to hear about until the next morning."

In addition, patients who were deemed as likely to receive better care than others included those who were socially engaging and interactive (as opposed to unresponsive or unpleasant), who had an illness not caused by bad habits (but rather, for example, "something genetic"), who were motivated to do whatever was necessary to improve their condition, and who were likely to make a full recovery. One trainee admitted that "I tend to connect more with patients that are more like me—young, educated, and are motivated to get better—I guess we just have more in common, and so I feel like I understand more what they're going through, and want to help them." As one third-year medical student observed, the vast majority of patients were treated with respect and received good care. However, "if something comes down to where the extra mile needs to be gone, or that extra something," the team spent time on patients with whom they "want to . . . not have to" care for.

Negotiating within the Moral Economy

Perceptions of patient worthiness in this study varied according to whether patients had a "curable" (i.e., not chronic) illness or an illness not caused by self-destructive behaviors, were pleasant and engaging, and were motivated to comply with the treatment advised by the medical team. Yet physicians-in-training are not simply passive recipients of the moral economic value judgments taught through the hidden curriculum; instead, the moral economy is arbitrated in and through physicians-in-trainings' efforts to operate within (and occasionally against) its structures. However, despite the efforts of some of the students in this study to deliberately reject the moral economic valuation of patient "worth" taught to them via the hidden curriculum, their efforts were confounded by the systemic requirements of the hospital to "move things along" and the hierarchical nature of medical education.

An intern described several contradictions in how medical school taught students to practice medicine and how it was actually practiced in clinical settings. "Ideally, you'd like to work things up from most probable to least probable over time in a rational way. . . . In practice, it seems like we throw the book at them and order as many tests—for anything we think is a remote possibility— just get it all done at once rather than ruling one thing out and then moving to the next." A fourth-year student agreed, saying, "It's kind of like moving patients through almost like a factory, like you're putting parts on them, but instead of parts you're throwing meds at them and running tests."

Learning how to work efficiently by making distinctions regarding patient worthiness is part of the clinical training process. Like other values and assumptions, these messages, explicit or implicit, are passed from senior to junior ranking members of a team. And because they work within a strict team hierarchy, physicians-in-training are heavily influenced by their superiors. In fact, as one resident explained, physicians-in-training are in some ways more heavily influenced by their superiors than they are by patients because, ultimately, their future medical career is dependent upon those who evaluate them.

> You sort of behave in accordance with the general attitude of the team. As a med student, you're evaluated qualitatively, and basically your grades

are a reflection of how much [your team members] like you, and you want to be liked, and that motivation is obviously there. And you're not graded by patients, you're graded by the team. So the desire to be liked more by your team than by your patients is real. And so if your team acts like a bunch of donkeys, you feel compelled to act a little bit like a donkey to fit in and to get your good grades.

Many participants acknowledged the strong pressure to "fit in" with the rest of the team. Interestingly, however, some younger physicians-in-training identified interactions with groups of patients typically identified as "less worthy" of care as a mechanism for gaining a sense of agency and importance within the confines of the moral economy enforced by the strict hierarchy of medical education. For example, several participants pointed toward care of the elderly as providing a sense of professional worth in exchange for their care. An intern stated that "when I take care of a 30-year-old patient, and I'm a 26-year-old doc, they're like, 'Oh you're the resident' [using a dismissive tone]." But with older patients, "Even if you're a medical student, if you're taking care of them you're the doc. They'll listen to you. . . . Older people have that 'you're the doctor' kind of attitude."

As these examples indicate, the ability for trainees to negotiate within the structure of the moral economy and to invest time with patients that may be considered otherwise "unworthy" of care offers the potential reward of professional recognition and a sense of agency. However, the opportunities for this kind of exchange are limited by increasing demands on trainees to be more efficient and care for a greater number of patients in less time as their training progresses. Physicians-in-training are often aware of the ways that moral judgment impacts medical practice and struggle with the conflicts and tensions between what they are taught should be "ideal" care and care based on the moral economy. Yet, even for those who recognize the problematic nature of this conflict, the moral economy remains the only way to operate within the health care system.

Discussion

The physicians-in-training in this study learned from their superiors that certain patients are more deserving of care, and that certain tasks are less worthy of their time and should be delegated to nurses and ancillary staff. During the process of being taught how to be a physician, they were also taught the norms of reciprocity and how messages about the relative worthiness of patients are to be transmitted and reinforced among members of the team hierarchy. In addition, physicians-in-training frequently found that their efforts to resist making moral judgments about patients were confounded by the need to "move things along" as well as the hierarchical nature of medical education. They learned that it's acceptable to spend more time with nicer patients, and to devote more energy to potentially rewarding patients with "fixable" medical problems. Indeed, being unable to "fix" a patient may represent a challenge to a medical practitioner's ego or professional sense of self, and may play an important role in the categorization of patients as more or less deserving of care.

Students challenging this moral economy of care expose themselves to potential persecution or criticism from their superiors. However, regardless of the potential for criticism or poor evaluations and in spite of unprofessional conduct by medical educators, some medical students continue to challenge the value judgments and behaviors supported by the hidden curriculum. While it is clear that negative role modeling has a powerful impact on students, there is also evidence that students who have positive experiences with patient care and feel that their superiors support a patient-centered approach maintain a commitment to ethical clinical care (Krupat et al. 2009).

Yet, the very possibilities of care are defined by macrostructural constraints including the health care insurance system, academic training hierarchies, institutional policies, and the political economy of disease (Cohen, Cruess, and Davidson 2007; Hafferty and Levinson 2008). Thus, learning to categorize patients based on very little information becomes not only a way for physicians to conserve time, but ostensibly defines clinical efficiency and competency. The categories of patients who incurred the most moral judgment seemed to demand more expenditure than return on the physicians' resources. These same patients provided an opportunity for physicians-in-training to challenge the objectives of the hidden curriculum, yet ultimately trainees recognized the ultimate authority of using moral judgments to determine the behaviors of physicians toward their patients.

Discussions of professionalism within the medical community stress that physicians should "provide patients with the best possible care" while also acting "as a good steward of society's medical resources" (Dugdale, Siegler, and Rubin 2008, 550). Clearly, the students in this study, while cognizant of structural, economic, and social factors influencing patients' abilities (and desires) to follow the behaviors and treatments prescribed by health care professionals, generally relied on moral economic determinations of patient worth to decide which types of patients medical resources were "wasted" on or "worthy" of attention.

Despite the recent increased emphasis on the notion of patient autonomy in medical education and professionalism training, these negative judgments of patient worth and value continue to center on individuals whose behavior violates the power hierarchies and norms of the health care system. However, these deviant or rebellious patients were labeled as "less worthy" of care not because their actions or health decisions were considered morally wrong, but because they represented a poor investment of physician time and effort. While the rhetoric of patient autonomy is supported by physicians and physicians-in-training, in practice patients must comply with the goals and values of the hospital system to be "worthy of care."

NOTES

1 The term "hidden curriculum" was coined by Philip Jackson in 1968 to describe the attitudes and beliefs that children must learn as part of the socialization process in order to succeed in school. Hafferty was the first to adapt the concept to the area of medicine in 1994.

2 R. Higashi, an anthropologist, conducted all field research activities under the mentorship of three physicians (M. Steinman, C. B. Johnston, and M. Harper).

REFERENCES

Cohen, J. J., S. Cruess, and C. Davidson. 2007. Alliance between society and medicine: The public's stake in medical professionalism. *Journal of the American Medical Association* 298: 670–672.

Davenport, B. A. 2000. Witnessing and the medical gaze: How medical students learn to see at a free clinic for the homeless. *Medical Anthropology Quarterly* 14: 310–327.

Dugdale, L. S., M. Siegler, and D. T. Rubin. 2008. Medical professionalism and the doctor-patient relationship. *Perspectives in Biology and Medicine* 51: 547–553.

Fineman, N. 1991. The social construction of noncompliance: A study of health care and social service providers in everyday practice. *Sociology of Health and Illness* 13: 354–373.

Hafferty, F., and R. Franks. 1994. The hidden curriculum, ethics, teaching and the structure of medical education. *Academic Medicine* 69: 861–871.

Hafferty, F., and D. Levinson. 2008. Moving beyond nostalgia and motives: Towards a complexity science view of medical professionalism. *Perspectives in Biology and Medicine* 51: 599–615.

Jackson, P. W. 1968. *Life in Classrooms.* New York: Holt, Rinehart & Winston.

Kishimoto, M., M. Nagoshi, S. Williams, K. H. Masaki, and P. L. Blanchette. 2005. Knowledge and attitudes about geriatrics of medical students, internal medicine residents, and geriatric medicine fellows. *Journal of the American Geriatric Society* 53: 99–102.

Kohli, M. 1987. Retirement and the moral economy. *Journal of Aging Studies* 1: 125–144.

Krupat, E., S. Pelletier, E. K. Alexander, D. Hirsh, B. Ogur, and R. Schwartzstein. 2009. Can changes in the principal clinical year prevent the erosion of students' patient-centered beliefs? *Academic Medicine* 84: 582–586.

Schensul, S. L., J. J. Schensul, and M. D. LeCompte. 1999. *Essential ethnographic methods: Observations, interviews, and questionnaires.* Walnut Creek, CA: Alta Mira Press.

Sprinkle, R. H. 2001. A moral economy of American medicine in the managed care era. *Theoretical Medicine and Bioethics* 22: 247–268.

Wear, D. 1998. On white coats and professional development: The formal and the hidden curricula. *Annals of Internal Medicine* 129: 734–737.

How Doctors Think

Clinical Judgment and the Practice of Medicine

Kathryn Montgomery

The Complexity of Clinical Rationality

Given the radical uncertainty of clinical medicine as a science-using practice that must diagnose and treat illnesses one by one, the complex reasoning physicians use requires a richer concept of rationality than a spare, physics-based, positivist account of scientific knowing. Kirsti Malterud argues that traditional medical epistemology is an inadequate representation of medical knowledge because "the human interaction and interpretation which constitutes a considerable element of clinical practice cannot be investigated from that epistemic position."[1] In view of this misrepresentation of clinical knowing, Eric Cassell has called instead for a bottom-up, experience-based theory of medicine:

> Knowledge . . . whether of medical science or the art of medicine, does not take care of sick persons or relieve their suffering; clinicians do in whom these kinds of knowledge are integrated. . . . [M]edicine needs a systematic and disciplined approach to the knowledge that arises from the clinician's experience rather than artificial divisions of medical knowledge into science and art.[2]

Such experienced knowing is clinical judgment, the exercise of practical reasoning in the care of patients. It is essential to medicine and its characteristic tasks: first (as Edmund Pellegrino enumerates them) to diagnose the patient, second, to consider the possible therapies, and finally to decide what is best to do in this particular circumstance.[3] By their nature, these are complex

Kathryn Montgomery, *How Doctors Think: Clinical Judgment and the Practice of Medicine* (New York: Oxford University Press, 2005), 37–41. Reprinted by permission of Oxford University Press, USA.

and potentially uncertain tasks, no matter how advanced the science that informs them, and the phronesis or clinical judgment they require is the essential virtue of the good physician. It is the goal toward which clinical education and the practice of medicine strive.

Complexity and uncertainty are built into the physician's effort to understand the particular in light of general rules. If physicians could be scientists, they surely would be. The obstacle they encounter is the radical uncertainty of clinical practice: not just the incompleteness of medical knowledge but, more important, the imprecision of the application of even the most solid-seeming fact to a particular patient. The development of epidemiology and strategies for its use with individual patients such as clinimetrics, clinical epidemiology, medical decision making, and evidence-based medicine (EBM) have reduced this uncertainty and vastly improved patient care. Following on decades of clinical research, the Cochrane Collaboration's evaluation and reconciliation of the results of disparate, apparently incommensurable studies has encouraged the sense that by using the strategies of EBM, invariant precision—real certainty—in dealing with human illness may be just around the corner.[4] Although EBM has never claimed that, its impossibility is no reason not to work toward greater reliability in diagnosis, treatment, and prognosis. But, like the distance between Achilles and the tortoise, the gap between invariant, reliable, universalizable laws and the variable manifestations of illness in a particular patient remains. That is the nature of a science of individuals. We want it to be otherwise, especially when those we love or we ourselves are ill. But despite medicine's miracles—and they are legion— clinical knowing is not certain, nor will it ever be.

Scientific advance will not change this. In that ideal future when the pathophysiology of disease is thoroughly known and the epidemiology of every malady established, and both are at the fingertips of the experienced practitioner, medicine will remain a practice. Diagnosis, prognosis, and treatment of illness will go on requiring interpretation, the hallmark of clinical judgment. Physicians will still be educated and esteemed for the case-based practical reasoning that is situated, open to detail, flexible, and reinterpretable, because their task will continue to be the discovery of what is going on with each particular patient. Even with the last molecular function understood, the genome fully explicated, and cancer curable, the care of sick people will not be an unmediated "application" of science. People vary; diseases manifest themselves in varying ways. The individual patient will still require clinical scrutiny, clinical interpretation. The history will be taken, the body examined for signs, tests performed, and the medical case constructed. Patients will go on presenting demographically improbable symptoms of diseases; some will require toxic therapy, and sometimes treatment will come too late. Tests will have to be balanced between their sensitivity to marginal cases and the specificity with which they can identify disease. Therapies of choice will be second choice for some patients and will never cure quite everyone. The attentive focus on the particular patient that is the clinician's moral obligation will continue to compel the exercise of practical reason.

Because the practice of medicine requires the recollection and representation of subjective experience, physicians will go on investigating each clinical case: reconstructing to the best of their ability events of body, mind, family, and environment. For this task scientific knowledge is necessary and logic essential, even though the task itself is narrative and interpretive. Clinicians must grasp and make sense of events occurring over time even as they recognize the inherent uncertainty of this quasi-causal, retrospective rational strategy. Piecing together the evidence of the patient's symptoms, physical signs, and test results to create a recognizable pattern or plot is a complex and imprecise exercise. It is subject to all the frailty of historical reconstruction, but it remains the best—the logical, rational best—that clinical reasoners can do. It is not science, not in any positivist sense, nor is it art.

The Misrepresentation of Clinical Rationality

Why does medicine collude in the misrepresentation of its rationality? One obvious explanation is that medicine's status in society depends in large part on the scientific character of much of its information. To claim to be a scientist in our culture is to stake out authority and power. But physicians suffer the ill effects of this hubris: as patients and as citizens, we expect them to be far more certain than either their practice or the biology on which it is based can warrant, and, for many reasons, they are likely to take these expectations for their own. Malpractice suits that arise more from anger over misplaced expectations and perceived neglect than from genuine mistakes are the result.[5] As for power, it arises more strongly from human need in time of illness than from science. A widespread appreciation of clinical judgment would provide physicians a human and fallible but still trustworthy authority.

A more interesting, less obvious reason for describing medicine as a science is a practical requirement of clinical medicine, its need for certainty when taking action on behalf of another human being. Hans-Georg Gadamer describes such a need (though not the accompanying claim to science) as characteristic of all practice. "Practice requires knowledge," he writes, "which means that it is obliged to treat the knowledge available at the time as complete and certain."[6] Certainly one of medicine's chief strategies for minimizing the inescapable uncertainty of its practice is to regard—though always with skepticism—the best available information as real, dependable, and absolute, and these qualities are held to be characteristic of science. This practical strategy makes sense of an odd phenomenon: physicians' lack of interest in the late twentieth-century debate about the status of scientific knowledge or its representation of reality. Despite stereotypes about pre-medical students, many physicians have had a good liberal education, and all of them have met up with the assumption-rattling puzzle of quantum mechanics in the physics courses required for medical school admission. With their white coats off, they are likely to know as much about the history and philosophy of science as other college graduates. They nevertheless seem to need the honorific label "science" as a warrant for their clinical acts. Medical students who as undergraduates were immersed in philosophy or anthropology or cultural studies are no more likely to resist the science claim (with or without the art hedge) than those who majored in biomechanical engineering or economics. Once in practice, many physicians well educated in the biological sciences and keenly aware of the ineradicable uncertainty of their work still refer to medicine as a science—and without an apparent shred of epistemological doubt. It is as if, having embarked on a perilously uncertain practice, characterized by ungeneralizable rules and exceptions to those rules that proliferate like epicycles of the planets in Ptolemaic cosmology, they must cling for intellectual justification—beyond the need for social and interpersonal power—to the shards of a historical but by now metaphoric and inapplicable certainty.

Science is regarded as the "gold standard" of clinical medicine precisely because it promises reliability, replicability, objectivity—in short, what certainty is available in an uncertain practice. The metaphor of the gold standard, so widely used as an image of best practice and scientific certainty, is ironically apt—and just as unexamined as the science claim. Gold no longer backs any major world currency. It has gone the way of positivist science. Like science and the popular conception of rationality it stands for, gold is still available for the invocation of value, but it was long ago relativized, rendered conditional, and understood as in part the product of its social use.

One other reason for medicine's misdescription is an ethical one. Physicians argue that the belief that medicine is a science is essential to medical education. Clinical knowledge, although evolving, is at any given moment fixed and certain, and as teachers they want to foster in their students and residents a nearly obsessive attention to detail, a drive to know all that can be known, and a dedication to the best possible care for each patient. These are the marks of the good clinician. It might seem outrageous to ask them simultaneously to acknowledge clinical medicine's irreducible uncertainty— although, as I will show, covertly they manage to do exactly that at every clinical turn. Patients are resistant too. Do we want physicians to tell us as they enter the examination room that their knowledge is incomplete, its application to our case will be imprecise, and its usefulness uncertain? Not unless our complaint is very minor we don't. We want to think of them as powerful, dedicated, perfect figures. This rigid expectation carries over into the smallest details of education and practice. Work shifts for physicians and 80-hour weeks for residents have been resisted because they might limit their all-out dedication to patients. And patients, even when they know the assertion is necessarily suspect, still want to go on hearing "We've done everything possible." Few clinicians—or patients—have imagined changing this *folie a deux.*[7]

Is it possible to educate good physicians while recognizing that science is a tool rather than the soul of medicine? I believe it is, especially if that education were framed formally, as it now is tacitly, as a moral education, a long and scrupulous preparation to act wisely for the good of their patients in an uncertain field of knowledge.[8] A first step would be to scrap the unexamined description of clinical medicine as both a science and an art. The duality ignores all that medicine shares with moral reasoning and reinforces the contemporary tendency to split ethics from medicine. Moral knowing is the essence of clinical method, inextricably bound up with the care of the patient. In medicine, morality and clinical practice require phronesis, the practical rationality that characterizes both a reliable moral agent and a good physician.

Accounts of clinical medicine should celebrate clinical judgment and not the idea of science that physicians borrow from Newtonian physics. Nor should they appeal to a vaguely defined "art" to modify or enrich that outmoded idea of science. Clinical medicine is best described, instead, as a practice. Accounts of physicians' work, especially celebratory ones, should emphasize the exercise of clinical reasoning or phronesis, the deployment of clinical judgment on behalf of the patient. In equipping physicians to perform that essential task, medical education is necessarily a moral education, for it is training to choose what is best to do in the world of action. Its goal is the cultivation of phronesis, the practical reason essential to clinical judgment. The practice of medicine requires knowledge of human biology, a store of clinical experience, good diagnostic and therapeutic skills, and a familiarity with the vagaries of the human condition. Their intersection in the care of patients—the practice that makes physicians who and what they are—is neither a science nor an art. It is a distinctive practical endeavor whose particular way of knowing—its phronesiology—qualifies it to be that impossible thing, a science of individuals.

NOTES

1 Kirsti Malterud, "The Legitimacy of Clinical Knowledge: Towards a Medical Epistemology Embracing the Art of Medicine," *Theoretical Medicine* 16 (1995): 183–198; 183.

2 Eric Cassell, *The Nature of Suffering and the Goals of Medicine* (New York: Oxford University Press, 1991), xi. His *Doctoring: The Nature of Primary Care Medicine* (New York: Oxford University Press, 1997), an experience-based epistemology of medicine, describes the inadequacy of science—its "superficiality"—as a model and a source for clinical knowing.

3 Edmund D. Pellegrino and David C. Thomasma, *A Philosophical Basis of Medical Practice*, 125–143.

4 The Cochane Collaboration is available online at www.cochrane.org (accessed September 15, 2004).

5 Linda T. Kohn, Janet M. Corrigan, and Molla S. Donaldson, eds., *To Err Is Human: Building a Safer Health System* (Washington, DC: Committee on Quality of Health Care in America, Institute of Medicine, 2000).

6 Hans-Georg Gadamer, *The Enigma of Health: The Art of Healing in a Scientific Age*, trans. Jason Gaiger and Nicholas Walker (Stanford: Stanford University Press, 1996), 4.

7 Harold Bursztajn, Richard I. Feinbloom, Robert M. Hamm, and Archie Brodsky describe how it might be done in *Medical Choices, Medical Chances*, 2nd ed. (New York: Routledge, 1990).

8 Charles Bosk, *Forgive and Remember: Managing Medical Failure* (Chicago: University of Chicago Press, 1979). See also Pellegrino and Thomasma, *Philosophical Basis of Medical Practice*.

Healing Skills for Medical Practice

Larry R. Churchill and David Schenck

We thought we could cure everything, but it turns out we can only cure a small amount of human suffering. The rest of it needs to be healed.
—RACHEL NAOMI REMEN

At the center of medical ethics is the healing relationship.
—EDMUND D. PELLEGRINO

All physicians recognize that their relationships with patients can have healing effects. Compassionate, trusting relationships with patients are the chief delivery vehicle for the scientific interventions of modern medicine. Clinicians are concerned daily with convincing people to undergo physical examinations; accept probes into their private lives; endure diagnostic tests; or take medications that are inconvenient, sometimes painful, and occasionally incur risk. Relational skills are fundamental to success in these persuasive endeavors, and relationships themselves have potential therapeutic value— it is described in scientific terms as the "placebo effect"[1] or the "meaning response,"[2] as well as in ethical terms, as Pellegrino argues.[3] In addition, relationships with patients are a large part of the intrinsic rewards of medical practice.

Despite this recognition, relational skills are rarely studied systematically and are often consigned to the unscientific and mystified "art" of medicine. Although there are numerous books on interviewing[4-6] and studies of physician-patient conversations,[7] we know of very few empirical studies of how physicians build relationships that have healing potential.

Larry R. Churchill and David Schenck, "Healing Skills for Medical Practice," from *Annals of Internal Medicine* 149, no. 10 (2008): 720–724. Reprinted by permission of American College of Physicians.

Interviews with Expert Healers

We interviewed 50 practitioners from 3 states who were regarded by their professional peers as especially good at establishing and sustaining excellent patient relationships. Practitioners included 40 academic and community physicians across a wide range of specialties and 10 non-MD practitioners in complementary and alternative medicine. Interviewees ranged in age from mid-30s to late 70s, and 50 percent of participants were women. We conducted face-to-face, semistructured interviews and made audio recordings of the interviews anonymous. We then independently analyzed transcripts for core themes and content and reconciled any disagreements in our analysis through discussion. The institutional review board at Vanderbilt University Medical Center approved the study, and expert practitioners gave informed consent.

Eight Themes

In response to the basic questions of the interviews ("How do you go about establishing and maintaining healing relationships with your patients? What concrete things do you do to bring this about?"), eight fundamental themes emerged (box 1).

BOX 1 Eight Practitioner Skills That Promote Healing Relationships

DO THE LITTLE THINGS

Introduce yourself and everyone on the team
Greet everybody in the room
Shake hands, smile, sit down, make eye contact
Give your undivided attention
Be human, be personable

TAKE TIME AND LISTEN

Be still
Be quiet
Be interested
Be present

BE OPEN

  Be vulnerable
  Be brave
  Face the pain
  Look for the unspoken

FIND SOMETHING TO LIKE, TO LOVE

  Take the risk
  Stretch yourself and your world
  Think of your family

REMOVE BARRIERS

  Practice humility
  Pay attention to power and its differentials
  Create bridges
  Be safe and make welcoming spaces

LET THE PATIENT EXPLAIN

  Listen for what and how they understand
  Listen for the fear and for the anger
  Listen for expectations and for hopes

SHARE AUTHORITY

  Offer guidance
  Get permission to take the lead
  Support patients' efforts to heal themselves
  Be confident

BE COMMITTED AND TRUSTWORTHY

  Do not abandon
  Invest in trust
  Be faithful
  Be thankful

1. Do the Little Things

Small courtesies and congenial manners, such as smiling, shaking hands, acknowledging others in the room, and making eye contact, often turn out to be highly significant, especially at the beginning of a relationship.

One of the things that I routinely do is, when I enter the patient's room, I try to make eye contact and to shake the patient's hand. I will often acknowledge anyone else that they have in the room with them, their significant others. So there are just certain obvious social gestures that are common in any new relationship that I try to establish right away. (Interview 21)

At initial meetings, a small community is forming very quickly and under unusual circumstances. The practitioner has enormous power to set the tone and direction for this little community in the first encounter.

If someone feels connected, then you're miles ahead in terms of being able to affect some sort of positive results or impact on the patient, and so it's really establishing a positive and unique relationship where the patient remembers you. Touch is extremely important, so walking in and shaking hands—and a hand on the shoulder. Those sorts of things are very, very important. (Interview 5)

2. Take Time and Listen

Beginnings that are courteous may show themselves to have been mere formalities unless openings are followed by genuine presence. Patients typically wonder, "Will the doctor listen to me?" A practitioner's willingness to be still and quiet demonstrates to the patient that there is space.

So my first meeting is to try to get acquainted, and what I know is that it takes time. I may have a thousand things going, but I need to sit down and try to look relaxed. I might even take off my coat, and try to give them body language that [says] "I have time for you." (Interview 19)

Taking time makes it possible to listen with care to the patients' answers to practitioners' questions.

I start teaching in the first encounter, but I spend a lot of time listening to the answers to the questions that I ask, and then I try to let some silence take place, especially in people who are very concerned, so that they can tell me what they're concerned about. (Interview 8)

An important part of listening is listening for stories—for the narratives that give coherence to patients' lives.

I found out early on that being able to listen to their life story connected me better with that child and that family, and then we had a relationship. (Interview 3)

Listening is the most important thing, I believe. Asking about them, not just about their disease. Letting them tell their own story without too many interruptions. Caring about the aspects of that story. (Interview 31)

Through listening and caring about patients' stories, physicians can sometimes reinterpret key parts of these narratives. Stories of suffering can become stories of healing.[8,9]

3. Be Open

Patients bring their wounds, which Pellegrino[3] called their "damaged humanity," to the practitioner. It takes courage on the part of the practitioner to be willing to be open to this vulnerability, patient after patient. Yet, our informants argue that it is such willingness and courage that makes healing possible.

> You have to be honest. You might be able to help a lot of times—it depends, but listen to his story. You listen for the wound and you let them know that you have wounds. You are not perfect. (Interview 13)

Part of why this makes healing possible is that when the practitioner models such willingness and courage, the patient has permission to follow suit and offer the same. In this way, immense power is generated.

> You know, I might get tearful, or I might get upset, and so I think a lot of physicians, at that point, pull back, become more clinical, and move through it, but if you stretch a little bit, and you allow yourself to feel those emotions, it helps the patient tremendously. It actually is very rewarding, as much as it's difficult. (Interview 22)

4. Find Something to Like, to Love

"Love" here is not so much an emotion as it is a quality of "heart and soul," and it manifests most authentically and most powerfully in compassion and understanding. Seeking in every patient a quality, an achievement, or even just a mannerism that can be appreciated or admired mobilizes a healing capacity in caregivers.[10,11] This was a strong theme from our interviews. Yet this compassionate demeanor cannot be a matter of rote behaviors or gimmicks—it must be based in something real.

> I took a class with a famous psychiatrist who taught techniques of patient conversation, including recommendations to "lean forward" and to "sit

on the front edge of your chair." I asked: "Wouldn't it be better to just be interested in your patients?" (Interview 26)

For some practitioners, it is useful to imagine the patient as being like their parent or spouse or their child or grandchild, depending on the age and sex of the patient. Once the caregiver feels empathy and opens to compassion, another realm of care becomes available.

> I have a heart and soul which I can offer them, which is the way of bringing them some love. Love is a tough word to talk about when you are talking about doctor and patient relationships. Do you love your patients? I think you have to. Some people don't want to say that they do, but I think to really get to the point of healing you have to love. You have to be compassionate and understanding and willing to walk the wounded path with them. (Interview 13)

One practitioner spoke for many others we interviewed:

> We're in it for the moment where there's that double heart open connection of love and truth. It makes my practice doable. (Interview 43)

5. Remove Barriers

Our expert practitioners said that they seek to remove as many barriers to a genuine person-to-person encounter as possible. Barriers can be of many sorts: some are physical objects, others are attitudes.

> I never have anything between me and the patient. I've always had my desk up against the wall. (Interview 8)

Removing attitudinal barriers often involves an appreciation of power differentials between physician and patient and an element of humility.

> I'm not too good to open a door and roll a patient back into the room, and I'm not too proud to wipe the snot off a crying mother, or empty a trash basket . . . or to do any of those things that the lowest-ranked employee of the hospital does. (Interview 20)

> I like to have them understand that I am a human being, that I am not a god. I am a physician. (Interview 13)

Our informants insisted that patients are the best source of information on their condition, and that an essential part of healing is allowing patients' understanding of their illness to be spoken and received. This, in turn, provides the opportunity for a reinterpretation, which itself is often an essential part of healing. Open-ended questions seem particularly effective.

> A good way to get the patient started is just asking them what they understand about what's going on so far. And that's a very broad opening; it allows them to either be very scientific and talk about the tests that they've had, or it's an opening if the emotional piece is important to them at that time. It gives them an opportunity to frame it for what they need the most, rather than starting with specific questions about the medical side. (Interview 22)

Then the practitioner can speak back in the language and terminology that is understandable and meaningful to the patient.[12] As the patient talks, the caregiver looks for the opening, the place to insert a comment or an insight—the place to go to further the healing process.

> First, there's making comfortable and dropping my judgment, and second, there's listening, and then third, is waiting for the cues, to see where is the invitation? I'm talking to somebody, and you know when they're ready to hear something. You know, when I am listening, there is just a knowing of when the words can come, and so I wait for the opening. (Interview 39)

7. Share Authority

Many practitioners establish their expectation of shared responsibility for healing at the very beginning.

> One of the initial parts of my consultation with somebody is that I'll tell them, "Today's visit is all about ascertaining whether I can help you or not. I'll make some recommendations to you. [But] you will always dictate what you want to do." (Interview 6)

For this shared responsibility to become shared authority—a rather more difficult relationship to establish—the practitioner must view the patient as a "fellow expert."

What's often not recognized is the patient brings a particular level of expertise, too. Who knows more about them than them? And after all, it is about them and how they are able to get better. (Interview 40)

For the patient to be a full partner, however, the practitioner must have confidence that projects itself into the relationship.[2] Patients must trust the practitioner's ability to hold the healing space securely, and to provide guidance as they move together down the "wounded path."

And so, I think a lot of it, for them, is a sense of perceived confidence, and that has to do with the way you interact, the way you speak about options, the confidence that you have in your own skills. (Interview 22)

8. Be Committed and Trustworthy

Our expert informants repeatedly used the word "trustworthy" and connected it to a fear of abandonment. Hence, an intentional plan to sustain the relationship and carry it forward is almost always needed.

One thing I always, always try to do is make sure that every patient leaves with a plan. . . . I will tell patients [this] is one thing you can always count on. You always leave with a plan with me. Now it might not work . . . but as least you have a plan. (Interview 21)

But the plan, whatever it is, rests on a foundation of trust, which is often connected to the previous theme of hearing the patient's story (see "Take Time and Listen").

Healing is about connections, and connections are about listening to people's stories. Listening to people's story is what makes us trustworthy— and as we are found trustworthy, we are able to be more effective. (Interview 3)

The patient's story continues outside the consulting room or hospital. And the practitioner shows his or her recognition of and involvement in that story by promising not to abandon the patient as the story progresses.

Your patients have to trust you. They have to trust that you have their best interests at hand, and there's nothing that solidifies that trust like saying, "I value you as an individual. I value who you are, what you do, and what you contribute to my life, and because of that, you can explicitly trust me and what I recommend to you." (Interview 5)

Note the phrase "what you contribute to my life." One of the most consistent themes of our interviews was that finding meaning in medical practice is fundamentally connected to the capacity for forming patient relationships based on real trust, and that such relationships are the principal reward of being a physician.

Discussion

Although there is wide interest in healing, few empirical studies are available that provide details on how physicians build healing relationships. The Pew-Fetzer Task Force report of 1994[13] is an early effort at defining this area that includes some themes that our informants also identified, such as the centrality of relationships, appreciation of power differentials, and the importance of facilitating trust. Two more recent empirical studies are also worth noting. Hsu and colleagues[14] used focus groups of 28 patients and 56 clinicians to seek a definition of healing that would be concordant between these groups. They found some concurrence among the participants around emotional and spiritual dimensions. The importance of relationships was one of five key themes they identified. Scott and colleagues[15] conducted a study similar to ours, in which they interviewed six physicians, and two to five patients associated with each physician to identify "model components" of healing. They presented their findings as "healing processes," couched as ideals or such concepts as "presence," "partnering," and "healer competencies," and among the competencies, "self-confidence" and "emotional self-management." Advantages of our study include the number of physicians interviewed and the broad range of specialties represented; the inclusion of complementary and alternative practitioners; and a focus on practical imperatives to promote healing, rather than concepts.

Our study has several limitations. We encountered similar patterns of response repeatedly; however, our findings are preliminary, and we were working with a relatively small, selected sample. Our study also lacks comparison with practitioners who were not peer-nominated for having exceptional healing talents. Finally, patient interviews and perspectives were not a part of our study, and they might reveal a different set of core skills. Still, we believe that our interviews reveal a sound preliminary portrait of core relational skills from the practitioner's perspective. An important agenda for further work is to determine whether there is any connection between what practitioners perceive as important to healing relationships and the actual wellbeing of patients under their care.

Remen[16] reminds us that healing skills remain central to medicine, and Pellegrino[3] affirms that these skills are not just interaction strategies but are essential elements of medical ethics. The benefits of mastering these skills will repay the effort many times over, both in improved patient care and in the ability of physicians to find deeper meaning and fulfillment in their practices.

NOTES

1   Brody H. *Placebos and the Philosophy of Medicine*. Chicago: University of Chicago Press; 1980.

2   Moerman D. *Meaning, Medicine and the Placebo Effect*. New York: Cambridge University Press; 2002.

3   Pellegrino ED. *Humanism and the Physician*. Knoxville, TN: University of Tennessee Press; 1979:117–129.

4   Coulehan JL, Block MR. *The Medical Interview: Mastering Skills for Clinical Practice*. 4th ed. Philadelphia: FA Davis; 2001.

5   Billings JA, Stoeckle JD. *The Clinical Encounter: A Guide to the Medical Interview and Case Presentation*. 2nd ed. St. Louis: Mosby; 1999.

6   Mishler E. *The Discourse of Medicine: Dialectics of Medical Interviews*. Norwood, NJ: Ablex Press; 1984.

7   Cassell EJ. *Talking with Patients*, Vol. I: *The Theory of Doctor-Patient Communication*. Cambridge, MA: MIT Press; 1985.

8   Charon R. *Narrative Medicine: Honoring the Stories of Illness*. New York: Oxford University Press; 2006.

9   Charon R, Montello M. *Stories Matter: The Role of Narrative in Medical Ethics*. New York: Routledge; 2002.

10 Chapman E. *The Caregiver Meditations*. Nashville, TN: October Hill Press; 2007.

11 Groopman J. *How Doctors Think*. Boston: Houghton Mifflin; 2007.

12 Kleinman A. *The Illness Narratives*. New York: Basic Books; 1988.

13 Tresolini CP, Pew-Fetzer Task Force. *Health Professions Education and Relationship-Centered Care*. San Francisco: Pew Health Professions Commission; 1994.

14 Hsu C, Phillips WR, Sherman KJ, Hawkes R, Cherkin DC. Healing in primary care: a vision shared by patients, physicians, nurses, and clinical staff. *Ann Fam Med*. 2008;6:307–314. [PMID: 18626030]

15 Scott JG, Cohen D, Dicicco-Bloom B, Miller WL, Stange KC, Crabtree BF. Understanding healing relationships in primary care. *Ann Fam Med*. 2008;6:315–322. [PMID: 18626031]

16 Remen R. Quoted by: Tippett K. *Speaking of Faith*. New York: Penguin Books; 2007:213.

The Hair Stylist, the Corn Merchant, and the Doctor

Ambiguously Altruistic

Lois Shepherd

The AHP Code of Ethics requires members to serve the best interests of their clients, be clear and honest with them, and keep their secrets confidential. Members pledge to represent their skills and qualifications honestly and to make appropriate referrals to others more qualified when out of their depth.[1]

AHP stands for "Associated Hair Professionals," or hair stylists, but their Code of Ethics looks a lot like the Hippocratic Oath and the current Principles of Medical Ethics of the American Medical Association. All of these ethics statements emphasize honesty, confidentiality, competence, serving patients' (or clients') best interests, and willingness to refer to other qualified professionals. But it's not just doctors and hair professionals who have codes of ethics. The SPCP—Society of Permanent Cosmetic Professionals—requires its members to "maintain high professional standards consistent with sound practices," "conduct business relationships in a manner that is fair to all," and avoid false or misleading statements to the effect that the application of permanent makeup is not tattooing, not permanent, and not painful.[2] (Physicians might consider that last point—I'm grateful for the time my doctor once warned me, "This is really going to hurt.")

Some of us from the traditional, or "learned" professions—medicine, law, ministry, teaching—might take umbrage, thinking "they're not like us." But they are. We all have promises to keep—whether we made them individually or collectively, explicitly or implicitly, and whether we are bound

Lois Shepherd, "The Hair Stylist, the Corn Merchant, and the Doctor: Ambiguously Altruistic," from *Journal of Law, Medicine, and Ethics* 42, no. 4 (Winter 2014): 509–517. Reprinted by permission of Sage Publications, Inc., Journals, conveyed through Copyright Clearance Center, Inc.

by a professional code (often the result of our achieving monopoly status through government licensing—not a disinterested act by any means) or simply because we are neighbors as fellow human beings. The traditional professions are no more noble than any other legitimate occupation, and it is time to give up the illusion that they are. Not simply because it is not true but because—as I'll explain—it prevents us from carefully defining what actual responsibilities professionals do have and determining whether those responsibilities have been met.

The medical profession in particular has a tradition of presenting itself as ethically exceptional.[3] It has long claimed and still claims that as a whole its members are altruistic—and more so than other professionals and other people.[4] William Osler proclaimed in a 1903 statement often quoted by those advancing medical professionalism that "the practice of medicine is not a business and can never be one. . . . Our fellow creatures cannot be dealt with as man deals in corn and coal."[5] These words have special resonance for some today. It might be appealing to think that in the increasingly corporatized, commercial world of medical care,[6] physicians would take great care to distinguish themselves from the hair stylist and the corn merchant, and that they should do so in large measure by identifying themselves as altruistic.

This approach is mistaken. The claim that physicians are or should be more altruistic than others does not withstand scrutiny. And while the corporatization and commercialization of the medical world pose some threat to patient well-being and autonomy, so do recent expansions of doctors' conscientious refusal and growing attempts to further blend clinical research and care.[7] Appeals to altruism obfuscate rather than clarify physicians' roles; the medical profession would do better to hold true to their basic duties to patients and commit to honesty, and perhaps a measure of humility.

The Claim and Its Merits

Altruism often goes undefined in claims that the medical profession is, by definition, altruistic or that individual physicians are required, as an ethical matter, to be altruistic in a way that we do not expect of others. The editors of the *New England Journal of Medicine* declared in 2000 that "medicine is one of the few spheres of human activity in which the purposes are unambiguously altruistic—in itself, a remarkable achievement."[8] The statement was bald—without any explanation or support. Because the statement prefaced the editors' review of medical achievements of the previous millennium, a reader might have expected that some of those achievements would have to do with altruistic behavior, but they were all scientific, with scientific values and purposes.

In 1998, the American Board of Internal Medicine (ABIM), in its *Project Professionalism*, declared that "Altruism is the essence of professionalism."[9] Together with two other influential physician organizations, the ABIM adopted the "Physician Charter"[10] in 2002, which the editor of the *Annals of Internal Medicine* wrote he hoped would be a "watershed event in medicine."[11] In identifying the principle of primacy of patient welfare, the Charter states that "altruism contributes to the trust that is central to the physician-patient relationship." There is no elaboration of the concept, however.[12] Some members of the profession have pushed for an even more prominent recognition of the importance of altruism, and have recommended that altruism be consciously and systematically developed among medical students and identified in medical student applicants.[13] It is becoming increasingly important, then, to understand what is meant—or perhaps more critically for this essay, what is *not* meant by the term.

The virtue of altruism—outside of these statements about medical professionalism—is commonly understood to mean a disposition to act in the interests of others at a cost to the interests of oneself.[14] It is generally understood as involving actions that are beyond obligation, or duty. If one had a duty to act in the interests of others in a particular situation—say, because one had been paid to do so—then we would not call actions taken for the benefit of others to be altruistic. Glannon and Ross explain that when physicians act in the best interests of their patients, they are fulfilling their fiduciary obligations.[15] Such actions are not "optional and supererogatory, beyond the call of duty."[16] A claim that physicians are altruistic has to mean more than that they are, in the context of the physician-patient relationship, recommending, prescribing, and treating the patient in ways that serve the patient's interests and not the physician's interests—because that is their job, "their daily professional work."[17]

It is not much different from what we expect from a hair stylist. We would think a hair stylist to be acting unethically if he rushed and botched a haircut to increase production rates or applied hair coloring that suited his own preferences rather than the client's or threw in an extra, expensive product application without client approval. The AHP's Code of Ethics may be a helpful reminder of the standards of common morality in the stylist-client relationship, but those standards would exist without the written code. We would not consider the hair stylist altruistic for following these guidelines;

indeed, there are times when a stylist works with hair that is dirty, or matted, or contains lice, or readies a corpse for burial; the stylist isn't altruistic for doing his best under these circumstances either—these activities, too, can be part of his job.

Ethical obligations of one sort or another inhere in every human activity and therefore every occupation, and it can be helpful to clearly set out what those obligations are—as reminders of how one ought to act. In truth, codes of ethics often contain very basic obligations that we expect of everyone when acting in morally appropriate ways. Even the "man who deals in corn and coal," to quote Osler, has ethical (and legal) duties of honesty and fair dealing even if he does not have fiduciary obligations stemming from a relationship of trust. Moreover, if he wants repeat customers and a good business reputation, he will try to help the customer understand which good or product will best serve his or her needs; many merchants will do the same for a one-time, out-of-town customer just out of simple human consideration. Which is all to say that there is nothing terribly extraordinary or burdensome about expecting individuals who hold themselves out as experts to be competent in the subject matter of their expertise or for those who have invited the trust of customers/clients/patients to only recommend and perform services in the latter's best interests.

So what is behind the claim that physicians are uniquely altruistic? It cannot simply be that they will act in the patient's best interests, as hair stylists have a similar obligation to their clients, and we do not generally think of hair stylists as being uniquely altruistic.

Perhaps what is meant is that physicians, as a group and because of their profession, tend to be placed in situations in which extraordinary demands are made upon them. This is a bit of a different claim, and one I can probably accept. But it is still worth asking whether these sorts of demands are truly unique. To be sure, physicians sometimes have a lack of control over their time, or face risk of harm, and even make financial sacrifices. We tend to associate these demands with the medical profession (including nurses, who typically enjoy far less financial compensation), though we might question how exclusively.

With respect to time, there may occasionally be disruptive and demanding calls upon the physician—emergency room coverage in the middle of the night, or extra long hours to provide a hospitalized patient with continuity of care—but comparable demands are made of others—firefighters battling prolonged forest fires, journalists covering foreign conflicts, and even (perhaps an unlikely example) legislators, called into special session for midnight votes.

It is true that physicians are sometimes called upon to deliver medical services in their off-duty hours. For example, we expect a physician, when dining out, to come to the aid of a choking diner, or when walking along the street and seeing a bystander collapse, to stop and administer first aid. But, then again, we expect this of anyone capable of providing help—the hair stylist, the teacher, the lawyer, the person who deals in "corn and coal"—that they step in as needed but will step out of the way for the person with more expertise to take over. (Neither the physician nor the nonphysician in these situations has a legal obligation to rescue.)

The most extraordinary demand—and perhaps the strongest case for a profession-wide claim to altruism—may be the ethical requirement to care for those who are dangerously infectious. Medical professionals (again including, and perhaps especially, nurses) really are on the "front lines" in those circumstances. The divergence from hair stylists seems clearer here. But are the dangers any more immediate or the risks any more commonplace than those faced by police officers, firefighters, soldiers—who, not insignificantly, are often compensated at a considerably lower rate?[18]

Moreover, if physician attitudes about caring for HIV positive patients in the early days of the HIV epidemic are anything to go on, altruism of this nature is not a widely adopted norm among U.S. physicians. Despite the ethical guidance issued in 1987 by the AMA's Council on Ethical and Judicial Affairs that physicians could not ethically refuse care to patients who were HIV positive, substantial numbers of physicians (for example, two-thirds of orthopedic surgeons according to one survey) did not believe this to be the case.[19] I think they were wrong—that they did have an ethical duty to care for HIV positive patients, but I also do not think meeting that duty amounts to altruism. Providing care in such situations is the responsibility the profession—and thus members of the profession—took on when it received the exclusive license to practice medicine and prevented others from doing the same.

Finally, we seem to have a fondness in the U.S. for thinking that doctors are—or, some might think, used to be—willing to sacrifice financial gain in their pursuit of the good of the patient. In 2010, a Senate candidate from Nevada, Sue Lowden, proposed a less regulated health care market as an alternative to the Affordable Care Act, a market in which individuals negotiate and even barter with their doctor. In making this argument, she harkened back to times past when patients would pay a physician in chickens or offer to paint the physician's house. When her remarks were mocked as simplistic and out-of-touch, she responded, "I mean, that's the old days of what people would do to get health care with your doctors," she said. "Doctors are very sympathetic people. I'm not backing down from that system."[20]

But there is no reason to think of such practices fondly. They represent circumstances of abject dependency on the part of patients and lord-like power on the part of physicians. We can appreciate the willingness of a rural doctor to work for chickens—we might even consider it altruistic, but seeing a patient out of charity (which many doctors do—and many do not) is not by any means the daily way of the business of doctors or the medical profession generally. Nor should we expect it to be. We are moving, thankfully, toward recognition of a basic, universal right to access to health care. How to pay for that care for those who cannot afford it will require complex and iterative negotiations and even experiment. But physicians will not and should not bear a greater share of the burden of the costs of such care than others.[21] Doctors frequently offer their services at reduced rates, or gratis, as do lawyers, accountants, and mechanics; this is nearly always a good thing, but it is also the kind of occasional altruism that people of all occupations do from time to time—it is not systematic, nor is it required (with the exception, to some people's surprise, of lawyers, who sometimes do have state-imposed requirements for pro bono or reduced fee services for indigent clients[22]). And doctors do tend to make a good living—some, an excellent living—and feel they've earned it, and usually they have.

Sometimes physicians volunteer in challenging, resource-restricted, and even dangerous regions of the world with organizations such as Doctors without Borders; in these instances, they are being altruistic in the way we generally understand that term.[23] But these activities are not required of physicians, and we would not think of individual physicians as being selfish or morally insufficient if they did not do these activities. There are altruistic doctors just like there are all kinds of altruistic people. We admire those who do this kind of work, but it cannot redound to the whole profession.

What Is Troubling about the Claim?

So far I have tried to debunk the notion that physicians are required to be altruistic in order to be an upstanding member of the profession. I've also challenged the idea that the profession as a whole is more inherently altruistic than other professions. But one might respond that the claim to altruism is aspirational; that it does no harm and can only promote good. There are many temptations in the modern medical world for doctors to make more money or secure other advantages by doing things that are not good for patients; shouldn't we encourage their own insistence on the virtue of altruism to protect patients? Doesn't believing they are altruistic make them better doctors?

No. In fact, appealing to altruism can have the opposite effect. As Simon Blackburn has written in *Being Good*, a natural reaction to extreme, unrealistic demands of morality is to shrug off those demands, to ignore them in practice though we may continue to preach them.[24] It can also contribute to the inability of doctors, and others, too, to accept some of our more humbling, shared human failings—like making mistakes—and it can make it more difficult for us to recognize and admit to conflicts of interest.

I like the mechanic who takes care of my car. He knows what he is doing. He advises me against some of the "extras" that might make him more money but that I don't need. I know that he has carried more than a few paycheck-to-paycheck customers. He recently misdiagnosed a starting issue with my car and installed an unnecessary part that did not fix the problem. He admitted the error, returned the part, did not charge me for his labor, and made the correct repair.

It was the right thing to do. It was also good business—I will be back and I will tell my friends about his honesty and commitment to his customers. But what if he believed that by "taking care of" my car he was doing me a favor, that he was (even though I pay him) doing the work as much out of the goodness of his heart as out of professional obligation? That he was being altruistic. It would have been hard for me to question his misdiagnosis and errant repair if he had not owned up to it. And he might not so easily have accepted responsibility for his mistake.

And so it can be with doctors, good doctors; they too often believe that holding them responsible for mistakes they have made when their hearts are "in the right place" and "they are only trying to help" (save a life, perhaps) somehow casts aspersions on them. A surgeon once initiated a lengthy discussion with me about how unjust medical malpractice (i.e., tort) law was to physicians. He argued that it wasn't right for physicians to be sued when they had merely made "an honest mistake." "Everyone makes mistakes," he pointed out. When I asked whether patients who were harmed from a mistake like the one he was describing should be compensated, he said, of course.

There was obviously a disconnect here. As a lawyer, I was focusing on compensation for a patient's injuries, which would require proof of negligence and injury before being awarded and which would be paid by malpractice insurance, for which the (hypothetical) physician would have already paid the premiums. What the surgeon was focusing on was what the lawsuit appeared to say about the doctor's *character*. Further, he was sensitive to what a statement about the character of the doctor would do to the doctor—it would be psychologically devastating.

A similar vulnerability was apparent in the responses of many in the medical community in the Spring of 2013 to the controversy surrounding the SUPPORT Trial, a large multisite study of premature infants.[25] The bioethics community split over whether consent forms used in the study were inadequate under the federal research regulations because they failed to disclose to the parents of the infants enrolled reasonably foreseeable risks of serious harms.[26] The Office for Human Research Protections (OHRP) issued a determination letter in March 2013 to the University of Alabama, the lead site, asking its institutional review board (IRB) to take measures to improve consent processes in the future.[27] Despite the extremely mild nature of the OHRP's response (essentially, "be more careful next time;" federal funding was not threatened, for example) and the fact that its criticism was limited to the consent forms and did not question the study's value or design or the integrity of the investigators, the agency and those who supported its action were generally seen as attacking the character of the investigators.[28] The editors of the *New England Journal of Medicine* blasted the OHRP for damaging reputations and emphasized that the investigators were acting in good faith.[29] An open letter signed by 46 scholars in bioethics and pediatrics argued that the OHRP should not second-guess IRBs on whether research ethics standards have actually been met by investigators, but should confine its inquiry to determining whether IRBs are duly constituted and the like.[30] The message replayed over and over was that the SUPPORT investigators were *good people—unselfishly devoted to saving—and learning how to save more—premature babies.* Any comparison to earlier studies that are part of the U.S. collection of research "scandals" was off limits because those earlier studies were conducted by immoral researchers—by people not like them. (History has generally taught us otherwise—that many research ethics lapses occur despite the presence of a well-meaning and upstanding investigator—that is why we have research oversight.)

Questions about a doctor's actions, especially if those actions have some relationship to matters of ethics, are perceived as an almost existential threat. But whether we are asking if standards of care were met in respect to execution of a surgical procedure or if informed consent forms disclosed all relevant risks, physicians' actions cannot be immune from criticism. It is worth considering whether the shields physicians tend to put up to deflect scrutiny of their actions, and the actions of their peers, are needed because they have made themselves so psychologically tender to attack by expecting themselves to be "all good" all the time.[31]

The shield of altruism can be insidious. This is nowhere more evident than in the resistance among doctors to acknowledge when they have a conflict of interest. Here, perhaps more than in any other sphere, the ideal of an altruistic profession can blind professionals to the very real enticements of gifts, money, prestige, and acclaim.[32] To presume, as many do, that the good they do (and I must repeat, they *do good*) sets them apart, makes them better able than others to avoid violating duties because of troubling conflicts of interests *without requiring rules and policies against these conflicts* is naïve and, it must be said, somewhat arrogant.[33]

It was not long ago when our prescriptions were written with pens supplied by drug companies and our throats checked by doctors using tongue depressors bearing the name of a prescription drug. Drug companies, before adopting a voluntary ban in 2008, used to hand these out to doctors like candy. What is more troubling than that these items proliferated throughout our health care settings is that many physicians believed that they were above being influenced by them. Before a similar ban in 2002, doctors were being given vacations by drug companies under the guise of "conferences" in exotic locations. Doctors generally believed they would not be improperly influenced by such junkets.[34] A legislator who sought office only for the good of her nation might be subject to myriad conflicts of interest rules because we do not trust her to always be able to judge when she is being swayed by special interests, but somehow doctors did not need the same ethical stringency. They did, after all, pursue purposes that are "unambiguously altruistic."[35]

While free pens and vacations have gone by the wayside, the financial ties between drug companies and doctors are stronger than ever with consulting fees and contract research.[36] Doctors also own imaging facilities, specialty hospitals,[37] and patents. Nonfinancial conflicts of interest can be harder to recognize and are rarely acknowledged as a conflict of interest—such as wanting to avoid a patient "dying on my watch" or wishing to discover scientific advances not for financial gain but, as I am sure the SUPPORT investigators wished, in order to make future patients' lives better.[38]

While lawyers tend to think of conflicts of interest as "objective, structural, and rule-based," doctors see them "as relating to the individual's character and ability to resist temptation."[39] As Sandra Johnson has written, "Tell doctors that they have a 'conflict of interest' in relation to a proposed protocol for research with human subjects, and they believe that you have accused them of unethical behavior. . . . [D]octors tend to assume that a conflict of interest exists only when they actually have made a 'bad' decision motivated by their financial interest."[40]

This means that if a doctor actually does something *improper* because of the temptation posed by a personal conflict of interest, he is bad; otherwise, the conflict of interest is not a problem and often goes unnoticed. Seeing themselves and their peers as either "good" or "bad" makes them less able and willing to see, identify, and manage conflicts of interest—their own and those of their colleagues.

And conflicts of interests are even more difficult for patients to see. We have long been aware of the phenomenon of the "therapeutic misconception" in research, under which patients mistakenly believe, even if told otherwise, that "decisions about their care are being made solely with their benefit in mind."[41] A mother of an infant enrolled in the SUPPORT Trial explained at a public hearing that she did not understand that her child was in a research experiment; she was "under the impression this was more a support group."[42] "What mother would not want support?" she asked.[43] Even when subjects understand that they have enrolled in research, they can be surprised to find they were on the placebo arm of a trial because the subjects—also patients—believe that no doctor would put them in danger by taking them off medication.[44]

Similarly, a patient or family member would likely be surprised to learn that a physician might have an interest in ordering extra tests to boost revenues at the imaging facility in which he has an interest, or that a nursing home might benefit from higher reimbursement rates for maintaining a surgically implanted feeding tube over feeding by hand, a less invasive and more personal form of care.

While the hair stylist also has conflicts of interests, they are easier to see. There is a clear price for the services performed, and it is no secret that he or she is selling the hair care products at the front of the salon. The delivery of medical care is more ethically complex and more essential to human well-being, it is true. But the collective inability or reluctance on the part of physicians, patients, and the general public to identify, disclose, and determine how to manage threats to patient welfare and patient autonomy posed by conflicts of interest—and to make the delivery of medical care *less* ethically complex when possible by *eliminating* conflicts of interest—depends in large part, I suspect, on our image of doctors as altruistic.

We have a lot of work to do identifying more exactly what we mean when we say a physician has a duty to act in the best interests of the patient. That is where our attention needs to go—not in further exploration of what it means for a doctor to be altruistic, how to identify altruistic medical school applicants, or how to measure whether students have grown in their commitment to altruism through their medical school education. Abandoning the idea may relieve its members of unrealistic burdens that can distort their ability to engage in critical self-reflection. Besides, why would the profession want to hold itself apart? If what the profession really means when it talks about altruism is not self-sacrifice, but instead empathy, understanding, connection with patients and others—and that may be what some in the profession actually do mean when they talk about altruism—then isn't it far better to understand that no single occupation or group of people has a stronger claim to being called altruistic? Aren't we all in this together?

Conclusion

A recent story in the news told about an 8-year-old boy in New York who woke to discover fire in his grandfather's mobile home, where he was spending the night. After awakening and ushering out six relatives, including two other children, he went back in to try to help his disabled grandfather and his uncle get out. But when he did, he became overcome with heat and smoke, and he died. Tyler Doohan was a hero. And he was treated as one. He was given a firefighter's funeral, in which firefighters from around the state wore dress blues and white gloves, and fire engines lined the streets. Tyler was hailed for his courage, his bravery, his selflessness.[45]

Tyler Doohan was not just a hero, he was an altruistic hero. Though given the title of an honorary firefighter in death, he was not trained to fight fires or expected to attempt to rescue others from a burning building. People of all ages and talents and occupations go out of their way to help others at cost and risk to themselves, sometimes making the ultimate sacrifice. Altruism does exist, and we need to honor it. But doing so requires us to recognize what it is and what it is not.

About a week after the story of Tyler Doohan, there was another inspiring national news story about someone who had done something terrific.

An unexpected and severe snowstorm in Alabama had stranded a surgeon, Dr. Zenko Hrynkiwon, on his way from one hospital to another to perform emergency, life-saving brain surgery. When travelling by car became impossible because of blocked roads, he headed out on the 6-mile trek in 20-degree weather in his scrubs, a jacket, and operating room slip covers over his shoes. He received the patient's CT scan via text as he walked, was eventually given a lift by a passerby for the last bit of the journey, and was in surgery two hours after he set out. The patient was believed to have had a 90 percent chance of dying without the surgery. He lived. According to news reports, upon arrival to the operating room, the charge nurse told Dr. Hrynkiwon, "You're a good man.'" The doctor replied, "I'm just doing my job."[46] They were both right.

NOTES

1 Associated Hair Professionals, *Code of Ethics*, http://www.insuringstyle.com/hairstylists/membership/ahp-code-of-ethics (accessed September 29, 2014).

2 The Society of Permanent Cosmetic Professionals, *Code of Ethics*, http://www.spcp.org/information-for-technicians/spcp-code-of-ethics (accessed September 29, 2014).

3 R. M. Veatch, *A Theory of Medical Ethics* (New York: Basic Books, Inc., 1981): at 6, 92–107 (discussing the inadequacy of reliance on any profession to determine its own moral foundation through agreement among its members).

4 The 1847 AMA code states that "there is no profession, from the members of which greater purity of character and a higher standard of moral excellence are required, than the medical." Veach, *Theory of Medical Ethics*, 93.

5 C. R. MacKenzie, "Professionalism and Medicine," *History of the Human Sciences Journal* 3, no. 2 (2007): 222–227 (citing W. O. Osler, "On the Educational Value of the Medical Society," in *Aequanimitas, with Other Addresses to Medical Students, Nurses and Practitioners of Medicine*, 3rd ed. [Philadelphia: Blakiston, 1932]: 395–423).

6 L. R. Churchill, "The Hegemony of Money: Commercialism and Professionalism in American Medicine," *Cambridge Quarterly Healthcare Ethics* 16, no. 4 (2007), 407–414.

7 R. Faden, N. Kass, and S. Goodman, et al., "An Ethics Framework for a Learning Health Care System: A Departure from Traditional Research Ethics and Clinical Ethics," *Hastings Center Report* 43, no. S1 (2013): S16–S27.

8 Editors, "Looking Back on the Millennium in Medicine," *New England Journal of Medicine* 342, no. 1 (2000): 42–49.

9 American Board of Internal Medicine, *Project Professionalism* (Philadelphia: American Board of Internal Medicine, 1998), 5.

10 Project of the ABIM Foundation, ACP–ASIM Foundation, and European Federation of Internal Medicine, "Medical Professionalism in the New Millennium: A Physician Charter," *Annals of Internal Medicine* 136, no. 3 (2002): 243–246.

11 H. C. Sox, "Preface," *Annals of Internal Medicine* 136, no. 3 (2002).

12 For a discussion of the medical professional literature on definitions and invocations of professionalism and altruism, see F. W. Hafferty, "Definitions of Professionalism: A Search for Meaning and Identity," *Clinical Orthopaedics and Related Research* 449 (2006): 193–204. Hafferty notes that British definitions of professionalism "do not highlight altruism as a core concept or an organizing principle" (199).

13 H. M. Swick, "Toward a Normative Definition of Medical Professionalism," *Academic Medicine* 75, no. 6 (2000): 612–616; D. D. Gibson, L. L. Coldwell, and S. F. Kiewit, "Creating a Culture of Professionalism: An Integrated Approach," *Academic Medicine* 75, no. 5 (2000): 509; C. L. Bardes, "Is Medicine Altruistic? A Query from the Medical School Admissions Office," *Teaching and Learning in Medicine: An International Journal* 18, no. 1 (2010): 48–49.

14 French philosopher Auguste Comte coined the term in the nineteenth century to describe an ethical obligation "to live for others," renouncing self-interest. *Stanford Encyclopedia of Philosophy*, s.v. "Auguste Comte," http://plato.stanford.edu/entries /comte/#EthSoc (accessed September 29, 2014). *Oxford Living Dictionaries* defines altruism as "the belief in or practice of disinterested and selfless concern for the well-being of others." *Oxford Living Dictionaries*, http://www.oxforddictionaries.com/us /definition/american_english/altruism (accessed September 29, 2014). See also A. MacIntyre, "Egoism and Altruism," in D. M. Borchert, ed., *Encyclopedia of Philosophy*, vol. 2 (New York: Macmillan, 1967): at 442–466. MacIntyre explains that altruism is often considered the opposite of egoism and describes the resulting preoccupation with determining which of these two motives, or ways of living, govern our actions. He provides a contrary view, writing that "if I want to lead a certain kind of life, with relationships of trust, friendship, and cooperation with others, then my wanting their good and my wanting my good are not two independent, discriminable desires."

15 W. Glannon and L. F. Ross, "Are Doctors Altruistic?" *Journal of Medical Ethics* 28 (2002): 68–69. For discussion of physicians' fiduciary obligations, see M. J. Mehlman, "Dishonest Medical Mistakes," *Vanderbilt Law Review* 59, no. 4 (2006): 1137–1173; M. A. Rodwin, "Strains in the Fiduciary Metaphor: Divided Physician Loyalties and Obligations in a Changing Health Care System," *American Journal of Law and Medicine* 21, nos. 2–3 (1995): 241–257.

16 Glannon and Ross, "Are Doctors Altruistic?"

17 Glannon and Ross, "Are Doctors Altruistic?" Similarly, R. S. Downie writes that "Morality enters medicine through the quality of the individual doctor's work, not by the definition of that work." R. S. Downie, "Supererogation and Altruism: A Comment," *Journal of Medical Ethics* 28, no. 2 (2002): 75–76.

18 Glannon and Ross, "Are Doctors Altruistic?"

19 D. Orentlicher, "The Influence of a Professional Organization on Physician Behavior," *Albany Law Review* 57, no. 3 (1994): 583–605.

20 B. Montopoli, "Sue Lowden Stands by Chicken Health Care Barter Plan," CBS *News*, April 22, 2010, http://www.cbsnews.com/news/sue-lowden-stands-by-chicken-health -care-barter-plan (accessed September 29, 2014). For reporting and video footage of the original Lowden comment on bartering with physicians, see E. Kleefeld, "NV-SEN Candidate Sue Lowden (R): 'Barter With Your Doctor,'" TPM, April 12, 2010,

http://talkingpointsmemo.com/dc/nv-sen-candidate-sue-lowden-r-barter-with-your-doctor-video (accessed September 29, 2014).

21 For an early essay presenting a *moral* argument for understanding the practice of medicine as a business, see R. M. Sade, "Medical Care as a Right: A Refutation," *New England Journal of Medicine* 285, no. 23 (1971): 1288–1292. Sade compares the physician to a baker.

22 American Bar Association (ABA), *Model Rules of Professional Conduct*, Rule 6.01 ("Every lawyer has a professional responsibility to provide legal services to those unable to pay. A lawyer should aspire to render at least [50] hours of pro bono publico legal services per year.") Because the requirement to provide pro bono services is somewhat general, it would be difficult to enforce, even in those states that have adopted Rule 6.01 as part of the regulations governing the conduct of lawyers. New York, however, has recently adopted a rule "requiring applicants for admission to the New York State bar to perform 50 hours of pro bono services." New York State Uniform Court System, http://www.nycourts.gov/attorneys/probono/baradmissionreqs.shtml (accessed September 29, 2014). Moreover, courts can appoint lawyers to serve particular clients in a case and when they do so, the lawyers' compensation for such representation will be fixed by the court. See ABA *Model*, Rule 6.2 ("A lawyer shall not seek to avoid appointment by a tribunal to represent a person except for good cause.")

23 See Glannon and Ross, "Are Doctors Altruistic?"

24 S. Blackburn, *Being Good* (New York: Oxford University Press Inc., 2001): at 48–49. Millennial medical student graduates may not be as inclined to support and promote altruism as a core value. F. W. Hafferty, "What Medical Students Know about Professionalism," *Mount Sinai Journal of Medicine* 69, no. 6 (2002): 385–398. Hafferty writes that classroom discussion with medical students as part of a professionalism curriculum revealed little support for the principle that physicians should subordinate their own interests to the interests of others. The students expressed a need for "balance" in their lives, the importance of taking care of oneself in order to help others, and a lack of commitment to vague and general professional codes and oaths imposed by others. He writes, "Students certainly verbalized a commitment to doing good, but they were unremittingly clear that the who, what, when, where, and why would remain under the control of the 'do gooder.'" While some of these attitudes are not particularly problematic under the thesis of this article, we might nevertheless be concerned that once "altruism" is rejected or discredited as the lesson to learn, students may not be taught or may not understand and internalize what their true and more specific ethical and legal obligations are to patients. Most concerning is Hafferty's statement that the students "[m]ost clearly and emphatically . . . rejected the notion that they were obliged to do anything. Period" (391). See also Hafferty, "Definitions of Professionalism."

25 S. Coons, "The SUPPORT Trial: Risk and Consent Questions Divide the Clinical Research Community," *Research Practitioner* 14, no. 5 (2013): 112–117. G. J. Annas and C. L. Annas, "Legally Blind: The Therapeutic Illusion in the Support Study of Extremely Premature Infants," *Journal of Contemporary Health Law and Policy* 30, no. 1 (2014): 1–36. R. Macklin and L. Shepherd, "Informed Consent and Standard of Care: What Must Be Disclosed," *American Journal of Bioethics* 13, no. 12 (2013): 9–13.

26 Compare B. S. Wilfond et al., "The OHRP and SUPPORT," *New England Journal of Medicine* 368, no. 25 (2013): e36, doi:10.1056/NEJMc1307008, with R. Macklin et al., "The OHRP and SUPPORT—Another View," *New England Journal of Medicine* 369, no. 2 (2013): e3(1)–(3), doi:10.1056/NEJMc1308015.

27 Office for Human Research Protections, *Letter to the University of Alabama at Birmingham,* March 7, 2013, http://www.hhs.gov/ohrp/detrm_letrs/YR13/mar13a.pdf (accessed October 1, 2014).

28 See, e.g., J. D. Lantos, "OHRP and Public Citizen Are Wrong about Neonatal Research on Oxygen Therapy," *Bioethics Forum, Hastings Center Report,* April 18, 2013, http://www.thehastingscenter.org/Bioethicsforum/Post.aspx?id=6306&blogid=140 (accessed October 1, 2014); see also comments posted by K. Barrington, on June 10 2013, to L. Shepherd, "The Support Study and the Standard of Care," *Bioethics Forum, The Hastings Center Report,* May 17, 2013, http://www.thehastingscenter.org/Bioethicsforum /Post.aspx?id=6358&blogid=140 (accessed October 1, 2014).

29 J. M. Drazen, C. G. Solomon, and M. F. Greene, "Informed Consent and SUPPORT," *New England Journal of Medicine* 368, no. 20 (2013): 1929–1931.

30 See Wilfond, "The OHRP and SUPPORT."

31 See MacIntyre, "Egoism and Altruism" (writing about our misguided preoccupation with understanding actions as taken either in self-interest or benevolence, either with bad motives or good motives).

32 See M. H. Bazerman and A. E. Tenbrunsel, *Blind Spots: Why We Fail to Do What's Right and What to Do about It* (Princeton: Princeton University Press, 2011): at 20–21 ("[M]ost smart, well-educated doctors are puzzled by the criticism against them, as they are confident in their own ethicality and the 'fact' that they always put their patients' interests first. . . . But the more pernicious aspect of conflicts of interest is clarified by well-replicated research showing that when people have a vested interest in seeing a problem in a certain manner, they are no longer capable of objectivity.").

33 Although a full exploration is beyond the scope of this essay, paternalism is an additional concern that often flows from the best of intentions but, nonetheless, raises concerns about which a well-meaning physician may not even be aware. An overblown sense of altruism may, at least in part, contribute to the pernicious self-rationalization that the doctor always knows best.

34 J. P. Orlowski and L. Wateska, "The Effects of Pharmaceutical Firm Enticements on Physician Prescribing Patterns: There's No Such Thing as a Free Lunch," *Chest* 102, no. 1 (1992): 270–273; A. Wazana, "Physicians and the Pharmaceutical Industry, Is a Gift Ever Just a Gift?" *JAMA* 283 (2000): 373–380; G. Harris and J. Roberts, "Doctors' Ties to Drug Makers Are Put on Close View," *New York Times,* March 21, 2007, at A1.

35 See Editors, "Looking Back on the Millennium in Medicine."

36. J. Fisher, *Medical Research for Hire: The Political Economy of Pharmaceutical Clinical Trials* (New Jersey: Rutgers University Press, 2008); see Harris and Roberts, "Doctors' Ties to Drug Makers."

37 J. E. Perry, "Physician-Owned Specialty Hospitals and the Patient Protection and Affordable Care Act: Health Care Reform at the Intersection of Law and Ethics," *American Business Law Journal* 49, no. 2 (2012): 369–416.

38 See generally L. Shepherd and M. F. Riley, "In Plain Sight: A Solution to a Fundamental Challenge in Human Research," *Journal of Law, Medicine, and Ethics* 40, no. 4
(2012): 970–989 (discussing the physician-researcher conflict of interest).

39 S. H. Johnson, "Five Easy Pieces: Motifs of Health Law," *Health Matrix* 14, no. 1 (2004):
131–140, at 131.

40 Johnson, "Five Easy Pieces."

41 P. S. Appelbaum, L. H. Roth, and C. Lidz, "The Therapeutic Misconception: Informed
Consent in Psychiatric Research," *International Journal of Law and Psychiatry* 5, nos.
3 & 4 (1982): 319–329, at 321; C. W. Lidz, P. S. Appelbaum, T. Grisso, and M. Renaud,
"Therapeutic Misconception and the Appreciation of Risks in Clinical Trials," *Social
Science and Medicine* 58, no. 9 (2004): 1689–1697, 1691.

42 S. Cook, "Comments at OHRP Public Meeting on Matters Related to Protection of Human
Subjects and Research Considering Standard of Care Interventions" (August 28, 2013),
video recording, http://www.youtube.com/playlist?list=PLr17E8KABz1Gc_ndt9grGg80
_jE5G1RNC; transcript, http://www.hhs.gov/ohrp/newsroom/rfc/Public%20Meet
ing%20August%2028,%202013/support-meetingtranscriptfinal.html (accessed October 1, 2014).

43 S. Cook, "Comments at OHRP Public Meeting." See also M. Hochhauser, "'Therapeutic
Misconception' and 'Recruiting Doublespeak' in the Informed Consent Process," *IRB:
Ethics and Human Research* 24, no. 1 (2002): 11–12 (explaining how the ubiquitous "brand
names" of clinical trials contribute to a research subject's therapeutic misconception).

44 "Clinical Trial Subjects: Adequate FDA Protections?" Hearing before the Committee
on Government Reform and Oversight House of Representatives, 105th Congress
(1998): 152–153, http://www.gpo.gov/fdsys/pkg/CHRG-105hhrg49827/pdf/CHRG
-105hhrg49827.pdf (accessed October 10, 2014).

45 "Firefighters Line Funeral of Tyler Doohan, 8, Who Died Trying to Save Family from
Fire," *CBS News*, January 29, 2014, http://www.cbsnews.com/news/8-year-old-tyler
-doohan-who-died-trying-to-save-family-from-fire-gets-a-firefighters-funeral
(accessed October 1, 2014).

46 A. Dier, Newser, "Surgeon Walked 6 Miles in Ala. Storm to OR," *USA Today*, January 31, 2014, http://www.usatoday.com/story/news/nation/2014/01/31/newser-alabama
-snowstorm-surgeon/5078179 (accessed October 1, 2014); M. Griffo, "Doctor Walks
6 Miles through Snow Storm to Perform Emergency Brain Surgery," *Huffington Post*,
January 30, 2014, http://www.huffingtonpost.com/2014/01/30/dr-zenko-hrynkiw-6
-miles-brain-surgery_n_4697195.html (accessed October 1, 2014).

Necessary Accessories

Nusheen Ameenuddin

My starched white coat hung on a plastic hanger suspended from a gray steel bookshelf. Worn only once, two years ago at the White Coat Ceremony, an event that welcomed first-year students into the profession of medicine, the coat would now be used in a functional capacity for my first clinical experience. The rest of my ensemble had also been carefully prepared. My khaki pants were neatly pressed. As I admired them, I ran my fingers along their crisp creases, which rarely graced my daily wear. I left my loose-fitting, thigh-length black and beige dress shirt untucked so as not to define the shape of my body.

I took my white coat off its hanger and put it on, tugging at the stiff lapels in a vain effort to make them lie flat. The name tag above my upper left pocket read "Nusheen Ameenuddin, Student Physician." I balanced my hunter green stethoscope around my neck, letting its weight tame the intractable lapels and allowing the small golden pin embossed with the image of a heart-shaped stethoscope to be properly displayed. The pin, a gift from the medical school, symbolized compassion in medicine. I adjusted my hijab, a simple black cotton knit cloth that covered my head and neck, and tucked several stray wisps of hair underneath.

Before I left the room, I stopped for one last look in the mirror to make sure everything was right. I saw a woman who at last was able to face the public as both a medical professional and a committed Muslim. But I wondered whether others might find my appearance an unacceptable contradiction.

Without my ever saying a word, my white coat states what I do, while my hijab states who I am. Although I slipped into the white coat easily, it had taken me years to work up the courage to wear a hijab. During my junior year

Nusheen Ameenuddin, "Necessary Accessories," from *What I Learned in Medical School: Personal Stories of Young Doctors*, ed. Kevin Takakuwa, Nick Rubashkin, and Karen Herzig (Berkeley: University of California Press, 2005), 63–69. Reprinted by permission of University of California Press.

of high school, after years of wanting to express my religion more openly, I warned my friends that I was contemplating donning a hijab when I became a senior. When I returned to school in the fall without it, a Christian friend chastised me for failing to follow through with my commitment to my faith.

For the first few weeks of school that fall, I retained my identity as a "normal" high school student. I felt unprepared to deal with the reactions a hijab would provoke. Some might see it as interesting, even exotic, but I knew the hijab connoted "foreignness." Wearing it would make me stand out as different—intentionally different from the rest of American society. I knew that once I put it on I could no longer quietly hide Islam in my heart and choose to reveal my faith only when and to whom I wanted. To the outside world, Islam would become the accessory I wore on my head, the first and often the only thing people would see about me.

I finally decided to wear the hijab after I attended an Islamic convention. There, for an entire weekend, among other Muslims, I did not need to explain such things as why I wore long sleeves and slacks in the middle of summer (so that I did not expose my skin or appear as a sex object in public) or why I spent lunch periods in the library during the month of Ramadan (as a quiet sanctuary, it reminded me of my commitment to fasting and prayer). I did not have to worry about how to incorporate the five daily prayers into my routine. At first, I felt like a hypocrite, putting on a hijab just for the convention because I knew that it would help me to feel more a part of the group. No one would doubt my commitment to Islamic beliefs and practices. It struck me that the women around me wore their hijabs so comfortably. My first impulse was to ask the girls my age if they really wore hijabs in public and how they dealt with the negative reactions. This impulse died away as I spent more time openly acknowledging my faith among others who did the same. I no longer felt like a hypocrite or a coward. Now I resolved to live openly as a Muslim and wear my hijab in the larger community.

I returned to school wearing my hijab and waited to see what would happen. The same Christian friend who had previously chastised me now flashed me a thumbs-up. Another told me that she admired me for going against the norm. One freshman boy, who wore a Confederate flag on his backpack, teased me, calling me a "sheet head." But by the end of the year, he was chatting with me about a science project. Some people asked me about the hijab's significance, which gave me the opportunity to share a part of myself. What concerned me were the people who did not ask and who likely drew their own conclusions, accurate or not, about Islam and Muslim women. Even so, I reasoned that I had made it through the toughest time and that, beyond high school, people would be even more open, accepting, and educated.

As I became more comfortable wearing the hijab on a regular basis, I also became increasingly committed to the idea of practicing medicine. For me, words I had read in the Qur'an many times lay at the heart of what drew me to medicine: "Truly my prayer and my service of sacrifice, my life and my death are all for Allah, the Cherisher of the Worlds" (Qur'an 6:162).

Growing up, I was introduced to Islam as a peace-loving, service-oriented way of life. For Muslims, every good deed performed with the intention of pleasing God is considered worship, whether it is making a child smile, seeking knowledge, or joining the noble profession of medicine. Entering medical school was my way of fulfilling my religious duty and making my life on earth count. Like religious clerics who devote their lives to God because of a calling they feel deep in their souls, I felt a pull toward medicine and could not imagine doing anything else.

Islam also influenced my career plans because Muslims (who follow the example of the Prophet Muhammad) are exhorted to correct injustice. If we cannot take action, we must oppose injustice with speech. If speaking out is not possible, then we must feel it in our hearts. I believed that inadequate health care was an injustice that I could help to correct as a public health physician.

I was inspired by stories of my grandfather, who practiced medicine for decades in Mysore, India. Most of his patients had little money, yet he never turned anyone away from the clinic he operated out of his home. Instead, he would accept the occasional live chicken, a portion of rice, or nothing at all. In the evenings, he would check on many of his patients in their homes, often with my father or one of his five brothers in tow. For my grandfather, medicine was a service to Allah that required personal sacrifice, and I wanted to be like him.

I believed that my commitments to medicine and to Islam were inextricably linked, but I wondered whether wearing my hijab would cause others in the medical community to see a contradiction. In college, I had three advisers, two of whom warned that wearing my hijab would be a problem. They argued that growing up in a university town had sheltered me from bigotry and that citizens in some areas of our rural state were unaccepting of people who did not attend the local church. They discounted as naïve my belief that as long as I was comfortable with myself, others would accept me as a physician in their community. In fact, when I was in medical school, my hijab did at times overshadow my white coat.

Once, for example, I walked into an exam room without the benefit of an introduction from my supervising physician. When she saw me, my patient stopped in mid-sentence. Her eyes moved conspicuously from my head to my feet and then fixated on my head. Surprised by her response, I stumbled through my introduction and assured her that I was, indeed, in the right place and that I would, with her permission, be taking her medical history. She exchanged a worried look with her husband, and only after several minutes of small talk did she appear to relax. She was not the first patient, nor would she be the last, to so obviously object to my appearance. I realized that I would have to work much harder than my classmates to put my patients at ease, and even then I might never gain their trust.

My third adviser, in contrast, encouraged me to pursue my goal of working in a rural area, while wearing a hijab. A political science professor originally from India, she suggested that I try to use my difference to establish connections within the community. Her instincts proved accurate in my experience with Mrs. Mayflower, a patient I met while I was an undergraduate student volunteering at a medical clinic in rural Kansas.

Mrs. Mayflower came into the clinic after a minor car accident. Undaunted by my hijab, she chatted with me about how important it was to her to be able to drive, in order to maintain her independence at the age of ninety-three. At the end of her visit, she patted me on the back and wished me good luck in my career.

Because of subsequent medical problems, Mrs. Mayflower came into the clinic several more times over the next few weeks. I learned that she was a lifetime resident of this small town. Every morning, she drove herself and three other elderly ladies to Mass and then volunteered as a driver for Meals on Wheels. When the doctor attempted to dissuade her from driving, she resisted, telling him, "Those people need their meals."

I came to the clinic one day to find that she had been hospitalized with severe internal bleeding in her gastrointestinal tract. I rushed to her hospital room, where I watched from a corner as the doctor and nurses worked on her. A priest performed last rites while Mrs. Mayflower's son summoned the rest of the family.

I waited for a break in the activity before approaching her bed. I leaned toward her and whispered her name. She turned toward me and her mouth opened, but no sound came out. I smiled at her, hoping she would respond, but her head rolled back on the pillow and her eyes closed. Her shallow breaths produced barely a hint of steam in her oxygen mask. Her short white hair was unkempt. Her head tilted back; her face held no trace of expression.

She reminded me of the other elderly patients I had seen in the hospital, homogeneous, nameless. I was frightened. But when Mrs. Mayflower's daughter arrived, she greeted me warmly, though we had never met. "Mother told us all about you," she said.

Standing in her room with her family, as I watched what I believed were her last moments, I began a silent prayer for Mrs. Mayflower. I recited verses from the Qur'an, and I made a supplication, a *du'a*, asking God for help. But I left that night expecting that she would pass away by morning.

The next day, her doctor told me that the bleeding had stopped and that Mrs. Mayflower would live. I found her in her room, sitting up in bed eating lunch. Traces of dried blood lined her left nostril, where a plastic tube had been the night before. The pale, empty expression she had worn the previous day was gone. Now her mouth was set in a firm line as she asserted that the surgeon had no right to charge her for procedures that she had not requested. She had not lost her sense of humor.

I smiled and took her hand. "You gave us quite a scare," I told her.

"Well, I thought I was going on a trip." She paused. "You prayed for me, didn't you?"

I nodded. She knew that I had remembered her and that, despite our different religions, we turned to the same God, the One Creator. She beckoned me to lean in closer. Placing both hands on my face, she drew me in and kissed me on the cheek. "You will be a good doctor," she said.

Wearing a white coat produces a curious phenomenon. Other people seem to recognize me in a different way. After the White Coat Ceremony, as I was giving my parents a tour of the campus, a senior medical student dressed in green scrubs saw us from down the hallway. He smiled at me, and his eyes held mine for a few moments before he offered a nod of acknowledgment. The memory of his gesture stayed with me because I am not used to having people accept me so quickly, hijab and all. My white coat allows me to be instantly recognized as a member of one of the most elite societies in America.

I know that throughout my medical career the simple approval I get by wearing my white coat will contrast with reactions to my hijab, which can be deeper and more complicated, whether they are positive, as with Mrs. Mayflower, or negative, as with some other patients I've seen. And maybe this is how it should be, because while the white coat is just my uniform, the hijab represents my underlying reasons for putting it on.

The Critical Vocation of the Essay

Barry F. Saunders

Why should students of medicine write essays?

This is a good question—and it becomes more urgent as essays serve expanding roles in medical "professionalism" curricula. Professionalism tends to emphasize students' proper behavior and phased accommodation to client-service responsibilities. In some medical schools, students are being asked to document their normative development in portfolios of "essays" reviewed by faculty.

Essaying is more than writing nonfiction within particular length parameters. For Montaigne, sixteenth-century originator of the genre, the essay is about trying, from *essayer*—cognate with assay—so also, weighing, testing, being put to tests. Medical students are familiar with tests, but largely as means to an end: knowledge, or "competence." Essays, at their best, are about something else.

Essays that enticed me into medicine included physician Lewis Thomas's, from the *New England Journal of Medicine*, collected in *The Lives of a Cell*. There was a memorable meditation on endosymbiosis: Thomas fretted that his mitochondria were alien life forms, and that they might be running the show—*his* show. Strangers, comprising maybe half his dry weight, mocking his presumption of self-identity—"operating a complex system of nuclei, microtubules, and neurons for the pleasure and sustenance of their families, and running, at the moment, a typewriter."[1] What a marvelous inversion of anthropocentrism—and of competence!

Montaigne's essays were written in the first person, always enfolding personal experience—distinguishing the essay genre from the "compendium of adages."[2] They were written in French rather than Latin, reaching across class hierarchies. Their composition was unsystematic. They endorsed

Barry F. Saunders, "The Critical Vocation of the Essay—Even in Professional Development," from *Atrium: The Report of the Northwestern Medical Humanities and Bioethics Program* 11 (2013): 1–4. Reprinted by permission of the publisher.

inquiry over knowing. And they were constantly under revision. Revision and change were part of Montaigne's concept of self: to essay was to test himself, engage in dialogue with himself, encounter himself *in flux*. And not merely self: the essay staged a *conversation*—with a range of classical interlocutors on his library shelves, especially the Stoics, with his lost friend la Boetie, with death.

Montaigne's low opinion of physicians—"their dogmas and magisterial frowns"[3]—is famous. Medical students may rationalize this as a function of the sad state of medical knowledge in the early modern period, but we do well to consider his indictments of therapeutic presumption and iatrogenic illness in our historical moment as well. Montaigne was deeply skeptical about therapeutic intervention writ large, about its inevitable interference in experiences of change, suffering, and dying. "To philosophize," Montaigne observed (after Cicero and Socrates), "is to learn to die."[4] But both are difficult commitments to incorporate into today's potent institutional ethos of: not on *my* shift! In any case, the birth of the essay implicates some of the most potent critique of the medical enterprise ever written.

Since Montaigne, throughout modernity, the essay has renounced straits and rigors of disciplinary genres—eschewing systematicity, or pretensions to cumulative certainty.[5] The essay's thinking emerges from particulars rather than generalities.[6] Nor is there necessarily a narrative arc or *telos*: as cultural critic Theodor Adorno noted, in the "force field" of the essay, "[t]hrough their own movement the elements crystallize into a configuration."[7] Literary historian Georg Lukács called the essay "too . . . independent for dedicated service."[8] Adorno was more emphatic: "the law of the innermost form of the essay is *heresy*. By [its] transgressing the orthodoxy of thought, something becomes visible in the object which it is orthodoxy's secret purpose to keep invisible."[9] The "form" of the essay for Adorno is an unexpected constellation among objects and concepts that escapes protocol, resists dogma, draws back veils on received wisdom.

Why should the essay's resistance to protocol be of concern for trainers or trainees in medicine? The hospital, seat of so much medical training, is not merely a place with a few protocols. In sociologist Erving Goffman's comparative analysis, hospitals are—along with prisons, monasteries, and bootcamps—exemplars of "total institutions."[10] When Goffman coined this term in the 1950s, total resonated with "totalitarian." Total institutions dictate ways of thinking and behaving: all inhabitants have assigned roles, and all their needs are supplied. Medical professionals and trainees are among these inhabitants. "In most total institutions . . . most inmates take the tack of what they call playing it cool. This involves a somewhat opportunistic combination of secondary adjustments, conversion, colonization and loyalty to the inmate group, so that . . . the inmate will have a maximum chance of eventually getting out physically and psychically undamaged."[11]

Fortunately, Goffman articulated (elsewhere) another capacity for individuals functioning in organizations: "role distance." This names the ability we all have to resist being fully co-opted by our roles. Role distance is what an eight-year-old discovers on the merry-go-round when she affects standoffishness about her ride, feeling a little too old to *be* a princess clinging to her loyal horse in quite the enthusiastic way a four-year-old does. In Goffman's terms, to exercise role distance, at whatever stage in life, is to look at one's assigned role critically, skeptically. Even, for a moment, *with disdain.*[12]

So role distancing is a reflexive exercise, a form of self-examination and resistance. To think critically about one's role does not require attribution of malevolence to the powers resisted—though that can be helpful in total institutions. It can simply be a heuristic device, a claiming of flexibility and imaginative freedom. There is no index or metric of co-optation that calls it up. Claiming such distance might hinge on sensing a kind of danger—perhaps especially the danger of enthusiasms of conviction.

Thinking critically: what does this really mean? Political philosopher Judith Butler has written a lovely essay on critique, tracing some of its conceptual genealogies. Butler cites cultural historian Raymond Williams to clarify that critique is not, as is popularly assumed, mere fault-finding, and not a swift rush to judgment: rather, it entails suspension of judgment.[13] She cites Adorno in clarifying that critique is a mode of engagement with *particulars*—so, always situated, never an abstract position. Critique is a *practice*. Yet as practice, critique is not focused solely on the object of criticism (nor mere exhibition of the critic's expertise). For Butler, critique is, at its core, a questioning of the very categories that enable its own practice.[14]

This brings Butler to a reprise of philosopher Michel Foucault's essay "What Is Critique?," and what he refers to as "critical attitude." There are two features of this critical attitude to mention here. One is its relation to modalities of *government*: critical attitude names a disposition to ask "how *not* to be governed"—not to be an anarchist, to render oneself radically ungovernable, but to ask a more situated and engaged question: "How not to be governed *like that*, by that, in the name of those principles, with such and such an objective in mind and by means of such procedures, not like that, not for that, not by them."[15] The second feature is Foucault's assimilation of this critical attitude to *virtue*. This is something of an enigmatic claim. Foucault links this virtue to modalities of self-knowing and self-styling especially apparent in Reformation resistances to Churchly dogma and monastic discipline. "Critique is the movement by which the subject gives himself the right to question truth on its effects of power and to question power on its discourses of truth."[16] Foucault also links this virtue to the *courage* figured in the Enlightenment motto of philosopher Immanuel Kant, "dare to know"—which entailed inquiry into the conditions of knowing, the limits of knowing. In the knowledge regimes of medicine, such inquiry takes courage indeed!

Foucault's essay on critique reflected on Kant's famous essay "What Is Enlightenment?"[17] Enlightenment is, in Kant's formulation, a people's escape from tutelage toward free exercise of reason. This was among other things a claim about literate persons' privilege, and responsibility, to think in public. The functionary thinking on behalf of an employer or administrator is engaged in a "private" use of reason, and therein obliged to obey the rules. But in our "scholarly" vocation—as writers addressing a cosmopolitan readership in journalistic writing or in academic journals—we may engage in public exercise of reason, which must be free to question, to object, to propose improvements.[18] Of note, for Kant, "public" did not imply the state. The state is one of the sovereign powers that provide people with offices and official duties. In the University of Kant's day, the "higher" Faculties—of medicine, law, and theology—were constrained in their exercise of reason by agendas of state, monarch, and church. Only the "lower," "philosophical" Faculty was in Kant's view able to exercise freedom of thought, to think in and with a *public*—indeed, sometimes about how not to be governed—unfettered by external authorities and by the enticements of thought's private uses.[19]

Medicine today remains an institution of tutelage, bound to instrumental utilities of the state, deeply informed by dogmas and by priestly authority. So how can medical training comport with Kant's sense of public freedom? This is difficult. Doctors, like all professionals, are granted monopoly over their learned practice by the state, on condition that they serve social goods. Physicians and physician-scientists seek, indeed compete for, state and princely funding. Enticements and fetters that can easily privatize, in the Kantian sense, the critical exercise of reason.

Foucault's emphasis on questioning the conditions of our knowing echoes Kant but is also animated by the rather more Nietzschean project of daring to know otherwise. There is a radical embrace of uncertainty and of emergence here. How to put this into practice in the powerful knowledge regimes of medicine and medical training? This returns us to essaying.

Essaying is a familiar practice in humanities, in qualitative social sciences, in "human sciences." Yet how does the essay fit into teaching agendas in medical schools, into training regimes seeking compliance with norms of behavior and competence? Can essaying in medical training be a vehicle for, or extension of, experiences of role distance?

Fortuitously, one of the "competencies" medical schools have begun to seek is "critical thinking." Yet there isn't much agreement about what this means. Some of it is about skills of evidence-based practice—mastery of protocols for distinguishing good from bad evidence. Too little of it is about questioning how evidence and knowledge are historically conditioned, networked, and produced in agonistic fields—"questioning of power on its discourses of truth." And there is even less agreement about how critical thinking should be taught. Perspectives and methods from humanities and social science disciplines—Kant's "lower" Faculties—seem necessary. Fortunately, they do find service in many medical schools.

Various colleagues and I sometimes conduct seminars with medical students together with graduate students from other disciplines. MS2s and graduate students from fields such as literature, anthropology, and religious studies, and occasionally even other professional schools (law, education, social work), gather at the same table for a semester. Aspirants to "higher" Faculties alongside those to "lower." These seminars are challenging, but they often go remarkably well and are the most fun I have as a teacher. To find sharable language—crucial for a reading "public"—students must explain long words and special concepts to each other. Discussions bear a mix of skepticisms, pragmatisms, disciplinary frictions, and translations. The readings collated in a syllabus are, at the outset of a seminar, a kind of connect-the-dot puzzle whose contours only become clear in the force-field of the cross-disciplinary seminar table. Like an essay.

In these and most other humanities and social science classes in our medical school—and in many medical schools—students also write essays. Not treatises, not lists, not true/false choices, not causal chains, not tables of statistical correlation: essays. Apart from thinking out loud in conversation, essays may be the best way for students to demonstrate their capacities to combine and compare concepts, to weigh sources in terms of genre, rigor, and persuasiveness; to generate interpretations, frictions, and syntheses; to relate particulars to generalities; to embrace uncertainty; to qualify agreement or disagreement; to think reflexively. Faculty members who read these essays are listening hard for forms of critical engagement. Some students hate writing essays, of course. Some students yearn for the comforts of a multiple-choice exam—in service of positive knowledge. Some demand to know just how essaying will make them better doctors.

As if in answer to this last question, lately additional "reflective essay" assignments have multiplied within the clinical training of these same medical students. This is happening at many institutions. Short essay assignments crop up in clerkships, under the sign of "professionalism" especially—a quality that clerkship directors are at pains to demonstrate that they can both teach and evaluate. In some places these "essays" are as brief as a couple of paragraphs—a napkin-scrawl. And many are read rather glancingly, perfunctorily: how many clinical faculty members are trained to read student writing closely and provide substantive commentary? Some of these essays wind up folded into professionalism portfolios, as markers of normative professional development. It is hard to imagine these conditions are likely to foster the freedoms that are the essay's historical province. Essays of professional development are at high risk of being pressed into the service of "private" thinking, under the restricted tutelage of the "higher" Faculty of medicine and its evaluation-bureaucracy—not the fostering of role distance, not contributions to a more cosmopolitan and "public" sphere of critique.

If medical students are to learn to think critically—and "professionalism" to include the sense of an examined life—we may need to return to essaying in the shadow of Montaigne's suspicions of professional authority and his discovery of selfhood in wider conversation. How can medical trainees feel supported in expressing concerns about the profession itself, the cultures in which it operates, or the powers, limits, and risks of its ways of knowing? Some medical schools have close relations with their parent universities: perhaps we can make better use of these.[20] Perhaps we could recruit readers of "professionalism" essays from other, non-medical disciplines—or even from medicine's clientele, its laity. Perhaps we could expand the training offered in some places to these essays' more medicalized readers.[21] Perhaps we could develop our faculties' capacities to teach how we know, how at times we unknow, and how new knowledge and new mastery produce new uncertainty. In any case, readers of essays of professional development need to be able to put professional norms and proprieties in brackets occasionally—to become connoisseurs of sassiness, insubordination, and various other prisings of role distance that student essays might articulate. If student writings within a normative process of professionalization are to call themselves essays, they should be allowed and encouraged to make balky gestures, to be meandering, interruptive . . . to be revised . . . and to imagine, if not to find, readerships outside the guild—in a *public* space.

The vocation of the essay *is* critique. Freedom from tutelage. Emergence, not mastery, even for professionals in the making. Heresy.

ACKNOWLEDGMENT

Adapted from an essay published in *Atrium* (Northwestern Medical Humanities and Bioethics Program), Issue 11 (Winter 2013)—a festschrift collection for Kathryn Montgomery—and a lecture given at the 4th National Conference for Physician-Scholars in the Social Sciences & Humanities (Chicago, April 2011): "Essaying Critique in a Total Institution." Indebted to conversations with Ruel Tyson.

NOTES

1 Lewis Thomas, "Organelles as Organisms," in *The Lives of a Cell* (New York: Viking Press, 1974), 72.

2 Graham Good, "The Essay as Genre," in *The Observing Self: Rediscovering the Essay* (London: Routledge, 1988), 1–3.

3 Michel de Montaigne, "Of Experience," in *The Complete Essays of Montaigne*, trans. Donald Frame (Stanford: Stanford University Press, 1958), 835.

4 Michel de Montaigne, "That to Philosophize Is to Learn to Die," in *The Complete Essays of Montaigne*, 56–67.

5 Good, "The Essay as Genre," 4–6.

6 R. Lane Kauffman, "The Skewed Path: Essaying as Un-Methodical Method," *Diogenes* 36 (1988).

7 T. W. Adorno, "The Essay as Form," trans. Bob Hullot-Kentor and Frederic Will, *New German Critique* 32 (Spring–Summer 1984): 151–171.

8 Georg Lukács, "On the Nature and Form of the Essay: A Letter to Leo Popper," in *Soul and Form*, trans. Anna Bostock (Cambridge, MA: MIT Press, 1974), 15.

9 Adorno, "The Essay as Form" (my emphasis).

10 Erving Goffman, "On the Characteristics of Total Institutions," in *Asylums: Essays on the Social Situation of Mental Patients and Other Inmates* (Garden City, NY: Anchor Books, 1961), 1–124.

11 Goffman, "Total Institutions," 64–65.

12 Erving Goffman, "Role Distance," in *Encounters: Two Studies in the Sociology of Interaction* (Indianapolis: Bobbs-Merrill, 1961), 105–110. The merry-go-round example is his own.

13 Judith Butler, "What Is Critique? An Essay on Foucault's Virtue," in *The Political: Readings in Continental Philosophy*, ed. David Ingram (London: Basil Blackwell, 2002), 212.

14 Butler, "What Is Critique?," 213ff.

15 Michel Foucault, "What Is Critique?," trans. Lysa Hochroth, in Ingram, *The Political*, 193 (emphases in original).

16 Foucault, "What Is Critique?," 194.

17 Foucault, "What Is Critique?," 194–200.

18 Kant's essay was published as a newspaper article. See Foucault, "What Is Critique?," 194.

19 Immanuel Kant, *The Conflict of the Faculties*, trans. Mary Gregor (New York: Abaris Books, 1979). Compare Montaigne, two centuries earlier, disavowing any profession but self-inquiry: "I readily excuse myself for not knowing how to do anything that would enslave me to others." "Of Experience," 825.

20 Raymond H. Curry and Kathryn Montgomery, "Toward a Liberal Education in Medicine," *Academic Medicine* 85, no. 2 (February 2010): 283–287.

21 The imaginative capacities and tool kits of "narrative medicine" are important here—though the essay is not an intrinsically narrative genre. Indeed, the essay may have its strongest affinities with dialogue/dialectic—in principle open-ended, often meandering. See Kauffman, "The Skewed Path," 70, citing Pater.

The Art of Medicine

Asthma and the Value of Contradictions

Ian Whitmarsh

Asthma is an enigmatic entity in contemporary medicine. The condition is increasing worldwide, particularly in urban areas and countries undergoing rapid development. These statistics have elicited various explanations. The hygiene hypothesis suggests that more modern homes and lifestyles may result in lower exposure to infections and bacteria at a young age, and a consequent oversensitisation to allergens. An alternative explanation implicates the increase in pollution associated with modernisation. Some epidemiologists argue that increased attention to the disease among both medical practitioners and the public has resulted in a higher rate of diagnosis, not a higher prevalence. A similar explanation notes the changing diagnostic techniques over the past three decades. These competing accounts for the increase reveal a puzzling disease category.

Such discordance has historically been foundational to the category of asthma in British and American medical research. Since the end of the nineteenth century, asthma has been viewed as neurosis or physiological predisposition; caused by dust, pollution, heredity, parental emotions, the unclean modern home (carpets harbouring dust mites), or the continually cleaned modern home (underexposure to infections); and treated with stimulants and depressants, dieting, steroids, and various tonics. Yet despite this diversity, what is striking about modern medicine's approach to asthma is not the plurality of definitions, causes, and diagnostic techniques, but rather the attempt to reduce this plurality.

This compulsion towards finding a single locus of disease has a history. Before the eighteenth century, asthma in western medicine was humoral, a congeries of symptoms brought on by excesses in cold or moist tempera-

Ian Whitmarsh, "The Art of Medicine: Asthma and the Value of Contradictions," from *The Lancet* 376 (2010): 764–765. © 2010 by Elsevier. Reprinted by permission of Elsevier.

ment. This humoral approach began to be replaced in the eighteenth century by a nervous system approach, but the condition was still defined by its various symptoms, such as wheeze, unusual blood circulation, fever, and coldness of the extremities. In this approach, it remained unclear whether blood circulation caused rare respiration, or the reverse. Such a lack of spatial causality was no longer possible by the mid-nineteenth century, however, a period when the physical origin of a disease in the body constituted its definition. Medical texts on asthma from the mid-nineteenth century onward sought the locus of the disease—its single starting point. Each treatise during this time offered an unambiguous origin, resulting in a wealth of competing accounts: asthma was a disease of the nervous system, or the lungs, or the blood, each site exclusive of the others, and each constituting an unequivocal definition.

During the second half of the nineteenth century, technologies became increasingly involved in categorising asthma, for example, through the use of respirometers and microscopes. These instruments provided specific quantitative measurements about a condition that continued to be explicitly defined by contrast: as nervous because no pathological lesions were found or as allergic because no germ causes were found. In the early twentieth century, the allergic approach became widespread, bringing the older sites of the disease into new areas of research—the hereditary predisposition in the blood, the psychological causes of the neurosis, and the physiological response in the lungs.

This history of contestation continues to be foundational to the medical meaning of asthma today. Disciplinary boundaries offer different perspectives through which to examine and understand asthma—for instance, population demographics, lung response, immune system, or gene-environment interactions. Different approaches to diagnosis in research add to this complexity, including response to allergens and medications, self-reporting of symptoms, physician diagnosis, levels of allergen antibodies in the blood, among others. Severity is similarly assessed with different measures, such as self-reporting about frequency of symptoms, use of medication, changes in peak airflow, assessment of biomarkers, or frequency of emergency room admission, alongside consideration of environmental risk factors and other comorbidities. And the causes of asthma contain the same heterogeneity. The various asthma triggers—air pollutants, domestic pollutants, pollens, foods—implicate everything from housing conditions and neighbourhood exposure to urbanization and modern amenities.

The tremendous market for, and research into, asthma in the past few decades has accentuated this ambiguity. These efforts have focused on the variability of asthma definitions as itself constitutive. Some have adopted the multiple criteria of asthma diagnosis and severity to argue for the inclusion of more than one technique, each independently sufficient, creating an expansive diagnostic. In this context, response to the β_2 agonists is increasingly used to diagnose asthma. The disease is here defined in terms of the physiological effects of the medication—that is, a lack is designed into the condition; the need for the pharmaceutical is already part of the meaning of the disease. Other diagnostic criteria—IgE concentrations, wheeze, patient's self-reporting—suggest different sites of intervention: the space of the lungs versus the space of pollens, or proximity to pollutants and hazardous chemicals. This is relevant for that troubled area of medicine today, adherence. As medical research and policy increasingly turn towards chronic diseases—asthma, heart disease, cancer, diabetes—the daily taking of medications has become a major focus. In the case of asthma, efforts to increase adherence have often focused on the mother of the child with asthma.

Women have been central to asthma interventions since the middle of the nineteenth century. In the late nineteenth century, women were considered particularly prone to "nervous asthma," an oversensitive disposition requiring careful monitoring. By the early twentieth century, the shift to psychoanalytic explanations of asthma made women, and specifically mothers, into causes of such a disposition: particularly in the USA, an overprotective mother was imagined to create a delicate and sheltered child prone to asthma. With the contemporary turn away from psychological meanings of asthma in favour of a purely physiological understanding, the focus has shifted to the mother as caretaker of the home. Asthma education and outreach target mothers to reduce pollen and dust exposure and to administer medications to their children. The process of consuming asthma treatments from the doctor is a translation of medical meanings and practices. In this context, taking (or not taking) the inhaled steroid may reflect a patient's suspicion about what their doctor is hiding in his or her concern about the patient's possibly fearful attitude toward the pharmaceutical. With the prescription, parents and patients are accepting some part of the medical system of categorisation, giving some authority to it, while at the same time, by determining when and how they consume the prescription, are placing a part of it under their jurisdiction.

Conditions such as asthma reveal where inexpert interpretations adopt a plurality that modern expertise devalues. This can be seen in cultural meanings of "pollution." The ambiguity of "pollution" in societal use is not due to varying definitions, but rather a fundamental slippage in the category. Pollution can be dust from the highway, mould and cockroaches in apartment walls, workplace hazards, pesticides, cigarette smoke. Similarly "asthma" in general use can be an attack, or a condition, or a diagnosis. Cultural ambiguity means mutually inconsistent meanings can coincide, which is what gives rich terms their power.

Ambiguity denotes spaces of irresolution—unfinished, still to be understood and interpreted. Our modern approach to disease often disavows such ambiguity: one rereads cultural interpretations to find hidden or further meanings; why reread a diagnosis? The extreme consistency of the modern medical designation can be precisely what gives patients pause—a claim to certainty amid evident uncertainty that may lead some people to seek out other interpretations. The cultural contradictions of asthma go beyond a view of the condition as a spectrum, a concept of ambiguity that relies on a single criterion of differentiation. In the ambivalence of culture, contradictory meanings can not only be maintained but can also reinforce each other. To the question, "Asthmatic as an identity or as a temporary condition?," culture will answer: yes. In the ambivalence of culture, contradictory meanings keep each other in doubt. In the twenty-first century, some medical approaches to asthma have integrated this ambiguity and suggested the disease category for asthma is a syndrome or a misnomer for several conditions. Some patients work to bring such ambiguity back in when it is banished from the clinical interaction, and they do so with other sources of authority (family, health books, experiences, and so on). As modern medicine maps out our fate, it suggests the avenues of escape by following medical interventions, that is, adherence. In the contested diagnostic category comprised in "asthma," patients at times make adherence ambiguous too, a source of choice rather than a decree. The ambivalence of culture both facilitates medical categorisations and is the source of alternatives to them. Culture places medical categories into quotes as their limits are examined and criticised in ways that are constitutive of their significance; creating a space for inconsistency, culture allows asthma its long and continuing history of ambiguity.

Anon. A plea to abandon asthma as a disease concept. *Lancet* 368 (2006):705.

Boon, J. A. *Other Tribes, Other Scribes: Symbolic Anthropology in the Comparative Study of Cultures, Histories, Religions, and Texts*. New York: Cambridge University Press, 1982.

Jackson, M. *Asthma: The Biography*. New York: Oxford University Press, 2009.

Whitmarsh, I. *Biomedical Ambiguity: Race, Asthma, and the Contested Meaning of Genetic Research in the Caribbean*. Ithaca: Cornell University Press, 2008.

Script

Mara Buchbinder and Dragana Lassiter

On January 17, 2014, Catherine Eagles, a federal judge for the Middle District of North Carolina, struck down as unconstitutional a portion of North Carolina's 2011 Women's Right to Know Act. The portion in question would have required abortion providers in the state to perform an ultrasound and display and describe the images presented to every woman seeking an abortion. Eagles concluded that this so-called "speech-and-display provision" was "performative rather than informative" and therefore served no medical purpose. She determined this in part because the original text of the law suggested that women might choose *not* to look at these ultrasound images: "*Nothing in this section shall be construed to prevent a pregnant woman from averting her eyes from the ultrasound images required to be provided to and reviewed with her.*"[1] In a 42-page memorandum outlining her decision, Eagles wrote, "Requiring a physician or other health care provider to deliver the state's content-based, non-medical message in his or her own voice as if the message was his or her own constitutes compelled ideological speech and warrants the highest degree of First Amendment protection."[2]

Abortion rights advocates in North Carolina hailed the ruling as an important victory. Yet the remainder of the Women's Right to Know Act still stands: women must receive counseling with specific, state-mandated information at least 24 hours prior to an abortion procedure. To comply with the law, then, an abortion provider must "deliver a content-based, non-medical message in his or her own voice." In our ongoing project, we are examining how abortion providers in North Carolina have grappled with this legal mandate. We have been especially interested in the social, ethical, and communicative dimensions of scripted abortion counseling.[3]

Scripts play a key role in anthropology and science and technology studies. Foundational concepts like *cultural scripts* and *technological scripts* reflect

---

Mara Buchbinder and Dragana Lassiter, "Script," from *Somatosphere: Commonplaces* (November 17, 2014). Reprinted by permission of the publisher.

a disciplinary preoccupation with the ways in which certain domains of human social life are partially predetermined. Yet the potential for social actors to stray from the script to improvise new possibilities and create new modes of action is also embedded in these concepts. In other words, the very presence of any script implies its logical opposite: that we also speak and act in fundamentally unscripted ways. In this way, the script reflects longstanding tensions in contemporary theoretical debates—between structure and agency, determinism and emergence, constraint and possibility, compulsion and choice.

Scripts are ubiquitous in science and medicine. Hospital procedures, informed consent documents, experiment protocols, standardized therapies, and ultrasound technologies all rely on scripts to order work processes, guide thoughts, speech, and action, and specify roles and relationships.[4] As institutionally authored documents, scripts enact and shape worlds by conveying the author's intended meaning. Yet scripts do more than relay referential meaning. They also produce effects, sometimes unintended, through the ways that they are implemented and performed. Such productivity can help us to bypass the dualisms mentioned above and generate potential new sites of theoretical inquiry.

The script at play in state-mandated abortion counseling is a highly formalized version of a much broader techno-social category. Clinicians rely on various scripts in conversations with patients—for example, asking "What brings you in today?" A few things distinguish abortion counseling scripts from colloquial uses of scripts in medicine: their legally compulsory nature, their selection of particular speech elements, and their capacity to transform health care providers into agents of the state. The state, an amorphous political subject, has relatively little power to speak to citizens in everyday life. By compelling providers to speak its message, the state flips the script undergirding most clinical interaction.[5]

Most abortion providers in our study found both the state's intentions and the potential effects of the counseling script on patients to be objectionable. As one physician told us, "I find it very condescending. As if women aren't being given proper informed consent or decision making about their abortion care. While others, you know, like legislatures, are trying to take away their decision making and autonomy." Because of this disdain for the script, the many possibilities for undermining its content have been empowering and even liberating. Some providers prefaced the script with disclaimers and apologies. Others read the script "word by word" to show that the words were not their own. Still others set the script in front of the patient to distinguish it as a legal artifact that they viewed as falling outside of normal clinical practice. Each of these actions served to denounce authorship, disaffiliate speakers from the animated content, and invite patients not to listen.[6] Several providers noted that such strategies had the unanticipated consequence of fostering patient-provider rapport, revealing a misalignment between perceived legislative intent and the script's performance. This highlights how the rift between meaning and intent can cut both ways, working both for and against the author's agenda.

In our study, providers routinely distinguished scripted abortion counseling from the informed consent procedures that they were already doing prior to the law. As an enumeration of the risks and benefits associated with clinical treatment, drug research, or specimen donation, informed consent also relies on scripts. Providers distinguished the scripts used in state-mandated counseling and clinical informed consent on the basis of whether the content was medically relevant and necessary to women's informed decision making. This difference is also implicit in Judge Eagles's distinction between the performative (i.e., non-medically relevant) and informative functions of the search-and-display provision. In making this distinction, both Judge Eagles and our interlocutors attempted to frame the law as an illegitimate instance of script-flipping—that is, appropriating the language, format, and authoritative voice of informed consent for another purpose. Yet insofar as informed consent is both one of the most routinized scripts in medicine and a paradigmatic example of information delivery in health care, this distinction begins to break down. Informed consent assumes the genre of disclosure that many patients in the United States have learned to view as a legal performance, an institutional requirement necessary to move along one's clinical care.[7] In other words, informed consent procedures have both informative *and* performative dimensions. By distinguishing between state-mandated abortion counseling and standard informed consent procedures, the providers in our study reified informed consent as purely informative, neglecting the performative dimensions of this everyday scripted practice.

State-mandated abortion counseling is a specialized case of the use of scripts in medicine. Medicine relies on many other taken-for-granted and routinized scripts. One strength of the script for scholars of science and medicine is that it "reads" across the ethical and legal, as in the case of informed consent. In doing so, it shows how the medical and the legal are not separate professional domains but necessarily co-constituted.

1 For the full legislative text of the North Carolina Woman's Right to Know Act, see http://www.ncleg.net/gascripts/BillLookUp/BillLookUp.pl?BillID=H854&Session =2011.

2 For the full text of this memorandum, see http://dig.abclocal.go.com/wtvd/docs /utrasound_rluling_011714.pdf.

3 This work has been supported by grants from the Society for Family Planning and the Greenwall Foundation, in collaboration with Rebecca Mercier, Amy Bryant, and Anne Drapkin Lyerly.

4 Madeline Akrich, "The de-scription of technical objects," in *Shaping Technology/Building Society. Studies in Sociotechnical Change*, ed. W. Bijker and J. Law (Cambridge, MA: MIT Press, 1992); and Stefan Timmermans, "Saving lives or saving multiple identities?: The double dynamic of resuscitation scripts," *Social Studies of Science*, 26(4) (1996): 767–797.

5 Carr (2011, 191) suggests that script flipping is an example of what Bakhtin (1984) calls vari-directional double-voiced discourse, "in which one's speech has a semantic intent contrary to that which one mimics." See E. Summerson Carr, *Scripting Addiction: The Politics of Therapeutic Talk and American Sobriety* (Princeton: Princeton University Press, 2011). See also Mihkail Bakhtin, *Problems of Dostoevksy's Poetics*, trans. and ed. C. Emerson (Minneapolis: University of Minnesota Press, 1984).

6 Erving Goffman, *Forms of Talk* (Philadelphia: University of Pennsylvania Press, 1981).

7 Marie-Andrée Jacob, "Form-made persons: Consent forms as consent's blind spot," *Political and Legal Anthropology Review*, 30(2) (2007): 249–268. doi:10.1525/pol.2007.30.2.249

Ordinary Medicine

The Power and Confusion of Evidence

Sharon R. Kaufman

There is a hidden chain of connections among science, politics, industry, and insurance that organizes evidence making and drives the U.S. health care system. Hidden as well is the ethos that supports those connections and impacts governance.

The multibillion-dollar biomedical research engine, with its emphasis on the clinical trials enterprise, is where evidence making begins. The infrastructure and high value of evidence-based medicine and clinical trials prioritize thinking about what constitutes responsible health care. And they are the dominant apparatuses of truth making in medicine.

How does this work? Trial "findings" are converted into "best evidence for treatment." And then, that evidence generates treatment standards. This is how scientific innovation organizes physicians' work, health care finances, and patients' and families' expectations about what is normal and needed. The cultural capital of evidence-based medicine, clinical trials, and the standards they set creates a unique quandary in contemporary medicine: When, where, and how to draw the line between too much and enough intervention? And how should one live with the tools medicine offers?

Evidence-based medicine is itself complicated by three interrelated developments that permeate American life, which are inherent in the global biomedical economy and that control the quandary of drawing that line. First, there is the increased role and influence of private industry. In 1980, 32 percent of clinical research was funded by private pharmaceutical, device, and biotechnology companies. Today, 65 percent of biomedical research is funded by

Sharon R. Kaufman, "Ordinary Medicine: The Power and Confusion of Evidence," from *Medicine Anthropology Theory* 3, no. 2 (2016): 163–168. Reprinted by permission under the Creative Commons Attribution 4.0 International Public License, available at https://creativecommons.org/licenses/by/4.0/legalcode.

private industry, whose goal is always to increase market share. Second, all those clinical trials have generated more evidence of therapeutic value and an ever-increasing number of standard treatment options. Third, the United States' national priority of new technologies has influenced our collective perspective on the timing of death. Today in the United States, most deaths, regardless of a person's age, have come to be considered premature.

All of the outcome studies, practice guidelines, and teaching tools within the vast evidence-based medicine matrix have a single goal: to provide a stronger scientific foundation for clinical practice. Yet that "scientifically based" (and especially numerically based) matrix omits the social, nonscientific, and messy features of health care delivery that influence what doctors do and what happens to patients. Consider the following five decidedly non-scientific features:

- Physicians sometimes act against their own best judgment and recommend or prescribe interventions despite their known lack of efficacy.

- Patients and families ask for treatments that have not been proven to show benefit in studies, and physicians, not infrequently, acquiesce to their requests.

- The pharmaceutical and medical device industries are slow to remove drugs and devices from the marketplace that lack benefit (or that prove to be harmful), and doctors may be slow to refuse to use them.

- Once a treatment is reimbursed by Medicare, the dynamics of hospital and medical center economics and physician prescribing patterns make it nearly impossible for all concerned to say "no" to it. Medicare reimbursement thus shapes both standard making and ethical necessity. It becomes the ethics of managing life.

- Whether treatments that benefit some carefully selected trial participants will also benefit a more diverse group of patients, especially children and older persons, is always a question and often a troubling one for doctors.

All these factors weave through the framework of what we call evidence-based medicine, shaping the work of health professionals and the practices of patients and families.

So how does evidence-based medicine play out in the clinic and in real lives? I draw from the example of the implantable cardiac defibrillator, the ICD, a little tool like a pacemaker implanted under the skin, designed to correct a potentially fatal heart rhythm. This is a therapy that has shifted from being "unthinkable" a decade ago to being routine and standard for older persons in the United States today. It became thinkable, and doable, when two things happened: evidence from clinical trials showed good survival rates, and Medicare and private insurers began to reimburse for its use.

As devices such as ICDs become smaller and techniques for implanting them become safer, physicians and the public have learned to view them as standard interventions that one does not easily refuse. In the United States these developments produce a sense that life extension is open-ended as long as one treats risk. That is the prevailing, ordinary logic that drives so much treatment. But when do we stop treating risk?

The ICD was used sparingly until 2002 for those who had already survived a potentially lethal heart attack and were at high risk for another life-threatening cardiac event. Then its use began to rise substantially. Why? Nine clinical trials of ICD use were conducted between 2002 and 2005, each one showing varying degrees of benefit among patient populations that had not experienced a potentially life-threatening heart rhythm. Taken together, the findings from those nine trials provided increasing "evidence of benefit" of the ICD for survival, and that evidence led Medicare, in 2005, to expand the eligibility criteria for reimbursement to include primary prevention for those who had never suffered a potentially fatal cardiac rhythm. The floodgates opened.

Now these devices have become the standard of care for patients with moderate to severe heart disease. The important thing about the ICD is that, in treating a potentially lethal arrhythmia, it prevents sudden death (the silent heart attack in the night), the kind of death many say they actually want in late life. Yet the device is difficult to refuse, even in very late life. Why? Because evidence organizes its expanded use, and because it seems to go against medical progress and common sense to say "no" to it. It has become an ordinary part of the medico-socio-ethical landscape. The effects of this logic most affect the oldest patients.

Today, more than 110,000 patients in the United States receive ICDs each year. There is no question of the unequivocal "good" of this device for preventing young people from dying. Yet most people receiving ICDs are older and sicker, with underlying cardiac disease, and the electrical shocks from ICDs do not necessarily extend an older person's life or improve its quality. Indeed, the ICD transforms the immediate risk of death into the near certainty of progressive heart failure. The hope of this life-extending treatment comes up against a prolonged, unwanted kind of late life and dying.

Consider Sam Tolleson, who, like some other patients with ICDs, endured the pain of the device's shocks and the knowledge that his debility was being prolonged. At age eighty-eight, when I met him, Mr. Tolleson had been living with cardiac disease for twenty-five years. Tall and thin with piercing blue eyes and a shock of thick white hair, he used oxygen and walked slowly, bent over his walker. He graciously welcomed me to sit down in his apartment and chat. Following a second heart attack at age eighty, he awoke in the hospital and was told that physicians had implanted a pacemaker that included a defibrillator. The physicians were following standard practice, doing what was appropriate both to stabilize his heart rate (the pacemaker) and prevent sudden death from a future heart attack (the ICD). Mr. Tolleson noted that it wasn't until sometime after getting the defibrillator that he learned what it would do.

About two years before we met, when he was eighty-six, the ICD had begun to shock his potentially lethal cardiac rhythms back to normal. Over a period of several months, Mr. Tolleson was shocked fifteen times. "There is no question," he offered, "that those shocks extended my life. It's very likely that one of those episodes, without the defibrillator, would have been my last." The first ten shocks were, he reported, "spread out, over weeks." But when he received five shocks in one day, he decided that he had had enough. "They were more and more painful. The very thought that I was going to have another one—I couldn't take it."

So he made an appointment to have the defibrillator part of the device turned off. This choice is highly unusual. It simply does not occur to most patients or their families that the device, once placed under the skin, can easily be deactivated and that patients can make that choice. Most physicians never discuss that possibility with patients. Mr. Tolleson noted, "Both the doctor and the technician [from the device company] were reluctant to turn it off. But I convinced them . . . and that distressed my family too. The family was very upset with me. I have three children, and they all cried. I had to talk with them about it, and I felt terrible after I talked with them." He continued, "Perhaps I should just have done what they wanted me to do: keep the ICD. But life is getting harder all the time."

Mr. Tolleson died two days after our conversation.

Scientific evidence, routine reimbursement, standard of care, specialist expertise, industry's goal to sell devices, and medicine's mandate to extend life are all strong forces. Mr. Tolleson found himself needing to defend his decision to turn off the defibrillator, both to his family and to the medical staff. He had crossed the line he did not wish to cross.

Since 20 percent of those on the receiving end for the ICD are now over eighty, and the proportion over age ninety is growing (in some places greater than 10 percent), the device is reshaping the aging experience and the transition to death for significant numbers of people. It staves off death but does not improve health. It turns life-threatening disease into a chronic condition enabling people to grow older, in need of more intervention, more risk awareness, and more prevention—all at the same time. This is where evidence has come to rest in the case of the ICD: in the kind of death we are asked to choose, and in a new, uncomfortable engagement with one's own role in the timing of death.

To conclude: make no mistake, this technology extends wanted life for many people. That is, of course, the crux of the matter. It has also opened up an ever-expanding market for other cardiac devices, because when this one no longer does the job, one can graduate to the LVAD—the left ventricular assist device, or heart pump, which costs ten times as much. Each device triggers quandaries about how one can or should live in relation to medical treatment, especially as one ages. Nowhere am I seeking to make a case for or against the use of the ICD or any other therapy. Rather, the questions for me are: How have clinical norms and our very lives been caught up in the perfect storm of ordinary, evidence-based medicine? How and why do evidence-based therapeutics bring increasing numbers of patients and families, politicians, and indeed our entire society to face the quandary of drawing the line, and to complain loudly about the systems that create that line? How, as more of us come to want, need, or acquiesce to these treatments, do the profound effects of evidence on medical practice and everyday life organize our "postprogress predicament"?

"Ethics and Clinical Research"

The 50th Anniversary of Beecher's Bombshell

David S. Jones, Christine Grady, and Susan E. Lederer

Human-subjects research receives intense scrutiny today. Researchers, institutions, funders, and journals pay serious attention to ethical conduct. Yet controversies continue, whether about experimenting with oxygen levels in neonatal intensive care or with the duty hours of surgical residents.[1,2] Some commentators have even argued that anxiety over the ethics of Ebola research created delays that resulted in lost opportunities.[3]

Many researchers and bioethicists believe that serious discussions of research ethics began after World War II.[4–6] The actual history is longer and more complex. Nonetheless, Henry Beecher's "Ethics and Clinical Research," published 50 years ago, played an important role. Beecher warned researchers and the public about serious problems with research in the United States and exhorted researchers to reform.[7] Research regulations proliferated in the ensuing decades. However, as Beecher surely anticipated, new policies and procedures have not resolved every dilemma. Now, as in 1966, reasonable people disagree about research ethics.

Research Ethics before 1966: Regulate or Rely on Virtue

Humans have experimented on humans for millennia, and they have long been aware of ethical risks.[8] Human research expanded in the late nineteenth century as physicians tested new theories and technologies.[9] Ethical concerns remained paramount. Claude Bernard set a high bar in 1865: "The princi-

David S. Jones, Christine Grady, and Susan E. Lederer, "'Ethics and Clinical Research'—The 50th Anniversary of Beecher's Bombshell," from *New England Journal of Medicine* 374 (2016): 2383–2389. © 2016 by Massachusetts Medical Society. Reprinted by permission of Massachusetts Medical Society.

ple of medical and surgical morality consists in never performing on man an experiment which might be harmful to him to any extent, even though the result might be highly advantageous to science."[10] William Osler insisted that researchers experiment on patients only if "direct benefit is likely" and only with "full consent." Otherwise "the sacred cord which binds physician and patient snaps instantly."[11]

Some researchers heeded these tenets. Walter Reed solicited volunteers from American soldiers and recent Spanish immigrants in Cuba, offered them payment, and had them sign contracts certifying their awareness of the risks before exposing them to yellow fever. Other researchers triggered scandals by infecting patients, orphans, or asylum inmates with pathogens without their knowledge.[8,9] In 1916, Walter Cannon pushed the American Medical Association (AMA) to mandate informed consent for research.[12] The organization refused, arguing that misconduct was a problem of rogue researchers, not research itself. The AMA believed that trust, not regulation, would foster better research and clinical care.[9]

World War II prompted extensive human experimentation. American researchers were often scrupulous in their use of informed, consenting volunteers but sometimes pressured soldiers to volunteer without full knowledge of the risks and sometimes used institutionalized populations.[8,13–15] German and Japanese researchers went further, committing atrocities in the name of scientific research.[16,17] When allied authorities prosecuted Nazi physicians at the War Crimes Tribunal, they issued the Nuremberg Code, specifying that researchers should always recruit competent research subjects who understood the nature of the research and voluntarily consented to participate.[18,19]

The Code, however, had no binding legal authority, and American researchers responded in complex ways. Some government agencies issued new guidelines—in 1953, for instance, the secretary of defense mandated written consent in military research on atomic, biologic, and chemical weapons (though this policy was kept "top secret").[20] The same year, the National Institutes of Health (NIH) Clinical Center implemented peer review and informed consent for research on healthy volunteers. In other venues, however, much was left to researchers' discretion.[8,21]

Many U.S. scientists believed that the Code, a response to the work of experiments by Nazi researchers, did not apply to them.[22] Others understood the need for guidelines but sought to moderate the Code's strict language. For instance, as the World Medical Association drafted its 1964 Declaration of Helsinki, U.S. representatives, with funding from the pharmaceutical industry, blocked the requirement for informed consent in all cases, believing it would threaten placebo-controlled drug trials. They also blocked a ban on research on institutionalized children and prison inmates, who were widely used to test vaccines and drugs.[23] Similarly, when the Senate debated a 1962 amendment that would have mandated informed consent for research with experimental drugs, dozens of leading researchers protested. One described informed consent as "a snare and delusion": "it is for the most part impossible to achieve and is certain to do more harm than good." Henry Beecher worried that the provision would cripple the country's lead in drug research, in part by preventing research on children and the mentally ill.[24,25]

Scandals, however, raised questions about whether to trust U.S. researchers. In 1964, news broke that 22 patients at the Jewish Chronic Disease Hospital in Brooklyn had been injected with cancer cells without their knowledge. The media firestorm, hearings, and lawsuits raised fundamental questions about medical research. However, the researchers from Memorial Sloan Kettering who conducted the study received no serious sanction.[26]

"Ethics and Clinical Research"

By 1950, Henry Beecher, an anesthesiologist at Massachusetts General Hospital, had emerged as a respected researcher, having examined battlefield trauma, the safety of anesthesia, subjective experiences (e.g., pain, thirst, and nausea), and placebo responses.[4,8,22,27,28] He advocated careful research methods, including the use of placebo controls. He had also consulted for the military about the use of mescaline and LSD as "truth serums," research that involved discussions with Central Intelligence Agency interrogators and former Gestapo officials.[29] This work got Beecher interested in "certain problems of human experimentation."[30] In 1952, he asked Pentagon officials for their new policy on human research. In 1955, he wrote to an English colleague to learn about the Medical Research Council instructions for investigators and editors.[30]

In 1959 and 1963, Beecher published articles in *JAMA* about the role conflict faced by physician-investigators.[31,32] Neither generated much response. He then collected examples of troubling behavior by U.S., Canadian, and European researchers. For instance, he examined 100 consecutive articles in the *Journal of Clinical Investigation* (*JCI*) and concluded that 12 were "unethical or questionably ethical." He compiled a set of 50 articles on studies funded by government agencies, conducted at leading institutions, and published in leading journals. He took care to ensure that his critiques were fair. For instance, he queried *New England Journal of Medicine* editor Joseph Garland about the *Journal's* decision to publish a study of thymectomy in children; Garland admitted that the ethical review had been inadequate.[30] Beecher also recognized his own mistakes. He regretted a 1948 study in which researchers in his laboratory, without adequate consent, prolonged anesthesia "beyond that necessary" to study the effects on kidney function.[30,33]

Beecher then accepted an invitation to speak at a conference in March 1965. He delivered a "bombshell." After reviewing the Jewish Chronic Disease Hospital controversy, he proceeded, without naming names, to describe 17 additional cases in which researchers had failed to obtain consent or had harmed their research subjects: "what seem to be breaches of ethical conduct in experimentation are by no means rare, but are almost, one fears, universal."[30] Reaction from his colleagues was immediate. Thomas Chalmers and David Rutstein called a press conference to accuse Beecher of "gross and irresponsible exaggeration."[34] Beecher condemned their kangaroo court and accused them of defamation of character.[30] The exchange received extensive media coverage.

After an inquiry to *Science*, Beecher submitted his manuscript to JAMA in August. The editor rejected it, citing its excessive length (it described 50 research studies) and poor organization. Beecher submitted a revised manuscript to the *Journal* in November. Garland sent it "to some picked reviewers," expecting no serious problems. Six of the seven recommended against publication: there were too many cases; Beecher did not allow the investigators to tell their side of the story; many readers would recognize the "anonymous" cases; and his critiques had already received extensive media coverage. One reviewer supported publication, but only if the *Journal* obtained a legal opinion "regarding any possible problems."[30]

The editorial board voted to reject the submission, but Garland overruled them.[35] Blurring the line between editor and coauthor, he helped Beecher revise the manuscript. Beecher reduced the examples to 25 and provided Garland with their citations. Garland convened a "brain cabinet" (two colleagues) to assess Beecher's accusations; they settled on a final list of 22 cases. Garland also moderated Beecher's language: "I have tried to omit anything accusatory or especially critical, since what we want is not an indictment but a sober and undramatic presentation of what has been done and is being done in violation of basic ethics."[30] The *Journal* published the article in June with an editorial by Garland.[7,36]

The cases made for shocking reading. Beecher focused on human experiments in which patients were used not for their benefit, "but for that, at least in theory, of patients in general."[7] Researchers sometimes withheld known treatments. In the case Beecher considered most egregious, penicillin was withheld from 109 soldiers with streptococcal infections; acute rheumatic fever developed in two and acute nephritis in one. In some cases, patients experienced harm or risk of harm without benefit. In others, researchers had not obtained consent. The examples were not from a lunatic fringe.[4] Four came from Harvard Medical School, three from the NIH Clinical Center, and the rest from other prominent institutions. The cases had passed peer and editorial review at the *Journal* (five articles), *JCI* (five), *JAMA* (two), and *Circulation* (two).

Beecher insisted that the researchers not be named: "I have no wish to point a finger at individuals. I was pointing to an all-too-general practice."[30,37] Garland accepted Beecher's request and asked readers to trust the *Journal's* assessment of the veracity of Beecher's accusations. Beecher was besieged by requests to identify his sources but steadfastly refused. As he explained to Arnold Relman, then editor of *JCI*, "I am assured by a professor in the Harvard Law School that the individuals involved could be subjected to criminal prosecution, and I have no wish to invite such action."[30] Beecher had divided loyalties. Even as he drew attention to misconduct, he did not want researchers to suffer legal consequences.[4] Since he expected that many cases would be recognized by the research community, he might have hoped that the researchers would be shamed among their peers, if not publicly. Remarkably, when the researchers were unmasked in 1991, they received little attention.[8,38,39]

Reactions in 1966 varied widely. Medical researchers were often angry and defensive, clinicians were outraged by researchers' conduct, and the public piled on with their own accounts of physician misconduct.[28] The researchers responsible for one of Beecher's cases published a letter to the editor: "Dr. Beecher quotes out of context, oversimplifies and otherwise distorts the purpose and findings of our investigation."[40] Beecher dismissed them: "I do not believe this is so, and obviously neither did the 3 editors who checked my cases."[37] Eugene Braunwald, involved in three of Beecher's cases at the NIH Clinical Center, prepared a point-by-point critique, arguing that Beecher misunderstood the role of patients and healthy volunteers and the role of consent at the Clinical Center. But recognizing the value of some of Beecher's critiques, Braunwald decided not to respond.[41]

It was clear that thoughtful researchers could disagree. Beecher's list included studies at the Willowbrook State School, in which researchers had infected disabled children with hepatitis.[7,42] As he explained to one critic, "The thought that some would have agreed that deliberate infection was all right since the subjects were mental defectives gives me the Nazi shudders."[30] The study's defenders, however, appealed to other justifications. Geoffrey Edsall, from the Massachusetts Department of Public Health, told Beecher that "if I had a child in Willowbrook, and if I had had it clearly explained to me—as Krugman et al. did with the parents of his children—that my child was bound to come down with hepatitis sooner or later, as all the children do in Willowbrook; if I was then asked to permit my child to be part of an experiment which hopefully would be of benefit to man, I would be delighted to have that opportunity to allow the child to contribute." If ethical barriers were set too high, Edsall argued, they would disrupt "the trend of progress that all human beings want, and that the vast majority are willing to contribute to."[30]

The Aftermath

Despite Beecher's fervor, his goals were modest. He qualified his "troubling charges" with the affirmation that "American medicine is sound, and most progress in it is soundly attained."[7] He hoped that simply revealing problems would be sufficient to address them. As he told Garland, "most of the ethics errors are owing to thoughtlessness or carelessness, not a vicious disregard for the patients' rights. I am utterly convinced that calling attention to the ethical problems involved will lead to elimination of the vast majority of mistakes."[30] He did not recommend new regulations or formal oversight, instead emphasizing the importance of informed consent and "the more reliable safeguard provided by the presence of an intelligent, informed, conscientious, compassionate, responsible investigator."[7]

Beecher's exposé had immediate impact. Members of Congress wrote to the NIH inquiring about possible corrective actions.[8] Beecher's article provided support for a 1965 proposal by NIH director James Shannon to require peer review of research, protect the rights and welfare of participants, and ensure appropriate informed consent.[43] Historian David Rothman highlights 1966 as the start of a broad transformation of bioethics and the patient-doctor relationship, as patients, lawyers, and ethicists shaped medicine's moral code. Beecher, according to Rothman, had joined the ranks of Harriet Beecher Stowe, Upton Sinclair, and Rachel Carson.[8]

These changes, however, were not a response to a single article. Beecher had published repeatedly about research ethics. Maurice Pappworth worked in parallel in England to expose unethical research.[22] In February 1966, between Beecher's conference presentation and publication of the article, the U.S. Surgeon General requested that hospitals and universities establish review boards.[21] Many scholars joined the discussion after Beecher.[44] And scandals continued to emerge. The Tuskegee syphilis study, which seized public attention in 1972, was the most famous.[45] In response, Senator Edward Kennedy (D-MA) held hearings on human experimentation that led to the National Research Act in 1974 and the National Commission for the Protection of Human Subjects. The Commission's 1979 Belmont Report guided the systems that continue to regulate human research in the United States.[8,9]

Would Beecher be satisfied with current arrangements? He put his trust in two safeguards: informed consent and virtuous researchers. Informed consent is almost always obtained today, though it remains imperfect.[46] Investigator virtue is highly valued, yet ironically, the compliance culture of modern human-subjects protection assumes that investigators cannot be relied on.[47] Discussions of ethics have become ubiquitous in the research community, something Beecher would have applauded. However, researchers complain that institutional review boards have lost sight of their original purpose of protecting human subjects, focusing instead on bureaucratic minutiae.[48] And researchers still worry that excessive attention to ethics can hinder the research enterprise.

Are we—50 years after Beecher—better than our predecessors at recognizing and preventing unethical research? All Beecher's examples had been published in prominent journals, yet few had inspired an outcry. We assume that we are now more sensitive to ethical concerns than past researchers, and we may well be. We have well-established guidelines that did not previously exist.[49] But sensitivity to research ethics did exist, even if past researchers resisted formal regulation: many understood how they ought to behave toward research subjects and worried about their failures to do so. Nevertheless, ethical failures occurred throughout the twentieth century and continue in the twenty-first.

Three lessons are clear. First, ethical values change over time, and it is important to understand how and why. Second, there is not always consensus on what counts as ethical research, or who can be appropriate research subjects: thoughtful people often disagree. Articles like Beecher's play a crucial role in fostering debate that can lead to consensus about ethical values. Third, many interests—medical, personal, political, military, and commercial—have led researchers to conduct studies they knew to be transgressive. It would be hubris to think that such lapses could not happen again.

NOTES

1 Drazen JM, Solomon CG, Greene MF. Informed consent and SUPPORT. *N Engl J Med.* 2013;368:1929–1931.

2 Bilimoria KY, Chung JW, Hedges LV, et al. National cluster-randomized trial of duty-hour flexibility in surgical training. *N Engl J Med.* 2016;374:713–727.

3 Gericke CA. Ebola and ethics: autopsy of a failure. *BMJ.* 2015;350:h2105.

4 Rothman DJ. Ethics and human experimentation. *N Engl J Med.* 1987;317:1195–1199.

5 Faden RR, Beauchamp TL. *A History and Theory of Informed Consent.* New York: Oxford University Press, 1986.

6 Truog RD. Patients and doctors—evolution of a relationship. *N Engl J Med.* 2012;366:581–585.

7 Beecher HK. Ethics and clinical research. *N Engl J Med.* 1966;274:1354–1360.

8 Rothman DJ. *Strangers at the Bedside: A History of How Law and Bioethics Transformed Medical Decision Making.* New York: Basic Books, 1991.

9 Lederer SE. *Subjected to Science: Human Experimentation in America before the Second World War.* Baltimore: Johns Hopkins University Press, 1995.

10 Bernard C. *An Introduction to the Study of Experimental Medicine.* 1865; New York: Dover, 1957.

11 Osler W. The evolution of the idea of experiment in medicine. *Trans Cong Am Phys Surg.* 1907;7:7–8.

12 Cannon WB. The right and wrong of making experiments on human beings. *JAMA.* 1916;67:1372–1373.

13 "Ethically Impossible": STD Research in Guatemala from 1946 to 1948. Washington, DC: Presidential Commission for the Study of Bioethical Issues, 2011.

14 Smith SL. Mustard gas and American race-based human experimentation in World War II. *J Law Med Ethics.* 2008;36:517–521.

15 Smith SL. *Toxic Exposures: Mustard Gas and the Health Consequences of World War II in the United States.* New Brunswick, NJ: Rutgers University Press, 2017.

16 Weindling P. *Nazi Medicine and the Nuremberg Trials: From Medical War Crimes to Informed Consent.* New York: Palgrave Macmillan, 2004.

17 Harris SH. *Factories of death: Japanese Biological Warfare, 1932–1945, and the American Cover-Up.* New York: Psychology Press, 2002.

18 Weindling P. "No mere murder trial": the discourse on human experiments at the Nuremberg medical trial. In: Roelcke V, Maio G, eds. *Twentieth Century Ethics of Human Subjects Research: Historical Perspectives on Values, Practices, and Regulations.* Stuttgart, Germany: Franz Steiner Verlag, 2004:167–180.

19 Annas GJ, Grodin MA, eds. *The Nazi Doctors and the Nuremberg Code: Human Rights in Human Experimentation*. New York: Oxford University Press, 1992.

20 Advisory Committee on Human Radiation Experiments. *The Human Radiation Experiments*. New York: Oxford University Press, 1996:236.

21 Stark L. *Behind Closed Doors: IRBs and the Making of Ethical Research*. Chicago: University of Chicago Press, 2012.

22 Edelson PJ. Henry K. Beecher and Maurice Pappworth: honor in the development of the ethics of human experimentation. In: Roelcke V, Maio G, eds. *Twentieth Century Ethics of Human Subjects Research: Historical Perspectives on Values, Practices, and Regulations*. Stuttgart, Germany: Franz Steiner Verlag, 2004:219–233.

23 Lederer SE. Research without borders: the origins of the Declaration of Helsinki. In: Roelcke V, Maio G, eds. *Twentieth Century Ethics of Human Subjects Research: Historical Perspectives on Values, Practices, and Regulations*. Stuttgart, Germany: Franz Steiner Verlag, 2004:199–217

24 Podolsky SH. *The Antibiotic Era: Reform, Resistance, and the Pursuit of a Rational Therapeutics*. Baltimore: Johns Hopkins University Press, 2014:92–93.

25 Beecher HK. *Research and the Individual: Human Studies*. Boston: Little, Brown, 1970:231.

26 Lerner BH. Sins of omission—cancer research without informed consent. *N Engl J Med*. 2004;351:628–630.

27 Harkness J, Lederer SE, Wikler D. Laying ethical foundations for clinical research. *Bull World Health Organ*. 2001;79:365–366.

28 Freidenfelds L. Recruiting allies for reform: Henry Knowles Beecher's "Ethics and clinical research." *Int Anesthesiol Clin*. 2007;45:79–103.

29 McCoy AW. Science in Dachau's shadow: Hebb, Beecher, and the development of CIA psychological torture and modern medical ethics. *J Hist Behav Sci*. 2007;43:401–417.

30 *Henry K. Beecher Papers, 1848–1976*. Boston: Harvard Medical Library, Francis A. Countway Library of Medicine.

31 Beecher HK. Experimentation in man. *JAMA*. 1959;169:461–478.

32 Beecher HK. Ethics and experimental therapy. *JAMA*. 1963;186:858–859.

33 Burnett CH, Bloomberg EL, Shortz G, Compton DW, Beecher HK. A comparison of the effects of ether and cyclopropane anesthesia on the renal function of man. *J Pharmacol Exp Ther*. 1949;96:380–387.

34 Osmundsen JA. Physician scores tests on humans. *New York Times*. March 24, 1965.

35 Ingelfinger FJ. Joseph Garland, M.D., 1893–1973: the editor. *N Engl J Med*. 1973; 289:641–642.

36 Garland J. Experimentation on man. *N Engl J Med*. 1966;274:1382–1383.

37 Beecher HK. Human experimentation. *N Engl J Med*. 1966;275:791.

38 Gold JA. Review of: *Strangers at the Bedside*. *N Engl J Med*. 1991;325:1387.

39 Truop SB. Review of: *Strangers at the Bedside*. *JAMA*. 1991;266:851.

40 Scott JL, Belkin GA, Finegold SM, Lawrence JS. Human experimentation. *N Engl J Med*. 1966;275:790–791.

41 Lee TH. *Eugene Braunwald and the Rise of Modern Medicine*. Cambridge, MA: Harvard University Press, 2013.

42 Robinson WM, Unruh BT. The hepatitis experiments at the Willowbrook State School. In: Emanuel EJ, Grady C, Crouch RA, et al., eds. *Oxford Textbook of Clinical Research Ethics*. New York: Oxford University Press, 2008:80–5.

43 McCarthy CR. The origins and policies that govern institutional review boards. In: Emanuel EJ, Grady C, Crouch RA, et al., eds. *Oxford Textbook of Clinical Research Ethics*. New York: Oxford University Press, 2008:541–51.

44 Ethical aspects of experimentation with human subjects. *Daedalus*. 1969;98:219–604.

45 Reverby SM. *Examining Tuskegee: The Infamous Syphilis Study and Its Legacy*. Chapel Hill: University of North Carolina Press, 2009.

46 Grady C. Enduring and emerging challenges of informed consent. *N Engl J Med*. 2015;372:855–62.

47 Koski G. Getting past protectionism: is it time to take off the training wheels? In: Cohen IG, Lynch HF, eds. *Human Subjects Research Regulation: Perspectives on the Future*. Cambridge, MA: MIT Press, 2014:341–349.

48 Fost N, Levine RJ. The dysregulation of human subjects research. *JAMA*. 2007;298:2196–2198.

49 Emanuel EJ, Wendler D, Grady C. What makes clinical research ethical? *JAMA*. 2000;283:2701–2711.

HEALTH CARE ETHICS AND THE CLINICIAN'S ROLE

....

III

....

Glossary of Basic Ethical Concepts in Health Care and Research

Nancy M. P. King

AUTONOMY · The principle of respect for autonomy and the right of self-determination are important concepts in health care ethics. "Autonomy" means the ability to govern oneself and the freedom to do so. "Self-determination" is often used to mean autonomy, especially in health care settings.

A person acts autonomously if that person acts intentionally, with understanding, and without being controlled by others. Both persons and their actions can be autonomous; autonomous people do not always act autonomously, and sometimes people who are not autonomous are able to make autonomous decisions or act autonomously in some instances. It is important to remember that no one is "fully" autonomous; we judge autonomy by the expectations we have of common human behavior, and we set a minimal standard of "substantial" autonomy by which to judge people and their actions.

In health care, respecting autonomy does not mean simply laying out all the options and telling the patient, "You decide." Respecting patients' autonomy often includes promoting an individual's ability to deliberate effectively, for example by providing a recommendation and discussing the reasons behind it.

Autonomy is not the same as freedom, and usually we view autonomy as including some responsibility for the consequences of one's actions. Now that society has become especially concerned about the interests or rights of communities, there is much disagreement about the boundaries between an individual's autonomy and the legitimate rights or interests of others.

Competence and decisional capacity, concepts related to autonomy, are defined below.

BENEFICENCE/BEST INTERESTS · The principle of beneficence, or the best interests of the person, is often contrasted to autonomy. There may, for example, be times when a health care provider believes that what an autonomous patient wants is not in that person's best interests. Beneficence focuses on doing good. The crucial question is, who should be allowed to judge what is good? An individual, health care providers, family members, friends, and other authorities may all have different judgments about what is in the individual's best interests. Best interests may be defined narrowly, as in "best medical interests," or broadly enough to consider a wide variety of personal factors and values.

The Hippocratic maxim "Above all, do no harm" is technically an injunction to *nonmaleficence*—avoiding harm—rather than to beneficence—doing good. In health care, these principles are often closely related and considered together. If they are ranked in importance, nonmaleficence generally comes first; however, as you might imagine, health care providers and patients must often weigh the risk of doing harm against the chance of doing good when deciding about treatment.

How "harm" is defined and who defines it are problems for nonmaleficence, just as they are for beneficence. At least one significant difference exists between the two concepts: physicians and other health care providers sometimes assert the right not to cause harm by withdrawing from the care of a patient and substituting another caregiver. A parallel unilateral right to do good against the patient's will does not exist.

———

COERCION · Coercion is control of one person's behavior by another. It is always incompatible with autonomy and is therefore morally unacceptable, unless it can be justified by a principle or interest that is sufficiently compelling to outweigh autonomy under the circumstances—for example, the safety of other persons put at grave risk by an autonomous actor.

Actions may be coercive, but coercion is usually accomplished by threats. Many influences are loosely called coercive, but "coercion" should be reserved for influences that are intended to control behavior by means of a severe and irresistible threat. Coerced actions are intentional actions, but actions about which the actor "has no choice." Controversy can arise about coercion in two areas: Generally, how should we define and measure what is "irresistible"? And specifically, can *offers* be so irresistible as to be coercive? (For example, is the promise of parole for a prisoner who submits to medical experimentation so great an offer as to overwhelm the person's reasonable concerns about the safety of the experiment and inclination to say no?)

Sometimes people talk about coercive situations. Unpleasant circumstances can indeed make people feel that they have no choice, but only other people can be coercive, because only other people can intend to influence that person's behavior. For example, the situation of having a severe mental illness can make a person feel that s/he has no choice but to take a dangerous drug with unpleasant side effects. That person is not coerced by the situation. But if taking the drug is required as a qualification for receiving government assistance in housing or education, such requirements—since they are instituted with the intention of encouraging mentally ill people to stay on medication—may be (but are not necessarily) coercive.

Manipulation and persuasion must be distinguished from coercion. They are each defined below.

COMPETENCE · A legal term. Adults (people age 18 and over) are presumed competent until proven otherwise. Thus, a severely impaired adult who has not been legally determined to be incompetent is legally competent. The determination of incompetence is made in a legal proceeding and can be quite complex and detailed. A determination may be global or limited. Someone of limited competence may retain some legal decision-making rights while losing others. For example, a limited guardianship might be established for financial matters, but the person would retain the legal right to make health care decisions. Involuntary commitment is not the same as a determination of incompetence. "Competence" is often mistakenly considered synonymous with "decisional capacity," which is not a legal term. It is defined below.

CONFIDENTIALITY · Confidentiality is the duty, expectation, and/or promise that information exchanged within a relationship will not be spread beyond the boundaries of that relationship (that is, "keeping secrets"). Confidentiality causes problems because so many different relationships can be connected to a confidential relationship. Sometimes a potential need arises to protect others who might need to know confidential information (for example, landlords or employers). Sometimes the perceived need may be to share confidential information with others (for example, family or health care providers) who could benefit the person who expects confidentiality to be maintained. Sorting out and balancing these competing needs and interests can be extremely difficult.

Confidentiality is not the same as privacy, which is defined below.

CONFLICT OF INTEREST · A general term that calls attention to a variety of ethical problems in service relationships. People who find themselves caught in a conflict of interest may feel that they are trying unsuccessfully to serve two masters or that they have conflicting loyalties or duties to others. (For example, managed care has given rise to much concern about conflicts of interest, because physicians in managed care contracts have incentives to save money that may conflict with their duty of beneficence to patients. However, traditional "fee-for-service" medicine rewards physicians for delivering more services, which may conflict with the duty of nonmaleficence to patients.)

Often the first type of conflict we think of is financial, but there are many others. For example, a parent's decisions about one child may be affected by the needs of the other children in the family; a health care provider may be concerned about the competing needs of family members other than the patient, or about how to meet the needs of more than one patient when time is limited; and there are many others. The term "conflict of interest" helps us flag complicated situations and sort out the potentially competing needs and interests involved.

Conflicts of interest are common in life and at least some may be unavoidable. How they should be addressed depends on the circumstances. Sometimes they should be eliminated; other times, they may be "managed," for example, by an oversight mechanism; and sometimes, disclosing them may be sufficient to allow the persons potentially affected by them to respond appropriately to the risks they pose.

DECISIONAL CAPACITY · The ability to make substantially autonomous decisions. It is assumed that adults have it. When questions arise about someone's decisional capacity, it is measured using practicality and common sense, and with reference to the specific decision(s) at issue. For example, an impaired person might have the capacity to decide about going into a nursing home but lack the ability to choose between two treatments for a health problem because that requires greater reasoning skills.

Although sometimes with mental illness, decisional capacity may need to be assessed by an expert, such as a psychiatrist, in most cases an equally reliable determination can be made by those who know the person, have talked with him or her, and are familiar with the circumstances. The best test of someone's capacity to make a particular decision is going through the informed consent process. A variety of different standards can then be used; they range from very lenient (does the person appear to express a choice?) to the overly strict (does the person make the "right" decision for the "right" reasons?). A more appropriate standard is provided by the definition of substantial autonomy given above: Does this person seem to know that there is a choice to be made, and does s/he seem to be choosing intentionally, with understanding of the meaning and consequences of the choice, and without being controlled by others? Difficult questions can arise about when the nonlegal determination that someone lacks decisional capacity should be followed up by a legal determination about competence.

———————

JUSTICE · Justice is a significant ethical principle that has many different aspects. Generally speaking, we worry about justice on a larger scale than the individual—for example, for communities, special groups (women, minorities, disabled persons, etc.), and societies. Justice is roughly synonymous with fairness, but what is just or fair depends on the circumstances. Is treating everyone equally just? Or is affirmative action more just because it redresses past wrongs? Distributive justice addresses how social goods (like food, shelter, and health care) should be distributed. Once again, we might ask whether equality is a just principle of distribution, or whether "from each according to his ability, to each according to his needs" is more just. Fair procedures and fair hearings are also components of justice.

———————

MANIPULATION · Manipulation is the hardest category to grasp in the trio of coercion, manipulation, and persuasion. Manipulation falls in between the other two and can essentially be one of two things: an intentional and successful alteration of a person's available choices by means that are not coercive (for example, by a resistible threat or offer), or an intentional and successful alteration of a person's perception of those choices by means that are not persuasive, that is, not focused on reason (for example, by a successful appeal to emotion, or by psychological influence). A common health care example is when a provider mistakenly believes that persuasion is morally wrong, but believes that a particular choice is the right one for a patient, and therefore slants or selectively provides information, perhaps using language chosen for a particular emotional effect, in order to ensure that the informed consent process has the outcome desired by the provider. A common example outside of health care is advertising.

Manipulation is to a large extent a matter of degree and a question of context. It is not always incompatible with autonomy, but there are almost always alternatives that help to protect, promote, and foster autonomy, which manipulation definitely does not.

PATERNALISM · "Paternalism" is another term that is often loosely used. True paternalism, also called strong paternalism, occurs when one person overrides the autonomous choices and actions of another in the other person's best interests (for example, preventing a "rational suicide"). It is not paternalistic to override someone's actions or choices in order to benefit, or prevent harm to, third parties. It is also not paternalistic to override someone's actions or choices when that person is not acting autonomously (for example, preventing suicide by a person who is delusional), because then beneficence and autonomy are not in conflict. However, this is also often called paternalism, or weak paternalism. As the suicide examples given help to show, many occasions when "paternalism" is mentioned are instances where the autonomy and beneficence of the choices at issue are questionable or in dispute.

PERSUASION · Persuasion is the intentional and successful attempt to induce a person, through appeals to reason, to freely adopt the beliefs, values, attitudes, intentions, or actions advocated by the persuader. It is compatible with autonomy, and indeed often facilitates autonomous decision making, because it is based on reasoned discourse and shared communication and discussion. Education and persuasion are closely linked.

PRIVACY · Privacy has two meanings: a commonsense meaning and a legal meaning. The constitutional right of privacy can be confusing because it means freedom from governmental intrusion into certain decisions and actions relating to one's body, relationships, reproduction, speech, and ideas—a real grab bag of personal actions and decisions. (This meaning of privacy has been somewhat modified by the courts, from a "constitutional privacy right" to a "constitutional liberty interest.")

Commonsense privacy is a somewhat different grab bag. It refers to freedom from intrusions upon solitude (being eavesdropped upon, photographed, or spied on in circumstances where we commonly have an "expectation of privacy," such as at home) and freedom from having private facts made public or from unwanted publicity (again, this is measured against what society reasonably believes is private and what is public). The privacy of medical records (more properly, the confidentiality of their contents, but popular and legislative language have confused the two) is an issue of growing importance in this information age, and determinations about what may and may not be shared with others (such as employers, insurers, and information purchasers) depends on what is considered a reasonable expectation of privacy.

"Privacy" in any of its meanings is not the same as "confidentiality," which means keeping shared information within a relationship.

RIGHTS · The concept of rights in health care is overused and difficult to define, but it needs clarification. Beginning in the 1960s and 1970s, American society became accustomed to talking about the rights of comparatively disadvantaged groups, such as ethnic and racial minorities, women, and patients. More recently, physicians and other health care professionals have pointed out that they have rights too (paralleling the development of "victims' rights" to complement the rights of persons accused and convicted of crimes). As the uses of the term "rights" have become more extensive, its meaning has faded. There are many different types of legal rights, for example, so that the mere assertion of a right tells us little about its scope or effect. Much specificity is necessary in order to make a claim of right clear and meaningful.

The best way to think about rights (moral or legal) is that they are correlative to duties. Thus, if I have a right to do X, someone else—an individual or perhaps the state—has a duty to me, either not to interfere with my doing X or, in some instances, to assist me in doing X. I may also have a duty to exercise my right responsibly, so as not to interfere with the rights of others.

One common problem with rights language is the perception that everyone has rights and no one has responsibilities. Another is that rights belong only to individuals, so that the rights of individuals are pitted against the interests of communities. Rights language should be used judiciously to avoid these pitfalls.

VIRTUES · Many of the basic concepts of ethics take the form of *principles*, that is, rules of general application. Autonomy, beneficence, and justice are all examples of principles. Rights also play a prominent role in medical ethics because of the connections between ethics, policy, and law. But there are other ways of conceptualizing ethics. One way that is well known to most of us is through virtues.

Virtue language is the language of "being" rather than "doing." Whereas principles provide "rules" for "solving" ethical "problems," virtues describe the kind of people we aspire to be. They set standards of character and consider how different traits of character add up to a good person, or a good health professional. The moral language that many people use more closely matches virtues than it does principles. A principlist might say, "You're wrong," or, "It's the right thing to do." Instead, many people say things like, "I wouldn't feel right if I did that," or, "I'm not the kind of person who could do that." Many codes of ethics for health care professionals use virtue language, focusing on what it means to be a good doctor or a good nurse more than on rules and action guides (for example, "The nurse should be honest," rather than, "The nurse should tell the truth").

Virtue language is the language of many religious traditions and forms the basis of much of the moral instruction that families pass on to children, but the concept of virtue ethics also has roots in Aristotle. Any complete system of ethics will include both principles and virtues, seeing them as complementary rather than competing ways of conceptualizing ethics.

Ethics in Medicine

An Introduction to Moral Tools and Traditions

Larry R. Churchill, Nancy M. P. King, David Schenck,
and Rebecca L. Walker

Foreground Decisions in a Background of Relationships

In this volume the reader is confronted with a variety of complex ethical situations in medicine and health care. These situations are typically expressed
as problems requiring sharp-edged, either/or moral choices: Should a physician lie to a patient when the lie promises patient benefit? Is it good to
be candid about medical mistakes, and if so, whose good is served? Should
physicians administer life-saving therapies in opposition to patient directives to forgo such interventions?

This essay is a brief introduction to ethics in medicine. One of its aims is
to provide a sketch of the major ethical theories and moral traditions that
are commonly used as tools for analyzing and resolving complex moral
problems. Although moral problem-solving is an important part of ethics, it
is only a part. All moral problems exist in a background of understandings,
relationships, and experiences that prefigure and shape them. In this way,
ethics is also about the nature and quality of human encounters.

A physician who decides to lie to her patient to protect him from some
harm does so in the context of a history and a relationship marked by many
nondecisional elements, including the previous understandings between
them, the motivations for judgment and action, and some degree of trust.
The *decision* to lie is thus only a small part of "ethics" in this example. Assuming that their previous interactions were marked by honesty, the physician
who lies to her patient changes their relationship and redefines herself. Surrounding her decision are deliberations, imaginings, and intentions that pre-
cede, inform, follow, and inevitably alter who this physician is, and who she
is with and for this patient.

This complex, contextual background necessarily gives moral decisions a larger meaning, because responding to moral dilemmas requires decision makers to identify, critically assess, and prioritize their moral values in order to find actions that express these values. Yet this is no simple matter, for three reasons. First, moral actors may be unsure just which commitments they want to express. Often our deepest convictions are not transparent to us, and we may have to work to discover them. Second, putting our convictions and commitments into practice requires many different capacities and skills. Ethics is part logic (following an argument), part leaps of empathic imagination (stepping into someone else's shoes), part storytelling (weaving a coherent thread through our moral motives, means, and actions), and many other things. Ethics involves many faculties and capacities. It is not just a function of clear reasoning capacity or benevolent feelings, of having the right rules or principles, or of possessing good intentions or achieving good outcomes. Instead, ethics involves all of these human capacities in ways that require moral actors to understand that their whole selves are involved. Third, because ethical choices engage our most deeply held and self-defining expressions, no one terminology for describing ethics predominates. For example, in explaining the first two points above we have alternatively talked about "values," "commitments," and "convictions." This multifaceted language signals that ethics is more than aesthetic preferences or tastes, more than consumer-style choices or desires. Ethics is too large and important to be confined to one standard set of linguistic terms, and this variety can sometimes lead to confusion. We will return to this pluralism in ethical expression later in this essay, when considering ethical theories and the importance of an eclectic approach.

Ethics as Human and Humanizing

Ethics appears to be distinctively human. Many other animals seem to be capable of moral behavior—shame, loyalty, helping others—and practice it routinely. But it is the capacity to systematically and critically reflect on one's moral behavior that seems to be uniquely characteristic of ethics. Ethics is not simply skill in doing good, but knowing *why* what one is doing can be called "good," having self-consciously chosen it from among the alternatives. As far as we can discern, only humans practice ethics in this reflective sense.

Ethics is also a *humanizing* activity. Conversations in ethics require viewing others with respect and regard; an exchange in ethics begins with the assump-

tion that others are of value and are subjects of a rich and complex life, just as we are. This simple gesture of respect is humanizing because it means that moral actors are willing to set aside, at least for the moment, differences in power and status in order to engage in ethics discussion with another.

This suspension of status and power enables attention to the other person—and, reflexively, also to oneself. Thus, engaging in ethical deliberation means listening—paying attention—and draws upon our empathic capacity.

Ethics requires us, and empathy enables us, first to recognize other persons as sentient and reflective beings whose moral commitments are as important to them as our own values are to us, and then to vigorously and respectfully engage with others and their values. This engagement is not easy. Americans tend to be tolerant of differences and sometimes reluctant to discuss them. Often they fear disagreement and see it as counterproductive or polarizing, as if acknowledging divergence in moral convictions would make conversation difficult and consensus impossible. Yet this kind of tolerant reluctance can be as debilitating for ethics as is the hardened ideological positioning it seeks to avoid.

Genuine ethical inquiry arises from the rich human background we have been describing and is characterized by openness to and exploration of differences. This moral agnosticism stands in opposition to moralizing or proselytizing for one's position and also in opposition to the tolerant relativism that would avoid endorsing any position at all. It says, "I have strong convictions, but I also know that I alone do not possess the final truth." Such a demeanor seeks the best options through a careful examination of the ethical implications of all the possibilities and a careful probing of the larger meaning of these options. The assumption that all parties engaged have a morally significant human voice (if not finally a fully persuasive position on resolving an issue) is the basic condition for dialogue. This assumption can also make consensus easier and the larger task of community building possible.

Engagement with others in moral discussion is humanizing in yet another way. The mutual empathy and respectful regard for differences that lets values emerge in an exchange is also a mode of interacting that is vastly less harmful for the participants. Anyone who has been involved in a situation that threatened to turn violent will immediately grasp the importance of this humanizing function. Ethical discussion can be thought of as a way of dealing with differences—one that is superior to many other modes of handling disagreements, such as shouting matches, holding grudges, filing lawsuits, or shooting people. Ethical skills become especially important and useful in a cultural environment of polarization and villainizing of those with different views.

Perhaps most important, the assumption of the moral importance of multiple voices makes community possible both before and after decisions have been made. Because moral dialogue is a mode of mutual recognition and respect, it has a positive effect on human bonding and community building even when it fails as a mechanism of problem solving or consensus. Ethics has intrinsic value, not just instrumental value as a means to an end. It is sometimes said that virtue is its own reward. This means not only that the virtuous should not necessarily expect to become rich and famous but also that being virtuous teaches one a better set of rewards than money or fame: the benefits of integrity, compassion, and self-respect. Engaging others in moral dialogue inherently advances personal and communal life in ways that have little to do with decisions, outcomes, or consequences. Thus, while it may lead to better decisions and outcomes, ethics as an activity is also its own reward.

Practicality, Expertise, and Common Moral Wisdom

In one sense ethics is eminently practical. It is about how to live our lives, what choices to make, and ultimately who we are, individually and relationally. A number of moral theories and traditions commonly invoked in medical ethics are discussed later in this essay. Sometimes moral agents, in the throes of a difficult choice, become impatient with theories and seek to bypass or ignore them. Yet theories often have practical utility. This utility arises in part because theories often contain some portion of distilled wisdom about what is good or right. In addition, the activity of theorizing can also be a very helpful way to locate inconsistencies in our thinking, precisely because it requires us to take a step back from the particular context of decisions and choices to ask *how* moral issues are being framed, what assumptions we are making, and what would count as a good reason for doing something. Moral theorizing is important because as humans we inevitably seek intellectual coherence for our lives.

Given its complexity and practical importance, ethics might be (indeed, has been) thought to be a field for experts. In the past, physicians, priests, and sometimes lawyers were thought to be the experts in medical ethics. In contemporary society, bioethicists and moral philosophers are often assigned that role. While there is a place for consulting authorities and moral expertise—

and real benefit from studying Hippocrates, Aristotle, Kant, and Nietzsche, not to mention Freud, Jung, Gilligan, and dozens of others—the insights of these scholars and the traditions and theories they represent can be made accessible to anyone. The practical skills of ethical discernment, reflection, and deliberation are already available to those who take the time to be thoughtful and not reactive in moral judgments. And with some study, the tools of various traditions and theories can be available as well. A major task of ethical deliberation is determining just which parts of these traditions and theories are useful tools for moral discernment in particular cases.

Ethical decisions can be very challenging for a variety of reasons. Sometimes what makes them challenging is a matter of inadequate theories, or a poor grasp or application of theoretical constructs. At other times the challenge arises from insufficient attention to the concrete dynamics of moral encounter, that is, to the settings and relationships in which specific ethical problems develop. Sometimes we do need better theories or better judgment about how to apply them. Sometimes it is more helpful to seek better modes of human engagement—to create and maintain a "moral space" (Walker 1993) within which we may safely encounter ourselves and each other. In short, ethical discussions that become unproductive or polarized can embody failures of several sorts: failures of empathy, failures of imagination, failures of logic and analogical reasoning, or, too often, multiple malfunctions.

The final aim of ethics is more than good decisions; it is a good life, a life marked by moral wisdom acquired through experience and reflection. Developing and consulting that reservoir of moral wisdom is a lifelong task. We are not morally transparent to ourselves; finding and critically affirming our values takes real work and the help of conversation partners. This was one of the most important lessons of Socrates. Moral traditions and theories can assist us in the work of locating, articulating, and testing the value-laden components of our experience—especially when they are thought of as tools, rather than as recipes for action or answer books.

Moral Traditions and Ethical Theories: A Beginning Inventory of Tools

Thus, being an ethically literate person means knowing what tools are available, and being a good doctor means having a working acquaintance with the traditions and major theories that are likely to be helpful in the situations physicians typically face. In Western moral tradition, theories of ethics can be roughly grouped into two domains: principle and virtue. Principle-based theories of ethics are currently dominant, but virtue-oriented approaches were synonymous with ethics until roughly the European and North American Enlightenment period (the eighteenth century), and they still play an important role. In contemporary thought, Eastern moral traditions, such as Confucianism and Buddhism, are usually thought of as virtue-based.

———————

PRINCIPLE-BASED THEORIES · Reasoning through principles is very familiar in Western thought; it is quasi-mathematical in style, seeking to deduce right choices from the application of norms. Principle-based reasoning forms the basis of much of American law and public policy, and it has strongly influenced modern medical ethics. Many recent professional codes of ethics are composed of principles, and some of the legal principles underlying the Bill of Rights—freedom of speech, freedom of religion, liberty and privacy, due process, and equal protection of the laws—have become thoroughly identified with health care ethics as a result of their importance in defining the rights of patients. The triumvirate of particular principles that shape most discussions of medical ethics—autonomy, beneficence, and justice—has been the centerpiece of medical ethics theory for several decades (Beauchamp and Childress 2012).

The principle of autonomy, or more fully, respect for autonomy, is the principle most often associated with patients' rights. Honoring the autonomy of patients means according them self-determination by viewing their decisions and choices as worthy of respect; it means not interfering with them (the "negative" right to be left alone) unless their actions injure others; and it also means assisting them in the exercise of their autonomy (for example, by providing information about health care decisions and reasoning with them about the benefits and harms of potential interventions).

In contrast, the principle of beneficence focuses on the duty of health care providers to act in the best interests of the patient. Beneficence, which entails both "doing no harm" and trying to do good, is generally seen by health care providers as the most important moral principle in health care. Moral quandaries in health care are sometimes presented, somewhat superficially, as conflicts between the principles of autonomy and beneficence, which are then dichotomized and offered as either/or choices. An example is a patient's desire for a course of action that is contrary to doctors' duty to protect the patient's health. In these instances, it is important to recognize that a number of key concepts and issues in health care ethics—in particular, informed

consent, truth telling, and confidentiality—combine and weigh both considerations of respect for autonomy and duties of beneficence. Careful analysis
will uncover the relationships between them, so that these principles are best
understood not as inevitably competing but as potentially complementary.

Justice is usually understood to mean fairness, and it introduces a wider
social dimension to individual caregiver-patient relationships than those
aspects emphasized by autonomy and beneficence. Justice sometimes means
addressing questions about the distribution of health care resources, and
what it means to do so equally or fairly. It sometimes means considering
whether health care should have a role in remedying injustices, past or present. Justice also focuses on questions like whether health care is (or should
be) a right, and what that might mean. Growing recognition of the limits
of the financial and material resources that can be applied to meet health
care needs has helped to bring the larger political and social dimensions of
health care ethics into the forefront of discussion and concern. The meaning
of justice in health care, both domestically and globally, is a central concern
of that inquiry.

Many of the major moral theories that have been applied to medical
ethics are principle-based. The "deontological" or duty-based moral theory
of Immanuel Kant (1724–1804), which emphasizes treating persons as "ends
in themselves," rather than as objects to be used only as means for achieving the ends of others, has been influential in medical ethics' understanding
of the principle of autonomy (1985). Jeremy Bentham (1748–1832) and John
Stuart Mill (1806–1873) are the most important exponents of utilitarianism, in which right actions are those that result in the greatest welfare for
the greatest number. Utilitarian theories consider beneficence to be central
(but Mill also prescribes that actions that do not harm others should not be
interfered with by society, thus establishing autonomy as a utilitarian good).
These two theories—Kantian deontology and utilitarianism—are the ones
most often cited in health care ethics. Too often they are viewed as being
in opposition, but they can be and frequently are combined as the basis of
much law and public policy (Steinbock, London, and Arras 2013).

VIRTUE-ORIENTED THEORIES · Virtue (or character) is very different
from principle as a way of thinking about ethics. It is not quandary-focused
and does not present a set of rules or norms to apply to a problem. Virtue
theory looks at persons. Instead of taking a choice or decision as the unit of
analysis, virtue-oriented approaches insist that morality is first and foremost
about the moral actor. Instead of asking whether an action is consistent
with a principle, such as "What decision does beneficence require?," virtue

theorists are more likely to ask "What does it mean to be a trustworthy physician in this situation?," focusing on a character trait of the person. Health professionals' codes and statements of ethics are often cast in virtue language rather than, or in addition to, the language of principles (for example, "The nurse should be honest" instead of "The nurse should tell the truth"). Western virtue theory has Greek roots, with Aristotle's (384–322 BCE) ethics being the best-known exemplar.

The term "character" is often associated with virtue ethics approaches. It refers to the way a group of virtues creates a distinguishing feature of an individual moral actor, just as we speak of a character in a dramatic production. Patients often focus on virtue and character more than on principles; many religious traditions express their norms in virtue language, enjoining their adherents to lead lives characterized by "faith, hope, and love," or to "have compassion." And virtue-oriented character formation is the chief aim of much of the moral instruction that families seek to pass on to children. The familiar childhood moral instruction "Be good!" is virtue language. In part because of its familiarity and in part because it is more challenging to apply to problems—where modern medical ethics focuses its attention— virtue-oriented thinking has not been the dominant approach over the past 50 years. Yet its revival by philosophers like Alasdair MacIntyre (1984) has spawned a renewed interest in virtue approaches to medical ethics. Pellegrino and Thomasma (1993), for example, have systematically explored those virtues they see as essential to medical practice: fidelity to trust, compassion, phronesis (practical wisdom), justice, fortitude, temperance, integrity, and self-effacement.

Most people in their personal and professional lives mix the language of principles with the language of virtues. Most of us also mix moral theories together when we are addressing issues, testing their suitability for the problem at hand, rather than stuffing the problem into a box labeled "autonomy" or "utilitarianism" and cutting off the parts that won't fit. This almost instinctively eclectic approach to practical moral problem solving represents a problem only if one is in search of an all-encompassing and final theory of ethics. For the everyday business of moral reflection, dialogue, and problem solving, a broad pluralism of theories and traditions is beneficial, since it is open to new approaches and the rediscovery of forgotten ones. One such theoretical rediscovery is *casuistry*, an analytical method revived by Albert Jonsen and Stephen Toulmin (1988) from Catholic moral theology. Casuistry means, simply, reasoning by cases. It employs cases—not principles or virtues—as the unit of moral analysis, and reaches judgments on a case-by-case basis, rather than attempting to apply or extract general rules. Casuistry is particularly attractive for health care ethics because clinical medicine is case-focused.

Another theoretical innovation in ethics comes from recognizing that cases inevitably involve the weaving of a narrative, and *narrative ethics* has emerged to name a way of doing ethics that focuses not just on the case but on the story (Hunter 1991; Chambers 2010). Stories have storytellers, major and minor characters, relationships, dramatic structure, and history. Stories can also often be told from multiple viewpoints, employing frames of reference of varying sizes: family, institution, community, and society. Using a narrative theory of ethics emphasizes that "the facts" of a case are never neutral or standing alone; they must be seen in their context in order to be fully understood and appreciated. For example, the patient's history, as presented by the doctor according to the conventions of medicine, may be different in highly significant ways from the patient's story, told by the patient, even when the factual details of the patient's "chief complaint" are identical in both accounts.

Another cluster of moral theories, even more difficult to characterize, might be loosely called *difference ethics*. They challenge the definitive position of Western ethical theories and assert the superiority of moral traditions other than those derived from the Greeks, Western religious traditions, or the Enlightenment. Feminist theories of ethics, for example, champion an ethics of care, compassion, and relationship over a traditional ethics based on reason and justice. Other theories build upon cross-cultural differences, arguing, for example, that individual autonomy is less significant in non-Western cultures, where family and community are central or where religious traditions are not focused on the individual self. Some theories of difference ethics go on to make a deeper critique of moral philosophy in general by highlighting power and inequality as a central but undiscussed issue in moral relationships, both individual and societal, and by bringing questions about the uses of power to the foreground. Though most often associated with feminist ethics, power analysis is common also to the search for an African American perspective on bioethics and to inquiries about the relationship between ethics and ethnicity and culture (Prograis and Pellegrino 2007; Tong and Botts 2018). It also has visible roots in modern medical ethics. For example, the recognition of inequality of power and knowledge between patients and physicians formed the basis for the doctrine of informed consent as it developed in the 1950s and 1960s (Faden and Beauchamp with King 1986).

Is There a Distinctive Medical Ethic?

It is noteworthy that physicians have not been satisfied to apply whatever moral standards were available from religion, political philosophy, or the common morality of society, but have from the beginning of Western medicine insisted on their own code of ethics. In asking whether there is anything that could be called a distinctive medical ethic, we are asking whether the work of physicians *should* be governed by a special ethic, a set of norms that are particular to doctors because of the work they do. The definition of medicine as a profession is linked to the idea that physicians are in some sense set apart by the nature of their work, destined for a different, if not higher, set of standards. They are, after all, asked to do some difficult things, such as train in relative social deprivation over long hours for many years, perform tasks in which their own health and safety may be at risk, and work in contexts that require patients to be extraordinarily vulnerable, both bodily and in terms of personal identity. Does this work require a set of standards that are, if not higher, at least somewhat more demanding?

Physicians since the Hippocratics have thought so. The Hippocratic oath not only describes the moral aspirations of a small sect of ancient Greek physicians but also invokes standards that set these physicians apart from other kinds of healers on moral/spiritual grounds. When this oath was first recited, it was a radical statement of highly stringent behavioral standards for a priestly brotherhood. So it appropriately begins with a pledge to "Apollo, Asclepius, Hygieia, Panaceia, and all the gods and goddesses." Today, appropriately sanitized of ancient Greek deities, the oath has come to be seen as stating many commonly held medical values. The various codes and statements of principle that physicians have put forward since the Hippocratic oath also serve as indices of medicine's dominant moral sensibility, indicating medicine's view of which issues are important and what standards should govern physicians' actions. Moreover, these codes are testimony to the need of physicians to state their standards publicly, as a way to signal to society that physicians are "worthy to serve the suffering" (the motto of Alpha Omega Alpha, the national medical honor society, as it appears on the title page of the journal *Pharos*). Because physicians have thought of themselves as to some degree set apart for arduous and important work, graduating classes of doctors all over the United States typically recite an oath. Sometimes this is a revised version of the Hippocratic oath, with the pagan deities and some of the more problematic injunctions (such as the prohibition against using the knife) excised. For others the commencement ceremony includes an affirmation of moral commitments that is discussed and agreed upon by the graduating class itself, often including many of the Hippocratic restrictions (such as the duty to keep confidences), but adding norms that reflect contemporary problems, such as pledging to work for an inclusive system of health care coverage.

While it is clear that physicians and other medical practitioners have special obligations engendered by their social role in promoting and protecting the health of patients, this does not mean that there is a separate medical ethic. If we think of medical ethics as wholly distinctive in its requirements and motivations, we run a risk of isolating the moral code of physicians from that of the rest of society. This not only would raise problems in negotiating conflicts between "medical" ethics and "common" ethics, but would also risk stagnation in a medical ethics not subject to broader social modification. (See Shepherd's essay in this volume for more on this issue.) Perhaps the best perspective is to view medical ethics as somewhat distinctive, but not as a separate ethic, and to see medical ethics and common ethics as constantly in dialogue.

A small sample of historical and contemporary codes of ethics is included in this volume. The reader is invited to consider not only the implications of what is reflected and omitted in these various formulations, but also the implications of having a separate or special set of norms for doctors. Codes of medical ethics are not just individual action guides for physicians. They also serve an important function as an expression of the medical profession's contract with society, pledging trustworthy behavior in exchange for social trust and power. In this vein, it is useful to ask why such codes are always authored by physicians, rather than being collaborative products of medicine's dialogue with patients and the larger public. Also, since codes of medical ethics serve to frame therapeutic relationships, should there be a complementary list of moral expectations and responsibilities for being a patient? If so, would these merely address being a "good" individual patient while one is sick, or should they also address collective social responsibilities, such as the distribution of scarce medical resources?

Medical codes of ethics must be considered as one of the most important moral traditions available for medical ethics, simply because they have been passed forward for over 2,500 years. "Tradition" is a term that means literally to pass along, or hand over. Of course in the process of handing over, things change; this is how traditions stay vibrant and relevant to their times. The most basic ethical challenge for doctors and medical students is to recognize themselves as part of a long and complex moral tradition, with an obligation to reflect critically on what is being passed along, discarding what is no longer useful and creating new ways to articulate and embody what is as yet unknown and unsaid about moral life in medicine.

Using Tools to Approach Problems: An Illustration

To stress that many traditions and theories are important to medical ethics is to eschew the vision of a single all-encompassing moral framework. The idea that morality could be finally and definitively secured by discovering and then following some monolithic theory is not just a philosopher's dream but a common human aspiration. A simple, unified theoretical basis for ethics that could eliminate the endless disputes and the vexing uncertainty of medical ethics decisions, unambiguously identifying what is good and right, would clearly be comforting. All candidates for such a unifying system in the past have proved to be procrustean beds. In Greek mythology, Procrustes, a son of Poseidon, forces his guests to fit themselves into his bed, by either stretching or cutting off their legs. Ethical theories that claim universal scope do similar damage, lopping off important facets of cases and situations in an effort to make them fit the preconceptions of theory and denying to moral agents the all-important exercise of their own particular moral perceptions and judgments.

In the absence of such theoretical unity, the task becomes one of using the wide range of tools and traditions skillfully. To illustrate how some of the tools we have described might be put to use, consider the following simplified case.

A 23-year-old female is brought to the emergency department by ambulance following a motor vehicle crash. She is in hemorrhagic shock from a severe pelvic fracture requiring surgery, and is currently unconscious. She is a Jehovah's Witness and has signed a statement refusing blood products. Her husband is not a Jehovah's Witness and wants her to be given blood. The patient's parents are also present and insist that she would not want it. Her husband states that she signed the form refusing blood before the birth of her 10-month-old son, and that she would do anything to save her own life in order to care for her son.

Should this patient be given life-saving blood products, or not? This is the immediate question. In responding, we will focus on how moral traditions and theories help by bringing to prominence important facets of the situation and by posing questions to frame and shape our perspective. Here are some of the questions that would be emphasized in the various approaches we have discussed.

What would it mean to seek to treat this patient as an end in herself, and not just a means? Does the form she has signed constitute her autonomous choice, in this case made in advance of the actual situation? Would a utilitarian approach, emphasizing the greatest overall good, mean saving this patient's life in order to satisfy the needs of her son and husband, rather than her parents' assessment of her wishes? Which of the medical virtues is it important to enact here—fidelity to trust in respecting the patient's religious convictions? Or perhaps courage, in overriding her parents and doing everything to save this patient's life? (There are other possible manifestations of both trust and courage in this situation, too, some of which lead in different directions.) A feminist interpretation might highlight the power struggle between family members over a female patient, whereas a narrative approach would want to know who constructed this version of the problem, whose story it is that is being played out here. Can a better version of this problem be constructed? What would make it "better"—that it is a more accurate description of the ethical problems, or a more complete story, or that it might lead to a quicker or different resolution? These questions are illustrative, not definitive or exhaustive. Being skilled in ethics means knowing how to pick up the conversation and continue it.

Three points in summary. First, consulting a wide range of approaches can better equip moral actors to make decisions that they (and others) can live with over time, decisions that honor rather than suppress the complexity of both the issues and the relationships involved. Second, the key element in a good decision is making discerning judgments: surveying the available tools, selecting the right ones for the job, and using them with a modicum of skill. Having a wide range of tools is important; if one's only tool is a hammer, every problem may look like a nail.

But of course this analogy of selecting tools for a defined job, while helpful, is too simplistic and mechanical. As we have emphasized, sometimes just finding the decision point for action from within a complex web of persons, events, and relationships is a more challenging ethical task than reaching a decision. The hard work of ethics may not be what to decide, but discerning *how* to decide, or even realizing that no decision is called for. It is characteristic of different ethical theories that they provide us not only with differing ways to solve a problem, but also with differing definitions of the problem itself and divergent pathways for the exercise of moral agency, that is, different perceptions of the moral roles of the persons engaged in the decision.

While it is important to recognize a pluralism in the tools of ethics, it is also important that this pluralism does not simply become a way to avoid the hard thinking that moral choices demand. Seeking the best moral tools—such as the theoretical constructs we have discussed—means carefully considering relevance, application, and consistency in the use of these tools, not simply choosing a position we are already inclined to take. Pluralism does not excuse us from the hard task of reflective discernment.

Finally, whatever decisional apparatus we adopt (or reject) brings with it relational commitments, both spoken and unspoken. Recognizing and naming the unspoken commitments is an important nondecisional aspect of ethics. It is also a necessary step in moral maturity and wisdom.

Third, ethical decisions are synchronic moments in larger diachronic histories; they are only slices of moral life. In spite of their high drama, and the great weight and consequence they may have, especially in life-and-death settings, individual decisions may not by themselves be definitive in shaping anyone's moral identity. Sometimes difficult decisions are a matter of doing the best one can in tragic situations, where all the options are bad ones. When clear choices do not appear and satisfying resolutions seem unlikely, the challenge lies in choosing the "least worst" alternative and muddling through. In these cases, then, moral routines and habits take on considerable importance in shaping an ethical life or being a good doctor, because they make up the background of resources and relationships against which moral decisions are understood and made. Ultimately, ethics is about the shaping of moral identity and the development and application of moral wisdom throughout life. However urgently we need good decisions, good intentions, or good outcomes, none of those individual endpoints is truly achievable or sustainable apart from the larger effort of learning to live a good life. The models and tools of moral decision making serve that larger goal and are also served by it.

Conclusion: Getting Grounded

Readers may view this rich moral landscape, featuring many languages and approaches to ethical problems, and many theories behind these approaches, with apprehension or delight at the possible paths before them. Recognition of the wide range of methods and approaches possible in ethics can be empowering for some, yet for others it may seem paralyzing: Without a universal, overriding ethical framework, what is there to keep us from becoming adrift in relativism?

The fear of moral relativism has been a nagging, but misunderstood, problem for Western ethics since before Plato (427–347 BCE). Relativism is the assumption that since there is no universal and timeless, agreed-upon standard for ethics, then there are no standards at all—everything must be up for grabs. The choice is conceived as between ethical certainty and the moral abyss.

Without offering a full discussion here, we submit that the practical moral pluralism described in this essay, which draws from many moral theories and traditions, does not lead to relativism. A plurality of resources is no more problematic for ethics than for other disciplines. There are competing theories in economics, psychiatry, mathematics, and physics—to name just a few—and shifting theoretical viewpoints over time in all these fields, yet no one assumes that because economists or physicists disagree among themselves, and sometimes combine theories and approaches, these fields are riddled with relativism. And so it is for ethics.

The best protection against both absolutist and relativistic interpretations of ethics lies in the recognition that the whole of ethics is, after all, a human enterprise, with the effort of persons and their hard-won moral wisdom the only assurance we have for the integrity of the effort. Those who worry about relativism and become skeptical typically forget that the basic aim of ethics is not final answers, but practical guidance and continual moral learning from life's experiences and choices. The place we have to stand is not upon a universal foundation of eternal truth, but simply on the ground, on our own feet. There is no knock-down argument to refute the relativist or silence the skeptic. The answer lies in a commitment to use what we have to pursue that wisdom of which we are capable, and to do so honestly and persistently. Montaigne (1533–1592) put it with characteristic pungency: "We seek other conditions because we do not understand the use of our own, and we go outside ourselves because we do not know what it is like inside. Yet there is no use our mounting on stilts, for on stilts we must still walk on our own legs. And on the loftiest throne in the world we are still sitting only on our own rump" (Montaigne 1965). At the beginning of this essay we noted that ethics is often conceived simplistically as a series of sharp-edged questions requiring either/or decisions. We have sought to make it clear that the responses given to such questions must be nested in a far larger context than is at first evident. The question "Should a physician lie to a patient when the lie promises patient benefit?" is meaningless without considering the role and place of truthfulness in a therapeutic encounter. Likewise, "Is it good to be candid about medical mistakes, and if so, whose good is served?" must be posed in the larger context of the need for personal and professional forgiveness

(Arendt 1957), given that all physicians will make mistakes that cause harm. And, "Should physicians ever impose a life-saving treatment that patients have chosen to forgo?" resides within a larger inquiry about the place and purpose of medical care in the individual's pursuit of a "good" life. Ethics is personal and decisional because it is first social and relational. It inevitably entails probing into the larger meaning of choices and sounding the deeper reservoirs of our common human wisdom.

REFERENCES

Arendt, H. 1957. *The Human Condition*. Chicago: University of Chicago Press.

Aristotle. 1999. *Nicomachean Ethics*. Translated by T. Irwin. 2nd ed. Cambridge: Hackett Publishing.

Beauchamp, T., and J. Childress. 2012. *Principles of Biomedical Ethics*. 7th ed. New York: Oxford University Press.

Chambers, T. 2010. "Literature." In *Methods of Medical Ethics*. 2nd ed. Edited by J. Sugarman and D. P. Sulmasy. Washington, DC: Georgetown University Press.

Faden, R., and T. Beauchamp, with N. King. 1986. *A History and Theory of Informed Consent*. New York: Oxford University Press.

Hume, D. 1978. *A Treatise of Human Nature, Book III*. 2nd ed. Edited by L. A. Selby-Bigge and P. H. Nidditch. Oxford: Clarendon Press.

Hunter, K. M. 1991. *Doctors' Stories: The Narrative Structure of Medical Knowledge*. Princeton, NJ: Princeton University Press.

Jonsen, A., and S. Toulmin. 1988. *The Abuse of Casuistry*. Berkeley: University of California Press.

Kant, I. 1985. *Foundations of the Metaphysics of Morals*. Translated by L. W. Beck. New York: Macmillan.

MacIntyre, A. 1984. *After Virtue.*, Notre Dame, IN: University of Notre Dame Press.

Mill, J. S. 1979. *Utilitarianism*. Edited by G. Sher. Indianapolis, IN: Hackett Publishing.

Montaigne, M. 1976. *The Complete Essays of Montaigne*. Translated by Donald Frame. Stanford, CA: Stanford University Press.

Pellegrino, E. D., and D. Thomasma. 1993. *The Virtues in Medical Practice*. New York: Oxford University Press.

Prograis, L. J., and E. D. Pellegrino, eds. 2007. *African American Bioethics: Culture, Race, and Identity*. Washington, DC: Georgetown University Press.

Smith, A. 1976. *The Theory of Moral Sentiments*. Edited by D. Raphael and A. Madie. Indianapolis, IN: Liberty Classics.

Steinbock, B., A. J. London, and J. Arras, eds. 2013. *Ethical Issues in Modern Medicine: Contemporary Readings in Bioethics*. New York: McGraw-Hill.

Tong, R., and T. F. Botts, eds. 2018. *Feminist Thought: A More Comprehensive Introduction*. 5th ed. Westview Press.

Walker, M. U. 1993. "Keeping moral space open." *Hastings Center Report* 23, no. 2: 33–40.

Historical and Contemporary Codes of Ethics

The Hippocratic Oath, the Prayer of Maimonides, the Declaration of Geneva, and the AMA Principles of Medical Ethics

Oath of Hippocrates (Sixth Century BCE–First Century CE)

Assumed to have been written by Hippocrates, the oath exemplifies the Pythagorean school rather than Greek thought in general. The oath of Hippocrates is one of the earliest and most important statements on medical ethics. Estimates of its actual date of origin vary from the sixth century BCE to the first century CE. Not only has the oath provided the foundation for many succeeding medical oaths, for example, the Declaration of Geneva, but it is still administered by many medical schools to graduating medical students, either in its original form or in a slightly altered version.

I swear by Apollo Physician and Asclepius and Hygieia and Panaceia and all the gods and goddesses, making them my witnesses, that I will fulfil according to my ability and judgment this oath and this covenant:

"Oath of Hippocrates," trans. Ludwig Edelstein, from *Bulletin of the History of Medicine* 3, suppl. 1 (1943), reprinted by permission of Johns Hopkins University Press; "Daily Prayer of a Physician," trans. Harry Friedenwalk, from *Bulletin of the Johns Hopkins Hospital* 28 (1917); "Declaration of Geneva," adopted by the 2nd General Assembly of the World Medical Association, Geneva, Switzerland, September 1948, and amended by the 22nd World Medical Assembly, Sydney, Australia, August 1968, and the 35th World Medical Assembly, Venice, Italy, October 1983, and the 46th WMA General Assembly, Stockholm, Sweden, September 1994, and editorially revised by the 170th WMA Council Session, Divonne-les-Bains, France, May 2005, and the 173rd WMA Council Session, Divonne-les-Bains, France, May 2006, and amended by the 68th WMA General Assembly, Chicago, United States, October 2017; "Principles of Medical Ethics," from the AMA Code of Ethics, © 2016 by American Medical Association, reprinted by permission of the American Medical Association. All rights reserved.

To hold him who has taught me this art as equal to my parents and to live my life in partnership with him, and if he is in need of money to give him a share of mine, and to regard his offspring as equal to my brothers in male lineage and to teach them this art—if they desire to learn it—without fee and covenant; to give a share of precepts and oral instruction and all the other learning to my sons and to the sons of him who has instructed me and to pupils who have signed the covenant and have taken an oath according to the medical law, but to no one else.

I will apply dietetic measures for the benefit of the sick according to my ability and judgment; I will keep them from harm and injustice.

I will neither give a deadly drug to anybody if asked for it, nor will I make a suggestion to this effect. Similarly, I will not give to a woman an abortive remedy. In purity and holiness I will guard my life and my art.

I will not use the knife, not even on sufferers from stone, but will withdraw in favor of such men as are engaged in this work.

Whatever houses I may visit, I will come for the benefit of the sick, remaining free of all intentional injustice, of all mischief, and in particular of sexual relations with both female and male persons, be they free or slaves.

What I may see or hear in the course of the treatment or even outside of the treatment in regard to the life of men, which on no account one must spread abroad, I will keep to myself holding such things shameful to be spoken about.

If I fulfil this oath and do not violate it, may it be granted to me to enjoy life and art, being honored with fame among all men for all time to come; if I transgress it and swear falsely, may the opposite of all this be my lot.

Daily Prayer of a Physician ("Prayer of Moses Maimonides") (1793?)

Almighty God, Thou has created the human body with infinite wisdom. Ten thousand times ten thousand organs hast Thou combined in it that act unceasingly and harmoniously to preserve the whole in all its beauty—the body which is the envelope of the immortal soul. They are ever acting in perfect order, agreement, and accord. Yet, when the frailty of matter or the unbridling of passions deranges this order or interrupts this accord, then forces clash, and the body crumbles into the primal dust from which it came. Thou sendest to man diseases as beneficent messengers to foretell approaching danger and to urge him to avert it.

Thou has blest Thine earth, Thy rivers, and Thy mountains with healing substances; they enable Thy creatures to alleviate their sufferings and to heal their illnesses. Thou hast endowed man with the wisdom to relieve the suffering of his brother, to recognize his disorders, to extract the healing substances, to discover their powers, and to prepare and to apply them to suit every ill. In Thine Eternal Providence Thou hast chosen me to watch over the life and health of Thy creatures. I am now about to apply myself to the duties of my profession. Support me, Almighty God, in these great labors that they may benefit mankind, for without Thy help not even the least thing will succeed.

Inspire me with love for my art and for Thy creatures. Do not allow thirst for profit, ambition for renown and admiration, to interfere with my profession, for these are the enemies of truth and of love for mankind and they can lead astray in the great task of attending to the welfare of Thy creatures. Preserve the strength of my body and of my soul that they ever be ready to cheerfully help and support rich and poor, good and bad, enemy as well as friend. In the sufferer let me see only the human being. Illumine my mind that it recognize what presents itself and that it may comprehend what is absent or hidden. Let it not fail to see what is visible, but do not permit it to arrogate to itself the power to see what cannot be seen, for delicate and indefinite are the bounds of the great art of caring for the lives and health of Thy creatures. Let me never be absent-minded. May no strange thoughts divert my attention at the bedside of the sick, or disturb my mind in its silent labors, for great and sacred are the thoughtful deliberations required to preserve the lives and health of Thy creatures.

Grant that my patients have confidence in me and my art and follow my directions and my counsel. Remove from their midst all charlatans and the whole host of officious relatives and know-all nurses, cruel people who arrogantly frustrate the wisest purposes of our art and often lead Thy creatures to their death.

Should those who are wiser than I wish to improve and instruct me, let my soul gratefully follow their guidance; for vast is the extent of our art. Should conceited fools, however, censure me, then let love for my profession steel me against them, so that I remain steadfast without regard for age, for reputation, or for honor, because surrender would bring to Thy creatures sickness and death.

Imbue my soul with gentleness and calmness when older colleagues, proud of their age, wish to displace me or to scorn me or disdainfully to teach me. May even this be of advantage to me, for they know many things of which I am ignorant, but let not their arrogance give me pain. For they are old and old age is not master of the passions. I also hope to attain old age upon this earth, before Thee, Almighty God!

Let me be contented in everything except in the great science of my profession. Never allow the thought to arise in me that I have attained to sufficient knowledge, but vouchsafe to me the strength, the leisure, and the ambition ever to extend my knowledge. For art is great, but the mind of man is ever expanding.

Almighty God! Thou hast chosen me in Thy mercy to watch over the life and death of Thy creatures. I now apply myself to my profession. Support me in this great task so that it may benefit mankind, for without Thy help not even the least thing will succeed.

Declaration of Geneva (World Medical Association)

The Physician's Pledge

AS A MEMBER OF THE MEDICAL PROFESSION:

I SOLEMNLY PLEDGE to dedicate my life to the service of humanity;

THE HEALTH AND WELL-BEING OF MY PATIENT will be my first consideration;

I WILL RESPECT the autonomy and dignity of my patient;

I WILL MAINTAIN the utmost respect for human life;

I WILL NOT PERMIT considerations of age, disease or disability, creed, ethnic origin, gender, nationality, political affiliation, race, sexual orientation, social standing or any other factor to intervene between my duty and my patient;

I WILL RESPECT the secrets that are confided in me, even after the patient has died;

I WILL PRACTISE my profession with conscience and dignity and in accordance with good medical practice;

I WILL FOSTER the honour and noble traditions of the medical profession;

I WILL GIVE to my teachers, colleagues, and students the respect and gratitude that is their due;

I WILL SHARE my medical knowledge for the benefit of the patient and the advancement of healthcare;

I WILL ATTEND TO my own health, well-being, and abilities in order to provide care of the highest standard;

I WILL NOT USE my medical knowledge to violate human rights and civil liberties, even under threat;

I MAKE THESE PROMISES solemnly, freely, and upon my honour.

Principles of Medical Ethics (American Medical Association)

PREAMBLE · The medical profession has long subscribed to a body of ethical statements developed primarily for the benefit of the patient. As a member of this profession, a physician must recognize responsibility to patients first and foremost, as well as to society, to other health professionals, and to self. The following Principles adopted by the American Medical Association are not laws, but standards of conduct which define the essentials of honorable behavior for the physician.

I A physician shall be dedicated to providing competent medical care, with compassion and respect for human dignity and rights.

II A physician shall uphold the standards of professionalism, be honest in all professional interactions, and strive to report physicians deficient in character or competence, or engaging in fraud or deception, to appropriate entities.

III A physician shall respect the law and also recognize a responsibility to seek changes in those requirements which are contrary to the best interests of the patient.

IV A physician shall respect the rights of patients, colleagues, and other health professionals, and shall safeguard patient confidences and privacy within the constraints of the law.

V A physician shall continue to study, apply, and advance scientific knowledge, maintain a commitment to medical education, make relevant information available to patients, colleagues, and the public, obtain consultation, and use the talents of other health professionals when indicated.

VI A physician shall, in the provision of appropriate patient care, except in emergencies, be free to choose whom to serve, with whom to associate, and the environment in which to provide medical care.

VII A physician shall recognize a responsibility to participate in activities contributing to the improvement of the community and the betterment of public health.

VIII A physician shall, while caring for a patient, regard responsibility to the patient as paramount.

IX A physician shall support access to medical care for all people.

Enduring and Emerging Challenges of Informed Consent

Christine Grady

Informed consent is a widely accepted legal, ethical, and regulatory requirement for most research and health care transactions. Nonetheless, the practice of informed consent varies by context, and the reality often falls short of the theoretical ideal. Contemporary developments in health care and clinical research call for renewed efforts to address the enduring and emerging challenges of informed consent, such as what information should be disclosed, how it should be disclosed, how much the persons providing consent should understand, and how explicit consent should be.

The moral force of consent is not unique to health care or research. Integral to many interpersonal interactions and well entrenched in societal values and jurisprudence, consent can render actions morally permissible that would otherwise be wrong. For example, with consent it is fine to borrow a person's car or draw blood, but these actions without consent are considered theft or battery.[1] Recent research conducted by Facebook and OkCupid, which made use of user information and generated arguments about whether the general consent given when joining a social network suffices as consent for such research or whether express consent is required,[2,3] illustrates both how deeply rooted the idea of consent is in society and the changing landscape in which it may apply.

Christine Grady, "Enduring and Emerging Challenges of Informed Consent," from *New England Journal of Medicine* 372 (2015): 855–862. © 2015 by Massachusetts Medical Society. Reprinted by permission of Massachusetts Medical Society.

Ethical and Legal Foundations

Consent is a long-standing practice in some areas of medicine, yet only in the last century has informed consent been accepted as a legal and ethical concept integral to medical practice and research.[4] Informed consent, in principle, is authorization of an activity based on an understanding of what that activity entails and in the absence of control by others.[5] Laws and regulations dictate the current informed-consent requirements, but the underlying values are deeply culturally embedded—specifically, the value of respect for persons' autonomy and their right to define their own goals and make choices designed to achieve those goals.[5] This right applies to all types of health-related interventions, including life-sustaining interventions. An early President's Commission report noted, "Informed consent is rooted in the fundamental recognition . . . that adults are entitled to accept or reject health care interventions on the basis of their own personal values and in furtherance of their own personal goals."[6]

Although informed consent is widely accepted in the United States and in many other countries, this understanding—and, indeed, the focus on an individual right to self-determination—varies according to culture. Cultural differences manifest in both the practice of informed consent—that is, what is told to whom and who makes decisions—as well as in an understanding of the normative underpinnings of informed consent as respect for individual autonomy. Persons in many cultures, both in the United States and around the world, rely on their families and sometimes on their communities for important decisions, and this may be the norm in cultures that stress the relationship of individuals to others and the embeddedness of individuals within society. Commentators and empirical evidence have shown that culture influences moral values and that other key values, such as loyalty, compassion, and solidarity, may be more dominant than autonomy in some cultures.[7] Respecting persons includes respecting their cultural values and may require adapting the specifics of information disclosure or obtaining authorization for treatment or research accordingly. Yet respecting cultural values does not negate the need to respect the persons for whom care or research is being considered or the need to implement respectful and appropriate procedures. As Gostin points out, "Vast personal, cultural, and social differences will perennially pose challenges to meaningful dialogue among physician, patient, and family; it is the regard, consideration, and deference shown the patient that remains the hallmark of respect for persons."[8] The World Medical Association Declaration of Lisbon on the Rights of the Patient emphasizes that patients everywhere have a right to information and to self-determination.[9] The Declaration of Helsinki and other international codes of research ethics similarly emphasize the centrality of informed consent in the context of research globally.[10]

Gaps between Theory and Practice

Informed consent is a process of communication between the health care provider or investigator and the patient or research participant that ultimately culminates in the authorization or refusal of a specific intervention or research study. According to the American Medical Association, "Informed consent is a basic policy in both ethics and law that physicians must honor. . . ."[11] The process involves multiple elements, including disclosure, comprehension, voluntary choice, and authorization. In theory, physicians and investigators disclose understandable information to patients and research participants to facilitate informed choice.[4] These persons use this information to deliberate and decide whether the intervention offered is compatible with their interests and whether to authorize or refuse it. Persons should have the capacity to understand the information and should be in a position to make and to authorize a choice about how to proceed. Neither medical nor research interventions should commence until valid consent has been obtained, except under limited circumstances (e.g., emergencies). When a patient or research participant is a child or an adult who is not capable of providing informed consent, permission for medical care or research is often sought from a substitute decision maker, such as a parent or legally authorized proxy.

Most accept that in practice, particular aspects of informed consent vary by context, and both scholars and practitioners continue to debate these aspects—such as the scope and level of detail provided and the methods of disclosure,[12,13] whether and how to assess comprehension, what constitutes necessary and sufficient understanding for valid consent,[14] approaches to assessing persons' capacity to consent and steps taken when they lack that capacity,[15] how to know when choices are sufficiently voluntary,[16] and issues concerning the documentation of consent.[17] Consent for an elective surgical procedure differs from that for a simple routine blood test or from a complicated research study, for example. Cultural, socioeconomic, and educational factors can also influence the process and practice of informed consent, as can different decision-making practices and norms related to the role of individual autonomy.[18]

TABLE 1 Current Trends in the Health Care and Research Landscape That Have an Effect on Enduring and Emerging Challenges in Informed Consent

Selected Current Trends in Health Care	Emerging Questions and Challenges	Enduring Questions and Challenges	Proposed Strategies
Learning health care systems, pragmatic trials, and quality improvement	Should informed consent for these activities be more similar to research informed consent or clinical informed consent? How much information should be given to participants in advance? Under what circumstances (if any) is notification rather than express consent sufficient? When can consent be ethically waived or altered? What information is important to patients and research participants? Is it ethically acceptable for a patient or research participant to provide consent for an unspecified or broad range of activities?	What is the appropriate amount and detail of information for valid consent in various contexts? What is the best way to disclose or present information to be sufficiently comprehensive but not overwhelming? What are the contextual elements that determine the appropriate amount, complexity, and format of disclosure?	Integrated consent, shared decision making; consent to be governed, more evidence about what persons giving consent want to know, alternative strategies
Adoption of complex technologies, such as next-generation genetic sequencing	How should information be presented, and what level of understanding should be sought when obtaining consent for complex technologies (such as genetic sequencing) characterized by voluminous and complex information, substantial uncertainty (e.g., variants of unknown significance), incidental findings, and implications for blood relatives?	Empirical evidence shows that patients and research participants often do not understand the information provided to them. Complex information and interventions may be more difficult to understand, especially in the setting of limited health and science literacy.	Use of technology to present information; broad or dynamic consent; consent to be governed; enhancement of science literacy
Consent for future use of clinical data or biologic specimens	Is it ethically acceptable for a patient or research participant to provide consent for an unspecified or broad range of possible future research or to consent to a program or system of governance?	How specific does the information provided in the consent process need to be regarding future uses of data or specimens? Does the answer differ if the data or specimens are deidentified or if future projects are subject to oversight?	Broad consent; dynamic consent; consent to be governed; deidentification of data and samples

Selected Current Trends in Health Care	Emerging Questions and Challenges	Enduring Questions and Challenges	Proposed Strategies
Demographic changes with an aging population and increase in prevalence of dementia	Older age, diminished mental capacity, and dementia per se do not indicate that a person is incapable of consenting, yet the increasing numbers of elderly people and increasing prevalence of dementia and other disorders suggest that professionals in both clinical care and in research should consider a person's capacity to consent and be trained in how to assess capacity. There is a need for respectful and efficient tools and processes for assessing capacity, promoting decision making, appropriately involving families and friends, respecting cultural values, and using substitute decision makers when appropriate.	Capacity is assumed for adults, and the capacity to consent is only occasionally assessed. Capacity may be questioned only when a patient or research participant disagrees with the physician or researcher. The standards for substitute decision makers vary by jurisdiction and are different for clinical and research decisions.	Respectful and effective assessment of capacity and training of health professionals; creative approaches to presenting information; involving trusted friends and family members in consent discussions and decision making; studying new paradigms for substitute decision making

Furthermore, in practice, emphasis is often given to the written documentation of consent, despite wide agreement that consent requires more than a signature on a form. Faden and Beauchamp acknowledge that there are two common and starkly different meanings of informed consent: autonomous authorization by a patient or research participant and institutionally or legally effective authorization, determined by a complex web of prevailing rules, policies, and social practices.[5] The latter meaning, which is not necessarily accompanied by autonomous decisions, may overemphasize written documentation and risk communication, and it serves to help protect providers and institutions from liability.

A substantial body of literature corroborates a considerable gap between the practice of informed consent and its theoretical construct or intended goals and indicates many unresolved conceptual and practical questions.[19-22] Empirical evidence shows variation in the type and level of detail of information disclosed, in patient or research-participant understanding of the information, and in how their decisions are influenced.[23] Physicians receive little training regarding the practice of informed consent, are pressed for time and by competing demands, and often misinterpret the requirements and legal standards. Patients often have meager comprehension of the risks and alternatives of offered surgical or medical treatments,[24] and their decisions are driven more by trust in their doctor or by deference to authority than by the information provided.[25,26] Informed consent for research is more tightly regulated and detailed,[27] yet research consent forms continue to increase in length, complexity, and incorporation of legal language, making them less likely to be read or understood.[28,29] Studies also show that research participants have deficits in their understanding of study information, particularly of research methods such as randomization.[30] Research participants, who are often patients with illnesses, frequently misunderstand the way in which research is distinct from individualized clinical care, and some worry that this "therapeutic misconception" can invalidate informed consent.[31] The federal regulations require most research informed-consent documents to include a standard set of informational elements and to be approved by an institutional review board before use.[27] However, recent controversy over a study of neonates, the Surfactant, Positive Pressure, and Oxygenation Randomized Trial (SUPPORT) study, illustrates that even when these requirements are adhered to, reasonable people disagree about the adequacy of the information presented on the consent forms.[32,33]

Various strategies to improve patient understanding in informed consent have been evaluated. Studies show that patients understand risk better when physicians are taught communication strategies.[34,35] Decision aids and decision-making tools[36] and a focus on shared decision making also enhance patients' understanding and satisfaction.[37,38] When time is spent explaining information about the study, the participants' understanding of research seems to improve.[39] Practical strategies, such as synthesizing and simplifying information and using technological tools and nonphysician providers to explain the research, have been suggested as ways to help achieve the ethical goals of consent.[40] More provocatively, some suggest a need to revisit the concepts and the contours of acceptable consent, noting that current notions of informed consent may be outdated[41] or that we may be expecting too much of consent.[42] Clearly, there is a need for continued consideration of the normative and practical aspects of informed consent in an attempt to reconcile practice with the theoretical ideal. Several contemporary trends in health care and research accentuate this need, as described in table 1.

Informed consent is one among several important challenges that have arisen as health care institutions and practitioners adopt robust learning models that hybridize patient care with research and evidence generation to efficiently integrate improved prevention, treatment, and care-delivery methods. The models include the Institute of Medicine Learning Health Systems, continuous quality improvement, comparative effectiveness trials, pragmatic clinical trials, and practice-based research, among others.[43,44] Accompanying the adoption of these models are debates about how specific the disclosed information should be, about when express prospective consent is necessary or when routine disclosure or notification might suffice, and about how closely consent for these activities should resemble a research model of informed consent.[45,46] Conventionally, information disclosure differs between clinical and research informed consent in detail, formality, and level of prior review; these differences are often justified by differentiating the primary goal of clinical care—helping the patient—from the primary goal of clinical research—generating useful knowledge.[47,48] With more recently embraced learning paradigms, these goals are converging, or at least the boundaries are shifting.[49] Some argue that in the context of learning activities, "research-like" written informed consent may be ethically unnecessary, overly burdensome, and likely to thwart improvement efforts.[50,51] Disagreement remains, however, about the right consent model for these clinical and research learning activities, and high-profile cases have spurred controversy.[52,53] One argument against research-like consent presumes that many learning activities—for example, evaluating the importance of repeat laboratory tests or how well health care providers use a checklist—add little or no risk for patients already receiving care, involve details of slight interest to patients, and have overall goals that patients support. Some would extend to learning activities a "simple" consent or notification paradigm that is used for certain clinical interventions, usually when the risks are low and patients are not likely to have strong preferences between treatment options or when there is only one logical choice.[54] The SUPPORT study, for example, brought to the forefront the unresolved question of the extent to which research in which participants receive standard medical care or the care that they would routinely receive outside the study poses "research risks" that require review by an institutional review board and comprehensive disclosure of these risks in a research informed-consent process.[55–57] Further research and dialogue will help guide decisions about how much disclosure is necessary in different learning contexts, the extent to which risk to participants matters in these decisions, how we should think about risk presented by research involving standard medical interventions, the role of patient preferences, and which, if any, activities can proceed without explicit prospective consent. Crucially, these efforts should include identifying what patients, research participants, providers, and others care about in various contexts.

Consent and Emerging Technologies

A second challenge to informed consent emerges from the complexity and uncertainty of the information generated by advanced technologies and expanded research opportunities. For instance, next-generation genomic sequencing technologies, such as whole-genome sequencing, which allow the quick and increasingly inexpensive detection of variation in the human genome, are rapidly being adopted into clinical research and routine clinical practice.[58] Although the routine implementation of genomic sequencing into standard clinical practice may be premature, turning back may be difficult.[59,60] Many recommend a robust informed-consent process for the use of genomic sequencing technologies.[61-63] Yet the complexity, volume, and density of generated health information, the anticipated discovery of variants of uncertain significance and secondary and incidental findings, and the implications for blood relatives present substantial challenges.[64,65] Comprehensively explaining in advance the elements necessary for obtaining informed consent, such as the expected risks, benefits, and likely outcomes of sequencing, can be difficult because of the sheer volume and inherent uncertainty of the information generated. Further, the level and type of details presented in an informed-consent process may appropriately differ between the clinical and research contexts, as well as according to population or setting. For example, the type of information and the way it is disclosed to informed healthy consumers who purchase direct-to-consumer genomic analysis may vary from that for ill patients seeking clinical diagnosis and treatment.[66]

In all settings, determining how to present complex scientific information is further complicated by the low prevailing rates of science and health literacy.[67] It has been suggested that in certain circumstances, it may be acceptable to ask people to consent to an oversight mechanism that serves to evaluate specifics (i.e., consent to be governed) rather than to consent to specific details;[42] there may also be a need for ongoing communication processes that allow the incorporation of changing information and changed expectations over time.[43] Engaging patients in the identification of suitable consent mechanisms or in the development of mechanisms of dynamic consent are additional strategies that have been suggested.[68,69] Similar consent strategies have been proposed for research involving biologic specimens and data. Inspired by the story of Henrietta Lacks (whose tumor gave rise to HeLa cells but whose permission to use her tumor cells for research was not sought),[70] scientists and policymakers are investigating and discussing models of consent to identify those that are both ethically and practically suitable for the future use of samples and data.[71,72]

Changing Demographics

A third contemporary challenge to informed consent emerges from expected sociodemographic trends. The U.S. population will become considerably older and more racially and ethnically diverse over the next few decades, with an expected doubling of the number of persons 65 years of age or older and an even more dramatic increase in the number of the "oldest old" (85 years of age or older).[73,74] Persons older than 65 years of age generally use more health care services, have a higher prevalence of chronic diseases, and more often have declining physical and cognitive function than do those who are younger.[75] The number of people with Alzheimer's dementia is also expected to more than double by 2050 and to increase more dramatically among the oldest old.[76] Preparing for these realities and their effect on health care is critical. For informed consent, they suggest the need for respectful, effective, and efficient methods of both ascertaining whether persons have the capacity to consent for themselves and facilitating decision-making processes for those who do not. Although many elderly persons, including some with dementia, retain the capacity to give informed consent for certain treatment decisions, others do not. Clinicians, who often lack training in assessing capacity, do not always recognize incapacity and may question a patient's capacity only when they face a risky decision or when the patient disagrees with their recommendations.[77] Cultural understandings of health and illness can also sometimes play a role when patients disagree with clinical recommendations. Assessing capacity and identifying appropriate and legally acceptable alternative decision makers or processes take time and resources and often receive short shrift in a busy clinical or research setting. Assessing the reasoning capacities of persons from cultural backgrounds that are not well understood by clinicians can also pose considerable challenges. Clinicians and investigators should be taught to assess capacity and should be provided with validated and useful tools[78] and the resources to help resolve difficult or borderline cases. Joint decision-making approaches that support the existing capacity of each patient but involve friends and family members have been recommended, because even "autonomous" decisions are often made together with trusted loved ones.[79,80] Patients may have the capacity for certain decisions but not for others, and capacity can wax and wane, so patients should remain involved in treatment decisions to the extent that it is possible. Creative and applicable methods of information disclosure are also necessary for persons whose capacity is diminished, as well as for the increasing numbers of patients who are not primarily English speakers.

Despite the enduring and emerging challenges of informed consent in health care and research, consent is recognized as morally transformative authorization, making certain activities permissible that otherwise would be wrong. Assiduous efforts to clarify and fine-tune concepts, expectations, practices, and the critical role of context are necessary to bridge the gap between the realities of informed consent and the ideal. Continued exploration through research, public dialogue, and creative approaches will help address the ethical permissibility and public acceptability of new models of consent, such as allowing consent for a broad set of activities, sometimes with an explicit system of governance over specifics; recognizing the validity of joint approaches to consent and decision making; refining processes to respect those who cannot consent for themselves; and finding creative, practical, and respectful ways of presenting information and supporting decision making tailored to each context. Respecting and promoting the informed choices of patients and research participants or persons acting on their behalf remain of paramount importance, despite the challenges of varied and changing contexts, altered capacity, limited health literacy, complex interventions, and shifting boundaries between health care and learning. Continued persistent and thoughtful efforts to bring the theoretical and practical realities of informed consent closer together are essential.

NOTES

1   Miller FG, Wertheimer A, eds. *The Ethics of Consent*. New York: Oxford University Press; 2010.

2   Albergotti R. Furor erupts over Facebook's experiment on users: almost 700,000 unwitting subjects had their feeds altered to gauge effect on emotion. *Wall Street Journal*.

June 30, 2014. http://online.wsj.com/articles/furor-erupts-over-facebook-experiment-on-users-1404085840.

3 Kramera AD, Guillory JE, Hancock JT. Experimental evidence of massive-scale emotional contagion through social networks. *Proc Natl Acad Sci USA.* 2014;111:8788–8790.

4 Berg J, Appelbaum P, Lidz C, Parker L. *Informed Consent: Legal Theory and Clinical Practice.* 2nd ed. New York: Oxford University Press; 2001.

5 Faden R, Beauchamp T. *A History and Theory of Informed Consent.* New York: Oxford University Press; 1986.

6 President's Commission for the Study of Ethical Problems in Medicine and Biomedical and Behavioral Research. *Making Health Care Decisions.* Washington, DC: Government Printing Office; October 1982. https://repository.library.georgetown.edu/bitstream/handle/10822/559354/making_health_care_decisions.pdf?sequence=1.

7 Turner L. From the local to the global: bioethics and the concept of culture. *J Med Philos.* 2005;30:305–320.

8 Gostin LO. Informed consent, cultural sensitivity, and respect for persons. *JAMA.* 1995;274:844–845.

9 World Medical Association. WMA Declaration of Lisbon on the rights of the patient. October 2005. http://www.wma.net/en/30publications/10policies/l4.

10 World Medical Association. WMA Declaration of Helsinki—ethical principles for medical research involving human subjects. October 2013. http://www.wma.net/en/30publications/10policies/b3.

11 American Medical Association. Code of Medical Ethics, opinion 8.08: informed consent. http://www.ama-assn.org/ama/pub/physician-resources/medical-ethics/code-medical-ethics/opinion808.page.

12 McManus PL, Wheatley KE. Consent and complications: risk disclosure varies widely between individual surgeons. *Ann R Coll Surg Engl.* 2003;85:79–82.

13 Bottrell MM, Alpert H, Fischbach RL, Emanuel LL. Hospital informed consent for procedure forms: facilitating quality patient-physician interaction. *Arch Surg.* 2000;135:26–33.

14 Wendler D, Grady C. What should research participants understand to understand they are participants in research? *Bioethics.* 2008;22:203–308.

15 Appelbaum PS. Assessment of patients' competence to consent to treatment. *N Engl J Med.* 2007;357:1834–1840.

16 Miller VA, Reynolds WW, Ittenbach RF, Luce MF, Beauchamp TL, Nelson RM. Challenges in measuring a new construct: perception of voluntariness for research and treatment decision making. *J Empir Res Hum Res Ethics.* 2009;4:21–31.

17 Schenker Y, Wang F, Selig SJ, Ng R, Fernandez A. The impact of language barriers on documentation of informed consent at a hospital with on-site interpreter services. *J Gen Intern Med.* 2007;22(Suppl 2):294–299.

18 Krogstad DJ, Diop S, Diallo A, et al. Informed consent in international research: the rationale for different approaches. *Am J Trop Med Hyg.* 2010;83:743–747.

19 Candilis P, Lidz C. Advances in informed consent research. In: Miller FG, Wertheimer A, eds. *The Ethics of Consent: Theory and Practice.* New York: Oxford University Press; 2010:329–346.

20 Joffe S, Truog R. Consent to medical care: the importance of fiduciary context. In: Miller FG, Wertheimer A, eds. *The Ethics of Consent: Theory and Practice.* New York: Oxford University Press; 2010:357–373.

21 Leclercq WK, Keulers BJ, Scheltinga MR, Spauwen PH, van der Wilt GJ. A review of surgical informed consent: past, present, and future: a quest to help patients make better decisions. *World J Surg.* 2010;34:1406–1415.

22 Hall DE, Prochazka AV, Fink AS. Informed consent for clinical treatment. CMAJ. 2012;184:533–540.

23 McKneally MF, Ignagni E, Martin DK, D'Cruz J. The leap to trust: perspective of cholecystectomy patients on informed decision making and consent. *J Am Coll Surg.* 2004;199:51–57.

24 Falagas ME, Korbila IP, Giannopoulou KP, Kondilis BK, Peppas G. Informed consent: how much and what do patients understand? *Am J Surg.* 2009;198:420–435.

25 McKneally MF, Martin DK. An entrustment model of consent for surgical treatment of life-threatening illness: perspective of patients requiring esophagectomy. *J Thorac Cardiovasc Surg.* 2000;120:264–269.

26 Ruhnke GW, Wilson SR, Akamatsu T, et al. Ethical decision making and patient autonomy: a comparison of physicians and patients in Japan and the United States. *Chest.* 2000;118:1172–1182.

27 U.S. Code of Federal Regulations, at Title 45 CFR.46.116 and 21CFR.50. http://www.hhs.gov/ohrp/humansubjects.

28 Paasche-Orlow MK, Taylor HA, Brancati FL. Readability standards for informed-consent forms as compared with actual readability. *N Engl J Med.* 2003;348:721–726.

29 Beardsley E, Jefford M, Mileshkin L. Longer consent forms for clinical trials compromise patient understanding: so why are they lengthening? *J Clin Oncol.* 2007;25(9):e13–e14.

30 Mandava A, Pace C, Campbell B, Emanuel E, Grady C. The quality of informed consent: mapping the landscape: a review of empirical data from developing and developed countries. *J Med Ethics.* 2012;38:356–365.

31 Appelbaum PS, Lidz CW. Twenty-five years of therapeutic misconception. *Hastings Cent Rep.* 2008;38:5–6.

32 DHHS Office for Human Research Protections. Letter to the University of Alabama regarding the Surfactant, Positive Pressure, and Oxygenation Randomized Trial (SUPPORT). March 2013. http://www.hhs.gov/ohrp/detrm_letrs/YR13/mar13a.pdf.

33 Drazen JM, Solomon CG, Greene MF. Informed consent and SUPPORT. *N Engl J Med.* 2013;368:1929–1931.

34 Kinnersley P, Phillips K, Savage K, et al. Interventions to promote informed consent for patients undergoing surgical and other invasive healthcare procedures. *Cochrane Database Syst Rev.* 2013;7:CD009445.

35 Schenker Y, Fernandez A, Sudore R, Schillinger D. Interventions to improve patient comprehension in informed consent for medical and surgical procedures: a systematic review. *Med Decis Making.* 2011;31:151–173.

36 Stacey D, Légaré F, Col NF, et al. Decision aids for people facing health treatment or screening decisions. *Cochrane Database Syst Rev.* 2014;1:CD001431.

37 Woolf SH, Chan EC, Harris R, et al. Promoting informed choice: transforming health care to dispense knowledge for decision making. *Ann Intern Med.* 2005;143:293–300.

38 Krumholz HM. Informed consent to promote patient-centered care. *JAMA*. 2010;303:1190–1191.

39 Flory J, Emanuel EJ. Interventions to improve research participants' understanding in informed consent for research: a systematic review. *JAMA*. 2004;292:1593–601.

40 Schenker Y, Meisel A. Informed consent in clinical care: practical considerations in the effort to achieve ethical goals. *JAMA*. 2011;305:1130–1131.

41 Henderson GE. Is informed consent broken? *Am J Med Sci*. 2011;342:267–272.

42 Koenig BA. Have we asked too much of consent? *Hastings Cent Rep*. 2014;44:33–34.

43 Institute of Medicine. Best care at lower cost: the path to continuously learning health care in America. 2012. http://www.iom.edu/reports/2012/best-care-at-lower-cost-the-path-to-continuously-learning-health-care-in-america.aspx.

44 Institute of Medicine. The learning healthcare system: workshop summary. 2007. http://www.iom.edu/reports/2007/the-learning-healthcare-system-workshop-summary.aspx.

45 Faden RR, Kass NE, Goodman SN, Pronovost P, Tunis S, Beauchamp TL. An ethics framework for a learning health care system: a departure from traditional research ethics and clinical ethics. *Hastings Cent Rep*. 2013;43:S16–S27.

46 Faden RR, Beauchamp TL, Kass NE. Informed consent for comparative effectiveness trials. *N Engl J Med*. 2014;370:1959–1960.

47 National Commission for the Protection of Human Subjects of Biomedical and Behavioral Research. The Belmont Report. 1979. http://www.hhs.gov/ohrp/humansubjects/guidance/belmont.html.

48 Miller FG, Rosenstein DL. The therapeutic orientation to clinical trials. *N Engl J Med*. 2003;348:1383–1386.

49 Kass NE, Faden RR, Goodman SN, Pronovost P, Tunis S, Beauchamp TL. The research-treatment distinction: a problematic approach for determining which activities should have ethical oversight. *Hastings Cent Rep*. 2013;43:S4–S15.

50 Platt R, Kass NE, McGraw D. Ethics, regulation, and comparative effectiveness research: time for a change. *JAMA*. 2014;311:1497–1498.

51 Kim SY, Miller FG. Informed consent for pragmatic trials—the integrated consent model. *N Engl J Med*. 2014;370:769–772.

52 Miller FG, Emanuel EJ. Quality-improvement research and informed consent. *N Engl J Med*. 2008;358:765–767.

53 Shepherd L. The SUPPORT study and the standard of care: the Hastings Center Bioethics Forum. May 17, 2013. http://www.thehastingscenter.org/Bioethicsforum/Post.aspx?id=6358&blogid=140.

54 Whitney SN, McGuire AL, McCullough LB. A typology of shared decision making, informed consent, and simple consent. *Ann Intern Med*. 2004;140:54–59.

55 Magnus D, Caplan AL. Risk, consent, and support. *N Engl J Med*. 2013;368:1864–1865.

56 Hudson KL, Guttmacher AE, Collins FS. In support of SUPPORT—a view from the NIH. *N Engl J Med*. 2013;368:2349–2351.

57 Department of Health and Human Services, Office of Human Research Protections. Draft guidance on disclosing reasonably foreseeable risks in research evaluating standards of care. October 20, 2014. http://www.hhs.gov/ohrp/newsroom/rfc/comstdofcare.html.

58 Wade CH, Tarini BA, Wilfond BS. Growing up in the genomic era: implications of whole-genome sequencing for children, families, and pediatric practice. *Annu Rev Genomics Hum Genet.* 2013;14:535–555.

59 Feero WG. Clinical application of whole-genome sequencing: proceed with care. *JAMA.* 2014;311:1017–1019.

60 Chrystoja CC, Diamandis EP. Whole genome sequencing as a diagnostic test: challenges and opportunities. *Clin Chem.* 2014;60:724–733.

61 Presidential Commission for the Study of Bioethical Issues. *Privacy and Progress in Whole Genome Sequencing.* Washington, DC: Department of Health and Human Services; 2012. http://www.bioethics.gov.

62 National Human Genome Research Institute. Informed consent for genomics research. http://www.genome.gov/27026588.

63 Appelbaum PS, Parens E, Waldman CR, et al. Models of consent to return of incidental findings in genomic research. *Hastings Cent Rep.* 2014;44:22–32.

64 Morgenstern J, Hegele RA, Nisker J. Simple genetics language as source of miscommunication between genetics researchers and potential research participants in informed consent documents. *Public Underst Sci.* 2014; April 21. (Epub ahead of print).

65 Clarke AJ. Managing the ethical challenges of next-generation sequencing in genomic medicine. *Br Med Bull.* 2014;111:17–30.

66 Sanderson SC, Linderman MD, Kasarskis A, et al. Informed decision-making among students analyzing their personal genomes on a whole genome sequencing course: a longitudinal cohort study. *Genome Med.* 2013;5:113.

67 Kutner M, Greenberg E, Jin Y, Paulsen C. *The Health Literacy of America's Adults: Results from the 2003 National Assessment of Adult Literacy* (NCES 2006-483). Washington, DC: Department of Education, National Center for Education Statistics; 2006. http://nces.ed.gov/pubs2006/2006483.pdf.

68 Weber GM, Mandl KD, Kohane IS. Finding the missing link for big biomedical data. *JAMA.* 2014;311:2479–2480.

69 Kaye J, Whitley EA, Lund D, Morrison M, Teare H, Melham K. Dynamic consent: a patient interface for twenty-first century research networks. *Eur J Hum Genet.* 2014:1–6.

70 Skloot R. *The Immortal Life of Henrietta Lacks.* London: Pan Macmillan; 2011.

71 Hudson KL, Collins FS. Biospecimen policy: family matters. *Nature.* 2013;500:141–142.

72 Simon CM, L'heureux J, Murray JC, et al. Active choice but not too active: public perspectives on biobank consent models. *Genet Med.* 2011;13:821–831.

73 Census Bureau. U.S. Census Bureau projections show a slower growing, older, more diverse nation a half century from now. December 2012. http://www.census.gov/newsroom/releases/archives/population/cb12-243.html.

74 U.S. Department of Health and Human Services Administration for Community Living. Administration on Aging (AoA) aging statistics. http://www.aoa.acl.gov/Aging_Statistics/index.aspx.

75 Cherry D, Lucas C, Decker SL. *Population Aging and the Use of Office-Based Physician Services.* NCHS data brief, no 41. Hyattsville, MD: National Center for Health Statistics; 2010. http://www.cdc.gov/nchs/data/databriefs/db41.htm.

76 Hebert LE, Weuve J, Scherr PA, Evans DA. Alzheimer disease in the United States (2010–2050) estimated using the 2010 census. *Neurology.* 2013;80:1778–1783.

77 Sessums LL, Zembrzuska H, Jackson JL. Does this patient have medical decision-making capacity? *JAMA*. 2011;306:420–427.

78 Dunn LB, Nowrangi MA, Palmer BW, Jeste DV, Saks ER. Assessing decisional capacity for clinical research or treatment: a review of instruments. *Am J Psychiatry*. 2006;163:1323–1334.

79 Nuffield Council on Bioethics. Dementia: ethical issues, October 2009. http://nuffieldbioethics.org/wp-content/uploads/2014/07/Dementia-report-Oct-09.pdf.

80 Kim SY, Kim HM, Ryan KA, et al. How important is "accuracy" of surrogate decision-making for research participation? *PLoS One*. 2013;8(1):e54790.

Teaching the Tyranny of the Form

Informed Consent in Person and on Paper

Katie Watson

My colleagues and I in Northwestern's Medical Humanities and Bioethics Program teach medical students a textbook vision of informed consent. We know physicians don't always do it that way in practice, but we figure teaching how it *ought* to be done gives our students a fighting chance to decrease inevitable gaps between the ideal and the real.

In 2012 my father was diagnosed with terminal esophageal cancer, my partner and I both had minor surgeries, and a routine colonoscopy tore my mother's spleen all in the course of six months. My "Year of Medical Management" made me realize my teaching about informed consent wasn't just intentionally ignoring a theory-practice gap—it was ignorant of how the modern medical workplace separates consent conversation from consent documentation, and how the "Tyranny of the Form" can undermine the decision-making process in surprising ways.

My father was a healthy 75-year-old who played his 36th season of softball in the summer of 2011, but in the fall he developed a persistent irritating cough, and in mid-January testing revealed an enormous tumor. He was quickly admitted to the hospital to figure out what to do with his tumor's unusual fistula—a dye test showed that everything he swallowed went in (and mostly out of) a small gap in his tumor, creating an infectious pocket that would be fatal if it burst—and the high-stakes question was what to do about it. Multiple teams cycled through his room reporting their test results and differing assessments of risks and benefits for the various approaches they advocated. Every option included life-threatening risks in uncertain quantities, and there was no clear answer. The morning before the endo-

Katie Watson, "Teaching the Tyranny of the Form: Informed Consent in Person and on Paper," from *Narrative Inquiry in Bioethics* 3, no. 1 (2013): 31–34. © 2013 by Johns Hopkins University Press. Reprinted by permission of Johns Hopkins University Press.

scopic procedure, my dad and his oncologist reviewed the possibilities and collaboratively decided to act conservatively, deferring the possibility of an esophageal stent or a drain through his back for later, and going with radiology's recommendation of an exploratory scope of his esophagus to determine the origin of his tumor and inserting a feeding tube in his stomach in preparation for a low-dose palliative round of radiation and chemotherapy. It was a textbook-perfect example of option review and collaborative decision making among physician, patient, and family—score one for informed consent!

That afternoon a surgery resident came in to "consent" my father for the next day's endoscopy, and as he scanned the form, he rattled off that they were going to place a stent. "No, they decided not to do that," my dad says. "That's okay," the resident says, "go ahead and sign it and they'll work it out tomorrow." My dad looks to me from his bed, and I back him up. "There was a lot of discussion back and forth and it sounds like maybe surgery didn't hear the final decision. Why don't you check with Dr. D [Dad's surgeon] to make sure everyone's on the same page and the form lists the right procedures?" The resident waves the consent form in the air. "This isn't a legal document." I don't correct him: I am off the lawyer-ethicist-professor clock, today I am a daughter in jeans curled in an uncomfortable chair who can still barely believe her hearty daddy has been bedded in a hospital gown. "It's not a contract," he says dismissively. "Just because you sign it doesn't mean we *have* to do what's on here—if it's wrong we won't do it. And," he says hopefully, "you might want a stent later." I smile. "Well then you'd want to talk to him about that then. Signing something we already know is wrong seems bad for safety, you know? With all these different teams . . . double-check with Dr. D, okay?" The resident leaves.

An hour later Dad's oncologist calls my cell phone sounding confused: "I hear your dad refused the endoscopy?" I explain. She chuckles. "I'll speak to the young resident." Two hours later I walk into Dad's room and the resident is back, this time with a radically different demeanor. He'd *never* want us to sign something that wasn't right, he was just trying to figure out what was accurate so he could make a *corrected* form, does *this* look okay to Dad and me? *Wonderful.*

In *The Healer's Power* (1992), physician-philosopher Howard Brody analyzed the power of the workplace, because he thinks discussing ethical problems in terms of the tension between care and work brings to light ethically relevant features that aren't raised by more traditional ethics language or concepts.

In this situation, the workplace division of labor had one person get the actual informed consent (Dad's oncologist) and another get documentation of that consent (the surgery resident). When these roles are separated, the person sent to document consent invariably lacks full knowledge of the actual consent conversation. But what accounts for the resident's resistance to changing the form when the patient informed him of its error?

From a workflow perspective the resident was under asymmetric pressure: if he'd gotten a signature he probably wouldn't catch trouble for adding an inaccurate consent form to the chart unless it resulted in a surgical error. And, of course, revising the form lengthens his to-do list. But if it doesn't matter what the form says, why are we signing it at all? During my father's hospitalizations I came to think of the hospital as a "health factory" with a gravitational pull toward efficiency that can disempower both physicians and patients. As Brody observes, "[t]here is a direct conflict between the routine and power of the workplace and the goal of patient autonomy" (p. 68).

Brody invites ethicists to use the language of power, but he doesn't analyze the power of language. Consider the expectation embedded in the directive "go consent her"—converting consent to a verb establishes "yes" as the goal and constructs patient refusal as a failure of the person sent to get "consent." The emphasis on outcome in "go consent her" also suggests the physician has a stake in the patient agreeing with the recommendation, one strand of which could be beneficence ("I think this is best for you and am invested in your wellbeing"), another could be personal power ("rejecting my recommendation is an affront to me and/or my expertise"), and Brody's focus on workplace power suggests a third strand—the patient who says no disrupts the momentum of a very expensive assembly line. (Twenty years later, Sharon Kaufman's ethnographic research, *And a Time to Die: How American Hospitals Shape the End of Life* [2005], confirmed Brody's insight about the pressure to keep things moving in the hospital.)

I used to chafe at this language (Aren't they sent to get the patient's decision? Would the response to refusal change if the shorthand were "go decision her" or "go risk-and-benefit her"?). This experience made me rethink my objection: when a higher-up has already had the conversation and the "yes" is a done-deal, "go consent her" is an accurate affirmation of the separation of conversation and documentation. In that situation, the person who leaves the room without a signature has failed a clerical task. Sadly for this resident, a glitch in the assembly line put a faulty form in his hand. From a safety perspective he should have been rewarded for catching an error, but his behavior on both occasions suggests he could have been responding to punishment (feared or actual) for disrupting workflow.

In other instances, the two acts of American medical decision making—discussing the procedure with someone who knows about it and documenting your decision—are combined. That was the case two months later when I needed surgery to remove uterine fibroids. Five days before surgery I had an appointment with my doctor's Fellow to review the procedure. The Fellow did an exemplary job of explaining risks, benefits, and alternatives in plain language and answering my questions. I caught the professorial part of my brain thinking, "Now *this* is informed consent" as the Fellow spoke—I was genuinely impressed with her.

Then she handed me the consent form, which said: "If any presently unknown conditions are revealed in the course of the procedures named above which call for different or further procedures, I hereby consent to and authorize the performance of such procedures as well." I reflexively cross this out as I read it, and the Fellow looks startled. I explain that I always cross out blanket consent sentences because I'm not agreeing to any and all procedures, only the one we discussed. She responds in what I register as a patronizing tone: "What if you were dying? Wouldn't you want us to save your life?" I wince at the hint of antagonism, sitting up straight. "Yes. I would. And you'd be authorized to do that by emergency exceptions to consent. But if you found a nonemergent condition you recommended other procedures for, I'd want you to discuss it with my surrogate." She says nothing. Fine. I read on, reaching the parts that say I consent to assistance or observation by medical students. During our conversation I told the Fellow that my doctor was fine with my request to exclude students, and the Fellow agreed that made perfect sense given my teaching role. Now I'm more anxious, but with suspended pen I say, "So I should cross out the consent to students, too . . ." and she flinches. "No, no. You can't cross anything else out." "Why not?" "I'd just hate for it to hold up your surgery. People see something scratched out, then people have to talk about it. . . ." "But couldn't you just tell them it's alright? I just want the form to match what we said." "We can't *guarantee* no students will come in." "Then we should talk about that more!" "It's not that, they won't. . . . I'd just hate for your surgery to get held up to the point you had to come back another day." It's silent for a moment as I process my options. Then she adds, "At some point you just have to trust us, right?"

She's right: I shouldn't agree to have my naked body jacked open while I'm unconscious unless I trust the people doing so to take care of me. And medically, I do. But I was asking them to care for me personally when I asked them to keep my students from seeing me like that, and "at some point you just have to trust us" felt like a threat, the elbow that says I'd be safer if I traded formal protection (the form) for personal protection (her word, which she has just indicated can't be "guaranteed"), which frightens me because now I realize I need her to *want* to protect me. "Trust us" frames my desire to alter the form as an offensive expression of mistrust, and suddenly the negotiation is personal: when I'm unconscious, is she more likely to bar students because the form says so, or because I deferred to her need to avoid responsibility for a form kerfuffle in the workplace? As Brody observes, "In the hospital, it may, ironically, be the interns who are guilty of using what little power they possess against the patients instead of for them. . . . [P]atients who do anything untoward or unexpected present a threat to the intern's all-too-limited power to control his environment" (p. 68). I'm the epitome of the empowered patient (a lawyer on the hospital ethics committee being treated at her own institution!), yet I felt bullied into signing a form that didn't reflect our verbal agreement in the hopes my deference to her paperwork inspires her to protect my dignity when I'm helpless. Brody is correct: "Patients quickly pick up the usually unspoken message that they will get the best 'care' precisely to the extent that they facilitate and do not impede the flow of the workplace" (p. 68).

My "Year of Medical Management" offered many events that deepened my understanding of the practice of informed decision making, but these two examples translate most clearly to the classroom. In this small anecdotal sample there was no theory-practice gap—I was delighted these informed decision-making conversations actually met the textbook ideal I teach. It was the documentation of that consent that turned junior physicians into flummoxed functionaries. Our teaching isn't incorrect; it's incomplete. The textbook we use only remarks that asking house officers to obtain consent signatures "might be problematic" if the patient has questions the inexperienced physician can't answer (Lo, 2009).

But now I believe there are other ways in which house officer administration of forms can undermine consent. Dad's surgical resident was right that the form is not a binding contract, and wrong that it's not a legal document—consent forms are specifically created as evidence that will be admitted in court if memories of that conversation diverge. I never want one of my students to pressure a patient to sign an inaccurate form, and I want them to understand that saying "it doesn't matter what the form says" is disingenuous—if Dad underwent an incorrect surgical procedure he signed off on, the burden of proof would be on him to establish the conversation was different. In my case, perhaps the Fellow's understanding that what the form says *does* matter is part of why she didn't want to promise on paper what she had promised verbally. I want my students to keep the spoken and printed word in synch, never expediently agreeing to something they can't really commit to. And on an institutional level, I need to contemplate whether I should be teaching about workplace pressure on young doctors as an issue of organizational ethics.

REFERENCES

Brody, H. 1992. *The Healer's Power*. New Haven, CT: Yale University Press.
Kaufman, S. 2005. *And a Time to Die: How American Hospitals Shape the End of Life*. New York: Scribner.
Lo, B. 2009. *Resolving Ethical Dilemmas: A Guide for Clinicians*. 4th ed. Baltimore: Lippincott Williams & Wilkins.

A Terrifying Truth

Rebecca Dresser

My father died of cancer when he was 39 and I was 12. No one told me or my two younger brothers that he was dying. He went to the hospital in October and died in December. We saw him just twice during that time, for this was an era in which visiting children were unwelcome in hospitals.

Although no one explained what was wrong with my father, we knew it was something bad. My mother was never home and we spent many hours in the care of aunts and other relatives. Every so often, one of us would work up the courage to ask when our Dad was coming home. The vague replies we received were meant to reassure us, but had no such effect.

I'll never forget this unsettling time. The old world I could count on had disappeared. The adults around me acted as though everything was fine, but why was my mother crying in the middle of the night, and why were we eating casseroles prepared by our neighbors for dinner? The evening we learned that my father had died was horrible, but it was a relief to know the truth. I remember thinking, *Oh, so that's why everyone's been acting so strangely.*

This is the way I learned that people should tell the truth about serious illness. This is the way I learned that "shielding" people from bad news does them no service. And this is the way I became interested in medical ethics.

Cancer was my introduction to truth-telling in medicine, burdensome treatments, and end-of-life care. My childhood nightmare began a life-long fascination with topics like these. Years later, just before I started law school, the Karen Quinlan case was in the headlines. I followed the case closely and enrolled in every course I could that addressed legal and ethical issues in

Rebecca Dresser, "A Terrifying Truth," from *Narrative Inquiry in Bioethics* 3, no. 1 (2013): 10–12. © 2013 by Johns Hopkins University Press. Reprinted by permission of Johns Hopkins University Press.

medicine. I knew there weren't many law jobs in this area, but vowed to look for any opportunities that might be out there.

Through a combination of persistence and good luck, I found a position in a medical school's ethics center. I began teaching and writing about things like advance directives, surrogate decision making, and clinical trials. Although I always remembered the time of my father's illness, cancer became primarily a professional rather than a personal matter.

Then, 42 years after my father's death, cancer became personal again. After months of disturbing symptoms and doctor visits, I received my own cancer diagnosis. Like anyone else, I was stunned to learn that I had cancer. Yet I didn't completely lose my professional outlook. When I heard my diagnosis, I thought, *this doctor is breaking bad news*. I had studied and taught medical students about this physician responsibility, and now I was seeing it in action.

The rest of cancer was like this, too. I struggled through harsh chemotherapy and radiation treatment the same way that other patients do. But when I was able to step back from the demands of treatment, I marveled at how much I was learning about my professional field. Cancer was giving me a new understanding of patient autonomy, treatment decision making, relationships between patients and clinicians, and many of the other subjects that were the focus of my academic work.

Although my second cancer experience produced many of the same feelings I had had during the first one—disorientation, fear, and isolation— it was also very different. I knew much more about the world of illness and medical care than I did at that earlier time. Yet having cancer myself made me realize how much was missing from my professional understanding of that world.

I vowed to make use of my new knowledge, but didn't think I could do it alone. So when I went back to work, I got in touch with some medical ethics colleagues who had been through their own cancer ordeals. We met to talk about our personal experiences and eventually produced a book called *Malignant: Medical Ethicists Confront Cancer*. But the book couldn't cover everything we learned, and one thing it omits is what cancer taught me about truth-telling and serious illness. As a 12-year-old, I learned how frightening it is when people don't tell you the truth; as a patient, I learned how frightening it is when they do.

Knowing about a life-threatening diagnosis may be better than not knowing, but it is terrible knowledge. With it come impossible treatment choices—for me, the choice between surgery (possibly more effective, but more likely to leave me unable to speak and swallow) and chemotherapy (possibly less effective, but more likely to preserve speech and swallowing). I had no idea how to reconcile my desires to live and to protect what seemed to me essential physical functions. I needed my doctors' guidance to respond to the truth of my situation.

And once I made the decision to have chemotherapy, I evaded the truth. The truth was that treatment might be ineffective, but I didn't want doctors, nurses, or anyone else reminding me of that. I don't think I could have endured the pain, nausea, vomiting, and other side effects without some protection from reality at that time. Even now, as I approach my annual follow-up examination, I don't want to face the truth that my cancer could return. Indeed, since my diagnosis, I have never asked doctors to give me a specific estimate of my survival odds.

Truth-telling in medicine is necessary, but coping with the truth is more difficult than I ever imagined. I can see why my mother didn't want to tell her young children that their father was dying. Her effort to protect us was unsuccessful, but I now understand the heavy burdens that truth imposes. Before having cancer, I didn't realize how much help patients and families need as they deal with the truth. My mother needed clinicians who could talk with her about breaking the bad news to her children. I needed clinicians who could help me choose a treatment and then let me put aside the truth so that I could concentrate on getting through the months of debilitating chemotherapy and radiation.

Truth-telling is the least-worst action when serious illness occurs. But truth-telling is destructive, too. It inflicts a new and terrifying reality on patients and the people who love them. Besides telling patients the truth, doctors and nurses must act to diminish truth's destructive effects. Sometimes this means talking with patients about how they will convey the truth to their families and friends. Sometimes this means recommending a treatment to a patient overwhelmed by the truth. Sometimes this means downplaying the truth that a burdensome treatment could fail. Personal experience taught me how complex and delicate truth-telling in medicine can be.

For me, cancer began as a personal crisis. Then cancer became a professional interest. And then, once again, cancer became personal. Now, with my colleagues, I am trying to bring the personal and professional together. I do this with some trepidation—I'm not sure how to bridge the gap between the two kinds of understanding. But I am sure of one thing. The voices of the cancer patient's young daughter, and the cancer patient she later became, belong in the medical ethics conversation.

REFERENCES

Dresser, R., ed. 2012. *Malignant: Medical Ethicists Confront Cancer*. New York: Oxford University Press.

The Lie

Lawrence D. Grouse

Annie is from New Hampshire and came here to the foothills of the Blue Ridge Mountains for the horse show. The nurses and I carry her from the car into the emergency room and gently place her on the gurney. She was kicked in the abdomen by her horse and lay in a field for over an hour until friends found her and brought her to the hospital. Even though I am working in the emergency room of a small hospital, I am confident. The nurses know their jobs. Faced with a serious surgical problem, we work well together.

Within a few minutes we have inserted two IVs, one in a forearm vein, another in the external jugular; her blood pressure, however, remains marginal. The fluid from the abdominal tap is grossly bloody, and so is her urine. Annie remains calm. Her serious eyes are piercing; I hold her hand to reassure her, but also take her pulse. She is bleeding very rapidly into her abdomen. Nothing I do seems to help, and I am scared. She is in shock, yet she converses politely and inquires about her condition.

"Thank you for helping me," she says. "Really, it wasn't the horse's fault!"

"We're not worried about the horse, Annie," I say. "The horse is fine."

"Is it a serious injury?" She pauses. "Will I live?"

"Everything will work out, Annie," I tell her. "It may be a little rough for a bit, but it will work out."

"Are you sure?" she asks, gazing steadily at me. "Please, tell me honestly."

I don't answer for a moment. I look at her. I am already fond of her and I do not want to lie. I squeeze her hand and smile. I am unsure how she will do, but I say, "Yes, I'm sure."

After a third IV is in place, her blood pressure stabilizes. The general surgeon and the urologist arrive and plan their emergency workup and exploratory surgery. I breathe a sigh of relief as they take charge of her care.

Lawrence D. Grouse, "The Lie," from *Archives of Internal Medicine* 157 (1997): 2153. © 1997 by American Medical Association. Reproduced by permission of American Medical Association. All rights reserved.

Suddenly, we find that the door to the surgical suite in the emergency room has been inadvertently locked and the head nurse's key won't open it. Annie and a nurse are locked inside. There is a great deal of key rattling and doorknob shaking. The pitch of people's voices starts to rise. I break into a sweat. The head nurse yells orders into the telephone and almost immediately three burly maintenance men with crowbars appear.

"Get rid of that door! Now!" the head nurse bellows.

The door is splintered in 20 seconds. Annie is laughing, tells us not to worry, tells us that she is fine. She thinks it is the funniest scene ever.

At surgery, we find that Annie has a severely lacerated liver and a ruptured kidney. The liver is repaired; the kidney is removed, but when I wake up the next morning and look in on Annie, disseminated intravascular coagulation has developed and she is receiving heparin. Four nurses and two physicians have already given blood for her. The intensive care unit hosts a steady stream of staff who have helped Annie and who come by with a few encouraging words. Her parents have arrived. Annie's father is a college professor: a tall, angular man, feeling frightened and out of place. Annie's mother is a small woman with delicate features. The surgeon's wife accompanies them. By the following day, when I leave the hospital after my weekend shift, several of the staff, including the head nurse, have each given two units of blood for Annie.

Two weeks later—during my next shift—I am waylaid and hugged by a happy and ambulatory Annie.

"Everyone here has been so good to me," Annie beams.

As we sit over a cup of coffee, her parents timidly inquire whether Annie might have been close to death on her arrival at the hospital. I can't help bragging about treating Annie in the emergency room. As I launch into the story, I find that Annie remembers it all, and she chimes in with an exact rendition of our entire conversation on the day of the accident. I am amazed! She was in shock, and still she remembers every word I said. I finish my story with a flourish. "When I found that you had abdominal bleeding and I still couldn't bring up your blood pressure with two IVs, I have to admit that I thought you were a goner."

Annie seems shocked to hear this. She looks at me angrily and says, "Don't you remember? You said you were sure I would live. I remembered that promise all the time! I put a great deal of weight on what you said, and you. . . ." Suddenly, for the first time since the accident, and to everyone's surprise, tears are in her eyes and she is weeping; she is inconsolable because I lied to her.

Discharge Decisions and the Dignity of Risk

Debjani Mukherjee

Mrs. Smith's eyes filled with tears as she said, "I feel like I've done something wrong. Are they punishing me because I've been refusing therapy and won't go to a nursing home?" She acknowledged that she hadn't always listened to her doctors but said that she knew better now and wanted to go home and see if she could make it work. Many staff members at our rehabilitation hospital had explained their safety concerns to her, and some had enlisted her adult daughter, with whom she lived, to convince her too. The rehabilitation team had called on the ethics consultation service, of which I am a part, to help figure out whether Mrs. Smith had the capacity to make an informed refusal of discharge recommendations.

Mrs. Smith, who was in her forties, had had several strokes and had acute renal failure, diabetes, and left-sided weakness and obesity. Her past refusal to take her antihypertensive medication was a contributing factor in her most recent stroke. She needed hemodialysis three times a week, could not safely transfer from her wheelchair without the help of two to three people, and lived in a walk-up apartment. Every single member of our multidisciplinary rehabilitation team agreed that the only safe discharge was to a skilled nursing facility. But Mrs. Smith disagreed.

As a licensed clinical psychologist whose practice is informed by clinical psychology, bioethics, and disability studies, I frequently find myself mediating between the health care team and the patient during clinical ethics consults. The term "dignity of risk" often rings in my ears as I try to tease apart the complexities of cases like Mrs. Smith's. Robert Perske coined the term when he observed people with mental retardation in Scandinavia and the innovative programs there that he contrasted with programs in the United

Debjani Mukherjee, "Discharge Decisions and the Dignity of Risk," from *Hastings Center Report* 45, no. 3 (2015): 7–8. Reprinted by permission of John Wiley and Sons.

States.[1] "Overprotection," he wrote, "endangers the retarded [*sic.*] person's human dignity and tends to keep him from experiencing the normal taking of risks in life which is necessary for normal human growth and development" (p. 24). "Dignity of risk" has been used by people working with individuals with developmental, physical, and psychiatric disabilities and is used especially among the disability rights community. The concept it represents involves respect for persons, self-determination, and attempts to minimize paternalism or parentalism. If you combine common dictionary definitions of "dignity" and "risk" (like the ones below from *Merriam-Webster*), they help you to understand the term as conveying that individuals are "worthy of honor and respect" even when they make decisions that may increase "the possibility that something bad or unpleasant . . . will happen."

This concept was very much on my mind during the ethics consult. I had never met Mrs. Smith before. What was risky in her context? For instance, did she consider not taking her antihypertensive medication a risky behavior? The concept of risk itself is one that requires contextualization, assessment, and judgment and can be objective or subjective. Health care providers are often acutely aware of medical risks and have only a small clinical window into the complexities of a patient's life. What objective risks would Mrs. Smith open herself up to if she went home? Her apartment was inaccessible, she needed assistance to go up stairs, and she had to leave and enter her home at least three times a week for dialysis. But "natural helping systems" such as family members or neighbors often enable people to live at home. And how do the risks of going home compare to the risks of institutionalization? Some institutions lack in services, amenities, or most importantly, freedom. What about the social risk of isolation or the emotional risk of depression due to a lack of agency? One patient told me that he would rather "go to a morgue" than to a nursing home. In another case, a surrogate exclaimed, "You have your ethics, and I have my ethics," and her ethics would not let her "send a dog" to the nursing home that she had visited for her daughter. The risks are the patient's and the family's to contextualize and assume.

The culture in rehabilitation is generally a "can do" one: patients are encouraged to push themselves to their limits, meet goals, and focus on what they can accomplish. But the point of discharge marks a culture shift of sorts. The lists of issues delineated by our multidisciplinary team—from physical, occupational, and speech-language therapies and psychology, nursing, and medicine—are often daunting, and recommendations are framed around "deficits." For example, we often recommend that patients have 24/7 supervision because they are at high risk for falls or for aspirating. How that risk is defined—percentage of likelihood, potential harms, risk to self or others—often varies. We discharge people with lists of medications, follow-up appointments, and instructions that should continue to maximize the gains they have made in rehabilitation. And a patient or his or her surrogate has a right to make an informed refusal of medical recommendations, including the level of supervision following discharge. Moreover, the empirical data that support some recommendations (such as medications) are much more robust than data that support others (such as 24/7 supervision). Some patients fail at home and end up reinjured or rehospitalized, whereas others do well with less supervision than recommended.

Mrs. Smith was refusing recommendations for discharge, which is not uncommon. Our hospital has a relatively new informed refusal policy that the ethics team developed with input from a multidisciplinary group of staff members. We ask if the refusal in question is a low-, moderate-, or high-risk one. Does the patient have capacity to make this particular decision? Is the patient under duress or being coerced? If the patient lacks capacity, does the surrogate have the legal right to refuse? If it is determined that the patient has capacity to make this decision and understands the risks and benefits, then the refusal is documented. In some cases, the legal department gets involved and drafts a document for the patient or surrogate to sign.

Rehabilitation teams are usually very good at taking a patient's context into account. They train willing family members to provide care if full-time paid home health care is unaffordable, and they work hard to figure out a safe support system that will allow someone to go home rather than to a facility. But some cases, like Mrs. Smith's, involve very serious safety concerns. In these situations, respecting the patient's dignity of risk gets trickier, and staff members, including ethics consultants, become more concerned.

Mrs. Smith was adamant in her refusal of discharge to a nursing home. She felt as though she was being unfairly tested. And sitting in her room listening to her story, I could see why. She said that she didn't know when she was admitted that she'd have to prove herself to be able to go home. She assured us that with her family, friends, and a part-time caregiver, she would be fine. She said that she knew she could die if she missed dialysis appointments or had a serious fall, but she had never missed a dialysis appointment before. She said that this time she would follow her doctors' recommendations about medications.

After the consult, we, the ethics consultation service, conferred with the patient's treating psychologist and speech pathologist. They agreed with our assessment that Mrs. Smith's cognitive impairments from her stroke were not interfering with her problem-solving ability, although she was "inflexible" in her decision.

Her attending physician was concerned that she would be unable to make it to dialysis three times a week, and he asked for the legal department to draft a document specifying the risks of refusal. Ethics recommended that the team have a backup plan in place and, with Mrs. Smith's permission, have a skilled nursing facility ready to accept her if she needed admission. The discharge plan also included more intense follow-up.

In some settings, Mrs. Smith's stroke diagnosis would have been assumed to mean that she lacked capacity, and her daughter, who expressed serious doubts about her mother's plan to return home, would have made the discharge decision. In other settings, Mrs. Smith's refusal itself would have been proof of her incapacity. We honored Mrs. Smith's decision and recognized the dignity of risk, although all of the members of the health care team felt uncomfortable and worried about her choice.

When she was back in her home environment, Mrs. Smith ended up sharing our concerns. Within twenty-four hours, she decided that it wasn't safe and chose to go to the skilled nursing facility. We didn't initially think of our recommendation as a time-limited trial of discharge to home, but, as we had the backup plan in place, it essentially was.

Was this a situation where we failed to convince a patient of safety concerns or one in which we successfully respected her autonomy and allowed her the dignity to fail? Honoring informed refusal of discharge recommendations is not easy, especially when health care providers and family are in agreement. The Hospital Readmissions Reduction Program, which was established by the Affordable Care Act, focuses on readmission rates during the first thirty days after discharge, and hospitals may, in effect, be penalized if they respect patients' dignity of risk and the patients are subsequently readmitted. Another critical ethical issue is the lack of discharge options. I had no response to the relative who said, "I wouldn't send a dog to that facility," although it was one of the few facilities that the patient in that case was eligible for on public aid. Funding for paid caregivers in the home would alleviate some of these difficult discharge decisions, although in Mrs. Smith's case, she also needed an accessible apartment. Given our current health care and social service systems, we are left balancing patient preferences, safety, quality of life, and sometimes, lousy options for discharge. And we have to respect our patients and their choices, even if they change their minds later. Patients have made a series of choices before they enter a rehabilitation (or any) hospital, and at the point of discharge, health care providers, armed with a lot of medical facts, can easily focus on what we know best, rather than on what the patient knows and wants. The dignity of risk is a concept that we must keep in the forefront of our practice; the risks, after all, are our patients' to take.

NOTE

1 R. Perske, "The Dignity of Risk and the Mentally Retarded," *Mental Retardation* 10, no. 1 (1972): 24–27.

No One Needs to Know

Neil S. Calman

My indoctrination into the underworld of medical secrecy began 25 years ago during my first clinical rotation in my third year of medical school. The lessons learned were not a formal part of my medical school curriculum but are as indelibly etched into my brain as are the names of the body parts I studied in anatomy.

The voyage began with the care of a patient I will call Charles McNight. Just over 60 years old, he had come to the medical center to receive the care of our most highly skilled cardiovascular surgeons. They replaced two of his heart valves, put a graft on his aorta, and performed bypass surgery—all in one procedure. I do not recall the details of his cardiac pathology, but he sailed through the surgery, and his rapid recovery far exceeded our expectations.

I had gotten to know "Charlie" because I had been assigned to do his admitting history and physical, a typical job in those days for medical students. His thick, pure white, Santa-like beard and the warm smile beneath it instantly charmed all who met him. His wife and daughter were equally engaging. I became rapidly and intensely involved in his care, providing a human touch—a role that medical students often play on the hospital team in lieu of making medical decisions for which they are not yet prepared.

Crossing Boundaries

My care for Charlie was both fueled and complicated by my infatuation with his daughter, who was my age and unmarried. Her life as a single parent of a four-year-old daughter gave me ample substrate on which to build a

Neil S. Calman, "No One Needs to Know," from *Health Affairs* 20, no. 2 (2001): 243–249. © 2001 by Project HOPE / *Health Affairs*. Reprinted by permission of Project HOPE / *Health Affairs*. The published article is archived and available online at www.healthaffairs.org.

wonderful fantasy. It was simple, it seemed, to help bring Charlie home, get him well, fall in love with his daughter, and be a stepfather to her little girl. These fantasies kept me returning to his hospital room.

A few weeks after surgery, Charlie was ready to be discharged. He went home with instructions to return weekly to the hospital lab for blood tests needed to adjust his level of coumadin, a medicine he was taking to prevent blood clots. A few days after discharge I received a call from his wife inviting me to their home for dinner—a small way for them to thank me for the extra care I had given Charlie in the hospital. I accepted, yet acknowledged to myself my level of discomfort in doing so. I had clearly crossed the line I had been taught to maintain between doctor and patient; I had allowed myself to become personally involved in Charlie's life. Dinner took place almost a week after Charlie's discharge, and I offered to bring the necessary equipment to take his required blood tests and to transport the blood back to the hospital lab. Charlie was grateful; he lived quite a distance from the hospital and was not looking forward to making the trip.

Dinner was great. Afterward, Charlie and I went into another room where I drew his blood. I then excused myself for the evening. The results of the tests were fine, and Charlie was doing well until a few weeks later, when he began to experience some sweats and weakness and the sensation that something was going wrong. Hours later he developed a low-grade fever that, within twelve hours, raged to 104 degrees. He called me at home that night. I was very worried for him and told him to go immediately to the hospital. His wife helped him put on a robe, and Charlie left home for what would be the last time.

I lived only a few blocks from the hospital and arrived almost an hour before Charlie and his wife. I was exhausted by my anxiety. My rotation in cardiovascular surgery had since ended, so I was there as a friend—a role I was not supposed to be playing as a medical student. Yet I was clearly part of the institution that was now responsible for Charlie's life.

Charlie's wife pulled their car into the emergency entrance. I helped him into the hospital. Sweat was beading on his brow; he was so weak he could hardly stand. I took one of his hands in mine. It was cold and wet from perspiration. My other hand gently touched his back to support him; even through his robe and two shirts I could feel the thermal struggle his body was waging against some unknown infectious invader. Within moments it became clear to the cardiac surgery fellow on call that Charlie had an infection, and all too clear about its probable cause. "I am admitting you to the hospital in intensive care," he told Charlie, whose face looked close to death. "You have an infection, maybe on your aortic graft."

Slippery Slope

A shudder went through me. I had seen two similar cases while on the cardiovascular surgery service. In both cases patients had been discharged from the hospital, had returned with fever, and died. I had also heard that there might have been a problem with a batch of cardiovascular catheters that were in use in the hospital. Weeks after use, some had been suspected to have been contaminated, presumably by the manufacturer, with a fungus called candida. The patients who had been catheterized with these units were subject to postoperative infection with the fungus and seemed to be resistant to treatment.

By morning the surgical team that originally treated Charlie was by his bedside. Only one hope remained: They loaded him with antifungal drugs and took him to surgery to replace the infected graft. I changed my clothes and went into the operating room to watch. The thought of being able to answer his family's questions about the long and complex surgery was so powerful that it obscured the pain that developed in my feet as I stood, out of the way, on a tiny patch of floor in the OR.

The surgery went well and confirmed the infection. Charlie was back in the cardiosurgical intensive care unit, and I was by his bedside with his wife and daughter. The surgeon appeared shortly thereafter and briefly reassured the family that his team had replaced the infected graft and that Charlie had done very well in surgery. The surgeon walked away. I stood with Charlie's wife and daughter and explained what I could about what I had seen in the OR, leaving out any mention that the infection he had suffered might have been caused by the contaminated catheters. Minutes later, a bell sounded, indicating the end of visiting hours. I left with them, as if the bell was meant for me, too, and sat in the waiting area discussing with them my optimism about Charlie's future.

As Pavlovian as the family's response to the visiting hours bell, my response to the hospital's emergency paging system was equally well programmed. I had learned since starting my clinical rotations that the moment a voice began to ring out on the pager, all other incoming auditory signals were instinctively shut out. The "code" was called for the cardiac surgical intensive care unit. I froze in fear, listening to the announcement. I told Charlie's family I needed to respond to this, a total fabrication, and left. The crowd around Charlie's bed confirmed my fears.

I was immobilized by not knowing what to do, by my emotions, and by the people running in every direction with medications and equipment. A few minutes later the surgeon who had just completed Charlie's graft repair came to the bedside. There was no hope. All resuscitation attempts failed to restart his heart. As the code was called to a halt, a nurse hurriedly handed a STAT lab result to the surgeon. The patient's serum potassium had soared to a level that would have made anyone's heart stop. I looked over the surgeon's shoulder as he held the slip of paper with the lab result, staring in disbelief. Charlie had died of a simple mistake. His potassium had been allowed to go too high after surgery. This well-known deadly event was caused by the release of large amounts of potassium into the blood from cells damaged at surgery. The event is so common in cardiac surgical procedures that close monitoring of the potassium was a routine part of postoperative care. How could such a small oversight undo the months of heroic medical care that Charlie had been given by the most skilled surgeons in the region?

Entering the Dungeon of Deception

The surgeon looked at me and to my great surprise put his arm around my shoulder. I was unaware that he had given a moment's thought to my role in Charlie's care. "Son," he began, "I've been very moved by the interest and concern you have shown for this patient. I also know that you realize that nothing good would come out of the family's knowing about the catheter problems or what happened just now. No one needs to know." He tapped my shoulder twice and walked away.

In those few seconds it happened. I had been invited to join the underworld of medical secrecy—that territory where doctors tread and where no others may look in; where secrets about mistakes and problems are brought and where they reside forever hidden.

I stood motionless. A stream of contradictory thoughts flooded my brain. Was I Charlie's friend, and should friendship prevail? Should I tell his family everything I knew? Or was I a doctor, albeit in training, committed to keeping the secrets that lie beyond the patients' and families' grasp? Was I partially responsible for the future survival of the wife, daughter, and granddaughter Charlie had left behind? Had I done everything I could? I had little time to think, and I never really made a decision what to do. The surgeon left my side and went to the waiting room to tell the news to Charlie's wife and daughter. I knew I had to follow but didn't know if I should be standing next to the family or next to the doctor.

The surgeon offered his condolences to the family. He remained only briefly and then asked if I could stay with them for a while. He was deputizing me—an act that subconsciously sucked me deeper into the underworld. I was now responsible for maintaining the charade that "we had done everything we could." It was up to me to understand the importance of the statement, "No one needs to know."

I saw Charlie's family only once after that, at his funeral. His daughter introduced me to everyone there as one of Charlie's doctors who had taken such good care of him. I played the role well. Dressed in my only suit, I told them how much he had endured, how sick he had been, and how he kept all of our spirits high to the end.

I got in my car and drove home across the city in a pouring rain. That was the last time I saw Charlie's family. I could not remain in contact with them while being filled with the secrets I had been implored not to reveal: the contaminated catheters that might have caused his infection, and the elevated potassium level that caused his heart to stop beating. I would be living a lie each moment I spent with his family. Even the closeness I had felt to them, my thoughts of his daughter, and my continuing sense of responsibility for them were not strong enough to overcome my discomfort. I knew I could not violate the laws of the secret society of medicine into which I had just begun my initiation. Being invited into the sanctity of this dungeon of deception was part of the honor of becoming a doctor. It made me feel special—an entrusted colleague, a real doctor. But many questions flooded my mind.

Had anyone else died before Charlie as the result of fatally high potassium after surgery? Had anyone explored the need to change the systems by which such monitoring took place? Did the company that made the catheters know that some had been contaminated? Would lawsuits have forced them out of business, making these devices unavailable to others who would benefit? Would the hospital be forced to pay millions to those who died as a result, eroding the services it was providing to other patients? Would doctors be afraid to assume the challenges of critically ill patients like Charlie? Did Charlie's family deserve to be compensated for the errors that caused their loss? Would the benefits to that one family outweigh the damage that could be done to the physicians and the hospital?

I had no answers and thus did nothing. Today I am puzzled by how quickly I adapted to this new role of "keeper of secrets" and remain concerned that others entering medicine are still taught in the same way.

Unstated Obstacles to Openness

What keeps any doctor I have ever known from initiating discussion of medical mistakes with patients is a set of redoubtable barriers. First, there is tacit agreement among physicians that mistakes are an inevitable part of practicing medicine. I have made my own errors over the years, some with minor adverse outcomes, others with horrible results. When I discover another physician's mistake, I only discuss it if the doctor is employed by me or is formally under my supervision. We physicians are afraid to turn up the heat on others, lest we fry in our own fire.

Then we have the specter of medical liability lawsuits. Who would reveal errors to a patient and initiate the years-long process of defending a medical liability lawsuit? The financial burden of such an action and the public humiliation involved are insurmountable for most physicians and deter a more honest reckoning of medical errors among physicians and between physicians and patients.

Finally, like most doctors, I went into medicine to be a helper and healer. Scrutiny by colleagues and the process of discussing my mistakes openly with others compel me to relive, over and over, the pain of having played a role in injuring someone who entrusted me with his or her life. A prolonged probing of my errors would force a level of self-doubt that would affect future decisions and could prove immobilizing. With no grounds for comparing my abilities and practice skills with those of my colleagues, I would be left asking, "Do I make more mistakes than my colleagues? Would another doctor have done a better job taking care of this patient?"

The formal internal quality assurance discussions that have been implemented in some institutions take place in a protected environment and thus promote a more open review of the cause of medical errors. Such sheltered examination often results in fixing systemic problems and thereby protecting patients from a simple oversight like the one that killed Charlie McNight. But building a legal firewall between quality review processes and public scrutiny fails to create a mechanism for the legitimate compensation of patients who have been injured through medical mistakes. Studies have shown that only a small percentage of such injuries are compensated through legal actions, while most go unaddressed.

The process by which law and medicine have evolved to deal with medical mistakes must be drastically changed, both to compensate those injured and to encourage the disclosure of errors. At the same time, each of us, as physicians and teachers, must fight the continuing urge to hide our mistakes. We must teach the next generation of students to talk about medical errors as a part of medical practice that will always be with us. Most of all, we must teach each other that the biggest gaffe of all is to cover up our mistakes, thus perpetuating barriers to safe care.

Everyone needs to know.

DEATH, DYING, AND LIVES
AT THE MARGINS

....

IV

....

Forty Years of Work on End-of-Life Care

From Patients' Rights to Systemic Reform

Susan M. Wolf, Nancy Berlinger, and Bruce Jennings

More than 2.5 million people die in the United States each year, most of them from progressive health conditions. Facing death is a profound challenge for patients, their relatives and friends, their caregivers, and health care institutions. Nearly 40 years of intensive work to improve care at the end of life has shown that aligning care with patients' needs and preferences in order to ease the dying process is surprisingly difficult—although there has been some incremental progress. Early optimism that the establishment of patients' legal and ethical rights to make decisions about their own care would lead to more appropriate end-of-life treatment faded in the face of sobering data showing that declaring these rights was not enough to alter treatment patterns and that systemic issues loomed large. This history has demonstrated the need to attack the problem at all levels, from individual rights, to family and caregiving relationships, to institutional and health systems reform.

Securing Rights (1976–1994)

In 1976, New Jersey's highest court decided the groundbreaking case of Karen Ann Quinlan, whose father sought permission to discontinue mechanical ventilation when she was in a persistent vegetative state. The court found

Susan M. Wolf, Nancy Berlinger, and Bruce Jennings, "Forty Years of Work on End-of-Life Care—From Patients' Rights to Systemic Reform," from *New England Journal of Medicine* 372 (2015): 678–682. © 2015 by Massachusetts Medical Society. Reprinted by permission of Massachusetts Medical Society.

that although "the doctors say that removing Karen from the respirator will conflict with their professional judgment," Karen had a "right of choice" that could be exercised by her father as surrogate decision maker. Many cases followed in which courts recognized the constitutional and common-law rights of patients to refuse life-sustaining treatment and the authority of surrogate decision makers for patients who lacked decision-making capacity.[1,2] Courts also began to address decisions to forgo life-sustaining treatment in newborns.

In those early days of efforts to curb overtreatment at the end of life and to improve the dying process, establishing the ethical and legal right to refuse life-sustaining treatment was a priority. More challenging was establishing surrogates' authority to refuse care on behalf of incompetent patients, articulating standards for surrogate decision making, and reaching general agreement on limits to surrogate authority. Cases involving patients who were never competent to make decisions about care and involving the cessation of artificial nutrition and hydration were notoriously difficult, as was decision making for incompetent patients without surrogates.

As more cases reached the courts and public attention intensified, experts began analyzing the issues and generating recommendations. In 1983, the President's Commission on Bioethics issued a report advocating the right of patients to decide about their health care, while addressing moral and legal limits.[3] In 1987, the Hastings Center published comprehensive ethics guidelines regarding end-of-life care.[4] These guidelines focused on recognizing a patient's right to refuse unwanted life-sustaining treatment and on articulating a three-tier standard for surrogate decision making that prioritized following the patient's wishes when known but otherwise relied on the surrogate to decide on the basis of the patient's values or, absent information on those values, in accordance with the patient's best interests. The guidelines also recommended processes for designating surrogates for patients with no family or friends to serve in that role and proposed using time-limited trials of treatment to inform decisions. The document addressed the need to improve pain relief, recommended rejecting requests for treatment that could not accomplish its physiological objective, differentiated treatment refusal from physician-assisted suicide and euthanasia, and considered obstacles to individual rights.

In the 1990 case of Nancy Cruzan—a Missouri woman in a persistent vegetative state, whose parents wanted artificial nutrition and hydration stopped—the U.S. Supreme Court finally recognized a patient's right to refuse life-sustaining treatment, although the Court noted that states could restrict the authority of surrogates to make decisions for patients lacking decisional capacity. In her concurrence, Justice Sandra Day O'Connor cited the Hastings Center guidelines and suggested that a surrogate's authority would be better protected if the surrogate were appointed by the patient in an advance directive. The *Cruzan* opinion and the passage of the federal Patient Self-Determination Act in 1990 spurred efforts to promote advance directives.[5]

Facing Clinical Realities (1995–2009)

The establishment of patients' rights and the option to use advance directives proved necessary but far from sufficient to align treatment with patients' preferences. In 1995, investigators in the Study to Understand Prognoses and Preferences for Outcomes and Risks of Treatments (SUPPORT)—a multimillion-dollar effort by the Robert Wood Johnson Foundation to improve end-of-life care—began publishing findings showing that documented treatment preferences, even when championed by a nurse advocate, failed to change clinical practice.[6] As one commentator wrote, "Improving the quality of care generally requires changes in the organization and culture of the hospital and the active support of hospital leaders."[7]

Further studies attempted to identify potential routes to progress, including improved access to palliative care. Although Congress had added a hospice benefit to the Medicare program in 1982—to provide palliative and comfort care for patients nearing the end of their lives—barriers to hospice access remained, including the requirement that death be expected within 6 months and that curative treatment efforts be abandoned. Throughout the 1990s, professional societies including the American College of Physicians,[8] American Medical Association,[9] and American Nurses Association[10] issued papers and policies aimed at identifying obstacles to good care at the end of life and improving clinical practice. Nonprofit organizations mounted efforts such as the Project on Death in America, which funded research on impediments to compassionate end-of-life care.[11] In 1997, the Institute of Medicine (IOM) published *Approaching Death: Improving Care at the End of Life*, which analyzed research, educational, clinical, and policy challenges and emphasized the need for tools to measure quality and outcomes of end-of-life care.[12]

In the face of difficulty in improving end-of-life care and ensuring access to good pain relief and other palliative measures, the movement to legalize physician aid to terminally ill patients who wished to end their lives gathered steam. In a 1994 ballot measure, reconfirmed in 1997, Oregon became the first state to vote for legalization of physician-assisted suicide and enacted the Death with Dignity Act. The statute survived federal litigation over the authority of the U.S. attorney general to limit the practice (*Gonzales v. Oregon*, 2006). In 1997, the Supreme Court rejected arguments that state bans on physician-assisted suicide violated patients' constitutional rights, and the Court recognized states' authority to prohibit or legalize the practice within their borders (*Vacco v. Quill*, 1997; *Washington v. Glucksberg*, 1997). Washington State followed Oregon and has now been joined by Vermont; the Montana Supreme Court and a lower court in New Mexico have also issued rulings allowing the practice.

As work progressed to change the clinical realities of end-of-life care, focus turned to the barriers facing subpopulations, such as terminally ill children. In the 2002 publication *When Children Die*, the IOM described problems in pediatric care, including that of parents being forced to choose between life-prolonging treatment and hospice care for their children.[13] The IOM then detailed research gaps in *Describing Death in America*, which urged the use of Medicare records as an important data set.[14]

Meanwhile, there was growing controversy over decisions to end life-sustaining treatment in cases of long-term disability. People with disabilities raised concerns that such decisions were sometimes based on inappropriate assumptions about quality of life. Neurologic disabilities raised additional concerns, as research distinguished the minimally conscious state, in which patients retain some potential for cognitive recovery, from the permanent vegetative state (*Wendland v. Wendland*, 2001).[15] In 2005, the case of Terri Schiavo—a Florida woman whose parents rejected the medical conclusion that she was in a vegetative state with no potential for recovery and objected to her husband's decision as surrogate to terminate tube feeding—triggered national controversy, revealing that decades of progress on surrogate decision making could not avert conflict over the termination of artificial nutrition and hydration in an incompetent patient who was in a permanent vegetative state when family members disagreed with one another.

The politics of end-of-life care became even more divisive in 2009, when opponents of the Affordable Care Act (ACA) spread the false assertion that a proposed ACA provision meant to authorize the reimbursement of physicians for voluntary counseling about end-of-life planning would create "death panels." The provision was removed under political pressure, and a similar Medicare-reform proposal was subsequently withdrawn. Thus, a period that began with a sobering realization that the validation of rights was not enough to change clinical realities was marked by important research and innovation—yet growing controversy.

Reforming End-of-Life Care Systems (2010–)

In 2010, Congress passed the ACA, the largest attempt at reform of health care finance and systems in decades. With advances in systemic reform, efforts to improve end-of-life care have become increasingly focused on health care institutions, systems, and finance. In 2014, the IOM released a new report, *Dying in America*.[16] The report and related commentary analyzed research showing that current financial incentives do not support ready access to the care patients want and need near the end of life.[17] The integration of palliative care with treatment remains incomplete, despite ample evidence of benefit.[18] Although hospice use has increased, Medicare data reveal patterns of treatment escalation before hospice enrollment.[19] Medicare data also reveal regional variation in transfers from nursing homes to hospitals, which are associated with medically inappropriate feeding-tube insertion.[20] The aging of the baby boomers will mean a sharp increase in the number of U.S. patients with Alzheimer's disease, which will place new pressures on families and care systems.[21] As ACA implementation drives system changes, renewed efforts to improve end-of-life care at the system level are emerging, including funding for concurrent hospice and curative care efforts for seriously ill children and renewed efforts to fund conversations between physicians and patients for end-of-life care planning.

As policy initiatives have become more system-focused and encompassing, so too have ethics initiatives. In 2013, the Hastings Center produced a revised, expanded edition of the 1987 guidelines, addressing not only individual rights and the clinical realities of decision making but also institutional and systemic issues such as transfers between institutions, end-of-life care in the context of large and complex health care organizations, the role of cost in decisions, and health care access for uninsured people.[22] The revised guidelines reflect the reality that patients are rarely isolated rights-bearers; family members are usually involved in end-of-life decisions and care. Both patients and family members further depend on clinicians to anchor a process of setting goals and developing treatment plans. Although respect for autonomy remains essential to end-of-life decision making, appropriately including the patient's chosen constellation of relatives and friends and helping all of them navigate care systems have emerged as integral to ethical practice. Persons living with disabilities have also provided crucial perspectives on the management of chronic conditions and treatment decision making over time.

The new guidelines and the recent IOM report similarly frame the care of dying people as "patient-centered, family-oriented,"[16] and dependent on sound systems of care and finance. The IOM report calls for a "major reorientation and restructuring of Medicare, Medicaid and other health care delivery programs" to ensure quality care that meets the needs of dying patients and their families.[16] Both documents recommend core elements of high-quality care near the end of life, including palliative care, and emphasize the need for better clinician education.

Lessons from 40 Years of Work

Establishing individuals' rights to forgo life-sustaining treatments and the authority of surrogate decision makers were signal achievements in the first phase of work on improving end-of-life care. Uncovering clinical barriers to progress in the second phase was essential. But we now know that all these efforts must be nested in systemic reform. Important strategies have emerged for continued progress on all levels.

First, clinicians can be trained to inform and support decision makers. The prospect of death inspires powerful emotions in everyone involved, creating a potential for conflict. Communication training for all professionals who care for patients facing critical treatment decisions can help support informed decision making under stressful conditions. Essential skills have been identified and tools developed for use by care teams.[23-26] Role models and access to new tools (including electronic decision-making aids and "choice architecture" techniques to structure options) can help professionals explain the options and support decision makers.[27,28] Advance care planning and the POLST (Physician Orders for Life-Sustaining Treatment) Paradigm—developed in Oregon in an effort to ensure that patients' preferences were honored in a range of care settings, including care by emergency medical services personnel—provide structured processes to help professionals and decision makers establish goals, document preferences, and create care plans.[16] Training priorities include discussing care preferences with patients with early-stage Alzheimer's disease who retain decision-making capacity and engaging in shared decision making with cognitively impaired patients and their surrogates. Pediatric specialists' experience with shared decision making in caring for the 50,000 children who die in the United States each year may offer broader lessons on effective communication with patients and families.[29]

Second, systemic improvements can be designed to assist all professions involved in caring for patients who are facing decisions about life-sustaining treatment or nearing the end of life, in all relevant clinical and residential settings. Clinicians should have access to at least generalist palliative care training[30] and be trained to collaborate across shifts, during transfers, and with family caregivers during discharge planning. Evidence-based models for safe care transitions can support better systems for end-of-life care.[31,32]

Third, productive systemic and financing reforms can be enacted. Misaligned financial incentives work against dying patients' choices, interests, and safety. Problems include referrals of dying patients to the intensive care unit or for dialysis even when such services will result in limited benefit and high burden to the patient,[19,33] the nonbeneficial use of feeding tubes in patients with end-stage Alzheimer's disease,[20] cost-shifting transfers of dying nursing home residents and hospice patients to hospitals,[34,35] and late hospice referrals for patients with cancer.[36] Abundant evidence indicates that reimbursements and organizational patterns drive these problems, and fixing them requires attention to service-utilization mandates and pressures.[37] The 2014 IOM report recommends creating financial incentives for advance care planning and shared decision making, electronic health records to support ongoing planning, and care coordination to reduce hospitalizations and emergency department visits.

End-of-life care in accountable care organizations and Medicare Advantage plans should also be rigorously evaluated. Explicit discussion of cost is essential, both in choosing care options and in addressing cost barriers to desired care. When patients lack the means to pay for needed life-sustaining treatment, professionals can advocate for them. In oncology, for example, professionals are publicly challenging ever-escalating drug prices.[38]

Facing death will never be easy, and controversial cases are inevitable. Yet too large a gulf remains between the theory and the practice of end-of-life care. More work is needed at all levels—to protect patients' rights to choose care options, to improve the quality of clinical care and clinicians' responsiveness to patients and families, and to create well-functioning health care finance and delivery systems that make high-quality care genuinely available. Federal, state, and organizational authorities can formulate explicit standards that support this progress. Health care leaders, administrators, and clinicians can also identify and confront persisting care problems within organizations and implement systems of accountability at the bedside, in the clinic, and in health care delivery and finance systems. We can apply lessons from four decades of work in order to advance toward solutions. The millions of Americans facing life-threatening conditions deserve no less.

NOTES

1 Hafemeister TL, Keilitz I, Banks SM. The judicial role in life-sustaining medical treatment decisions. *Issues Law Med.* 1991;7:53–72.

2 Meisel A, Cerminara KL, Pope TM. *The Right to Die: The Law of End-of-Life Decisionmaking.* 3rd ed. New York: Aspen Publishers; 2004, and annual cumulative supplements.

3 President's Commission for the Study of Ethical Problems in Medicine and Biomedical and Behavioral Research. *Deciding to Forego Life-Sustaining Treatment: Ethical, Medical, and Legal Issues in Treatment Decisions.* Washington, DC: Government Printing Office; 1983.

4 The Hastings Center. *Guidelines on the Termination of Life-Sustaining Treatment and the Care of the Dying.* Bloomington: Indiana University Press; 1987.

5 Wolf SM, Boyle P, Callahan D, et al. Sources of concern about the Patient Self-Determination Act. *N Engl J Med.* 1991;325:1666–1671.

6 The Writing Group for the SUPPORT Investigators. A controlled trial to improve care for seriously ill hospitalized patients: the Study to Understand Prognoses and Preferences for Outcomes and Risks of Treatments (SUPPORT). *JAMA* 1995;274:1591–1598. [Erratum, *JAMA.* 1996;275:1232.]

7 Lo B. Improving care near the end of life: why is it so hard? *JAMA.* 1995;274:1634–1636.

8 American College of Physicians. Papers by the End-of-Life Consensus Panel. https://www.acponline.org/clinical-information/clinical-resources-products/end-of-life-care/papers-by-the-end-of-life-care-consensus-panel.

9 American Medical Association. AMA policy on end-of-life care. http://www.ama-assn.org/ama/pub/physician-resources/medical-ethics/about-ethics-group/ethics-resource-center/end-of-life-care/ama-policy-end-of-life-care.page.

10 American Nurses Association. Position statement: registered nurses' roles and responsibilities in providing expert care and counseling at the end of life. http://www.nursingworld.org/MainMenuCategories/EthicsStandards/Ethics-Position-Statements/etpain14426.pdf.

11 Aulino F, Foley K. The Project on Death in America. *J R Soc Med.* 2001;94:492–495.

12 Institute of Medicine, Committee on Care Near the End of Life, Field MJ, Cassel CK, eds. *Approaching Death: Improving Care at the End of Life.* Washington, DC: National Academies Press; 1997.

13 Institute of Medicine, Committee on Palliative and End-of-Life Care for Children and Their Families, Field MJ, Behrman RE, eds. *When Children Die: Improving Pallia-*

tive and End-of-Life Care for Children and Their Families. Washington, DC: National Academies Press; 2002.

14 Lunney JR, Foley KM, Smith TJ, Gelband H, Institute of Medicine. *Describing Death in America: What We Need to Know.* Washington, DC: National Academies Press; 2003.

15 Fins JJ. Rethinking disorders of consciousness: new research and its implications. *Hastings Cent Rep.* 2005;35(2):22–24.

16 Committee on Approaching Death: Addressing Key End-of-Life Issues. *Dying in America: Improving Quality and Honoring Individual Preferences near the End of Life.* Washington, DC: National Academies Press; 2014.

17 Care at the end of life. *New York Times.* October 4, 2014:A18.

18 Greer JA, Jackson VA, Meier DE, Temel JS. Early integration of palliative care services with standard oncology care for patients with advanced cancer. *CA Cancer J Clin.* 2013;63:349–363.

19 Teno JM, Gozalo PL, Bynum JP, et al. Change in end-of-life care for Medicare beneficiaries: site of death, place of care, and health care transitions in 2000, 2005, and 2009. *JAMA.* 2013;309:470–477.

20 Teno JM, Mitchell SL, Kuo SK, et al. Decision-making and outcomes of feeding tube insertion: a five-state study. *J Am Geriatr Soc.* 2011;59:881–886.

21 Hurd MD, Martorell P, Delavande A, Mullen KJ, Langa KM. Monetary costs of dementia in the United States. *N Engl J Med.* 2013;368:1326–1334.

22 Berlinger N, Jennings B, Wolf SM. *The Hastings Center Guidelines for Decisions on Life-Sustaining Treatment and Care near the End of Life.* 2nd ed. New York: Oxford University Press; 2013.

23 Schell JO, Arnold RM. NephroTalk: communication tools to enhance patient-centered care. *Semin Dial.* 2012;25:611–616.

24 Oncotalk: improving oncologists' communication skills. Seattle: University of Washington. 2013. http://depts.washington.edu/oncotalk.

25 The IPAL project: improving palliative care in the ICU. New York: Center to Advance Palliative Care. 2013. http://www.capc.org/ipal/ipal-icu.

26 Back AL, Arnold RM. "Isn't there anything more you can do?": When empathic statements work, and when they don't. *J Palliat Med.* 2013;16:1429–1432.

27 Barfield RC, Brandon D, Thompson J, Harris N, Schmidt M, Docherty S. Mind the child: using interactive technology to improve child involvement in decision making about life-limiting illness. *Am J Bioeth.* 2010;10:28–30.

28 Blinderman CD, Krakauer EL, Solomon MZ. Time to revise the approach to determining cardiopulmonary resuscitation status. *JAMA.* 2012;307:917–918.

29 Berlinger N, Barfield R, Fleischman AR. Facing persistent challenges in pediatric decision-making: new Hastings Center guidelines. *Pediatrics.* 2013;132:789–791.

30 Quill TE, Abernethy AP. Generalist plus specialist palliative care—creating a more sustainable model. *N Engl J Med.* 2013;368:1173–1175.

31 Williams MV, Li J, Hansen LO, et al. Project BOOST implementation: lessons learned. *South Med J.* 2014;107:455–465.

32 Naylor MD, Aiken LH, Kurtzman ET, Olds DM, Hirschman KB. The care span: the importance of transitional care in achieving health reform. *Health Aff* (Millwood). 2011;30:746–754.

33 Schmidt RJ, Moss AH. Dying on dialysis: the case for a dignified withdrawal. *Clin J Am Soc Nephrol.* 2013;8:1–7.

34 Teno JM, Mitchell SL, Skinner J, et al. Churning: the association between health care transitions and feeding tube insertion for nursing home residents with advanced cognitive impairment. *J Palliat Med.* 2009;12:359–362.

35 Pathak EB, Wieten S, Djulbegovic B. From hospice to hospital: short-term follow-up study of hospice patient outcomes in a US acute care hospital surveillance system. *BMJ Open.* 2014;4(7):e005196.

36 Goodman DC, Morden NE, Chang C, et al. Trends in cancer care near the end of life: a Dartmouth Atlas of Health Care brief. Hanover, NH: Dartmouth Institute for Health Policy and Clinical Practice; 2013. http://www.dartmouthatlas.org/downloads/reports/Cancer_brief_090413.pdf.

37 Feng Z, Wright B, Mor V. Sharp rise in Medicare enrollees being held in hospitals for observation raise concerns about causes and consequences. *Health Aff* (Millwood). 2012;31:1251–1259.

38 Experts in Chronic Myeloid Leukemia. The price of drugs for chronic myeloid leukemia (CML) is a reflection of the unsustainable prices of cancer drugs: from the perspective of a large group of CML experts. *Blood.* 2013;121:4439–4442.

Try to Remember Some Details

Yehuda Amichai

Try to remember some details. Remember the clothing
of the one you love
so that on the day of loss you'll be able to say: last seen
wearing such-and-such, brown jacket, white hat.
Try to remember some details. For they have no face
and their soul is hidden and their crying
is the same as their laughter,
and their silence and their shouting rise to one height
and their body temperature is between 98 and 104 degrees
and they have no life outside this narrow space
and they have no graven image, no likeness, no memory
and they have paper cups on the day of their rejoicing
and paper cups that are used once only.

Try to remember some details. For the world
is filled with people who were torn from their sleep
with no one to mend the tear,
and unlike wild beasts they live
each in his lonely hiding place and they die
together on battlefields
and in hospitals.
And the earth will swallow all of them,
good and evil together, like the followers of Korah,
all of them in their rebellion against death,

their mouths open till the last moment,
praising and cursing in a single
howl. Try, try
to remember some details.

Failing to Thrive?

Kim Sue

"Failure to Thrive"

I recently took care of an 80-year-old patient named Emma (a pseudonym), who was found down, unresponsive, in a large pool of bloody vomit in her apartment. She was described in her chart as an "80F admitted with fall, unresponsive, recent 30 lb weight loss." She lived alone and was considered lucky to be found relatively quickly by a friend who sometimes came to check on her. Originally from southern Europe, she had been living in Massachusetts for the past twenty years, and her closest family was in California. Emma was admitted to the intensive care unit and, with the ministrations of modern medical technology, including mechanical ventilators and medications to help keep blood pressures high, she lived. This was the second time in six months that she had been admitted to the intensive care unit after being found unresponsive in her home. In the intensive care unit, they found she had a very low blood count and discovered she had a gastrointestinal bleed. She had an extensive work-up, including an endoscopy and colonoscopy, and they still could not find the source. After she was transferred to the general medical floor, I came by on my rounds to check on her every morning. She was incredibly frail, sitting with her tiny legs propped up on a footstool. Every day she would deny having any blood in her bowel movements. "No blood, no pain, doctor. Can I go home today?" Or maybe it was, "Doctor, can I go home today?" "Not just yet," I'd reply, "one more thing to do."

What was the plan for this woman, whose diagnosis had evolved from a gastrointestinal bleed to "failure to thrive"? As I grappled with what was at stake for her, and had to deny her request to go home every single day, I

Kim Sue, "Failing to Thrive?," from *Medicine Anthropology Theory* 3, no. 3 (2016): 96–104. © 2016 by Kim Sue. Reprinted by permission under the Creative Commons Attribution 4.0 International Public License, available at https://creativecommons.org/licenses/by/4.0/legalcode.

thought about how increasingly common it is for medical practitioners to use this term "failure to thrive," shortened in our notes to simply "FTT."

"FTT" is a medico-legal term initially used in a pediatric population (discussed further below), but today's International Classification of Disease (ICD-10, published by the World Health Organization) includes diagnosis codes for hospital and clinical billing for both children (R62.51) and adults (R62.7). These are both grouped within the large diagnostic code 640: "Miscellaneous disorders of nutrition, metabolism, fluids and electrolytes." With regard to children, the clinical information notes that there is "substandard growth or diminished capacity to maintain normal function," at times "due to nutritional and/or emotional deprivation and resulting in loss of weight and delayed physical, emotional, and social development" (WHO 2016, n.p.). FTT can be of organic, inorganic, or mixed etiologies, in which the first is understood to be a problem within the patient, the second as a problem in the patient's environment, and the third a combination of two.

For adults, the ICD-10 definition is a "progressive functional deterioration of a physical and cognitive nature. The individual's ability to live with multisystem diseases, cope with ensuing problems, and manage his/her care are remarkably diminished" (WHO 2016, n.p.). In clinical practice, it can be used as a stand-in for unexpected weight loss. It can also be used as a proxy when clinicians and teams taking care of patients are faced with frequent admissions for patients with falls, failing to meet nutritional basic caloric needs to sustain stable weight, or otherwise existing in a tenuous or unstable living environment. It appears that within the common usage of the term FTT, medicine is actually grappling with the strong force of the social itself.

"Lassitude, Loss of Energy and Joie de Vivre"

Historically, the term "failure to thrive" emerged in the late nineteenth century. There was an ongoing contest of ideas about what precisely constituted failure: was it related to nutrition, particular vitamin deficiencies, maternal neglect, congenital abnormalities, or physiological development of essential organs? The various stances largely reflected the cultural and political ideas and biases of the groups forwarding them. The late Victorian era was dominated by both increased attention to child welfare as well as the emergence of the idea of public health as a discipline and a means of collective intervention.

In the United States, the term "failure to thrive" became popular in pediatric clinical medicine in the late 1960s, with robust use in the literature throughout the 1970s and 1980s. In the early use of the term, child psychiatrists associated the diagnosis with neglect between the mother and child (see Bullard et al. 1967) or to refer to an aberrant bond between the mother and the child (see, for example, Elmer 1960). Even then, it was a frustrating term to some; Henry Marcovitch (1994, 35) notes it was primarily a "descriptive term, not a diagnosis," marked by "evidence of lassitude, loss of energy and joie de vivre." Those working in inpatient hospital settings noted that "failure to thrive" could be diagnosed by weight below the third percentile "with subsequent weight [gain] in the presence of appropriate nurturing"; they felt that was "characteristic of the child with failure to thrive to have improvement of these symptoms with hospitalization" (Barbero and Shaheen 1967, 640), suggesting problems within the child's home environment.

Initially, there was a strong distinction between "organic" versus "nonorganic" failure to thrive (read: biological versus social). Altemeier and colleagues (1985, 361) described "nonorganic failure to thrive" as a "form of maternal neglect, because rapid improvement in both growth and development follows adequate nutrition and emotional support in the hospital." Yet increasingly pediatricians recognized the complex interplay between a child's position within growth curves and underlying medical conditions, parental behavior, poverty, and the overall home environment (Markowitz et al. 2008, 481).

Interestingly, the diagnosis of FTT has begun to fall out of favor. For pediatricians in particular, FTT is no longer en vogue. Parents dislike the term FTT for its vague all-encompassing nature and the implications of moral wrongdoing. There is stigma about being a parent of a child with FTT, and for that reason it is becoming increasingly abandoned as a diagnostic term in pediatrics.

But the inverse is true regarding FTT and adults. Over the past twenty years, FTT has become used in relation to the cadre of elderly people living alone who often go unseen or unheard until they arrive in the hospital in distress. As Robertson and Montagnini (2004, 343) write, "Failure to thrive describes a state of decline that is multifactorial and may be caused by chronic concurrent diseases and functional impairments . . . including weight loss, decreased appetite, poor nutrition and inactivity." In the hospital where I work, we see patients who are elderly, who are homeless, who are dying of AIDS or cancer, who are chronically malnourished; they all variously can be diagnosed with FTT.

Arriving at the hospital in the way that Emma did adds a certain immediacy and intensification toward the social worlds of such patients by both clinicians and the family members of patients. Physicians and care teams in hospitals are routinely tasked with addressing the fates of these patients, and the way they do so shapes the course of these individuals' lives. Emma is not unique. The *New York Times* profiled a person named George Bell, whose often lonely life and lonely death was chronicled in great detail, as an exemplar of an increasingly solitary, aging population (Kleinfeld 2015). Sociologist Eric Klinenberg (2001) writes about this phenomenon in his article "Dying Alone: The Social Production of Urban Isolation," which analyzes the 1995 Chicago heat wave that killed over seven hundred mostly elderly, isolated Chicago residents, and which was followed by his book, *Going Solo: The Extraordinary Rise and Surprising Appeal of Living Alone* (2012). The appeal of being alone and living alone is woven into the American ethos of self-determination, autonomy, and independence, including the freedom to live and die in circumstances of our own choosing.

Hospitals are places where people who lack a social safety net, like Emma and George Bell, are brought. In fact, we routinely admit and discharge patients like them every day. What is my ethical obligation as a physician to these patients—to do no harm, to promote safety, to ensure the best chances of health and well-being—versus my moral obligation to honor and respect another person's autonomy? Is it my obligation or right to deny Emma the opportunity to die in the time and place of her own choosing, as a direct result of what some might deem to be failures of self-care but in the conditions of her own determining? Sharon Kaufman (2005, 1) argues from her ethnographic work on dying in hospitals that as human beings and as physicians we have a "deep, internal ambivalence about death"; she argues that the process of hospitalization extends and indelibly alters the process of the "gray zone at the threshold between life and death."

I am faced with this dilemma with Emma. Her hospitalization poses significant existential questions about the quality and quantity of her life and the inevitability of her death. I am faced with the immediacy and stakes of another's life; I am implicated in either action or inaction. What am I compelled to do with the private, intimate knowledge of another's pathology laid bare in the hospital records? As physicians every day we confront these realities of messy lives and deaths so often hidden away: "We stand in the thick of human experience, in the space of human problems, in the real-life local places where people live in the face of dangers, grave and minor, real and imagined" (Kleinman 1998, 376).

As anthropologists, we maintain faith in the belief that we can access someone else's lifeworld, that at the very least, we can recognize the shifting beliefs and narratives that ground experience. But my professional obligation as a physician, by an uncodified, implicit, bioethical stance, is to assure as much safety as possible, to create the conditions for physical flourishing even at the expense of happiness and autonomy. Yet very rarely do our thought processes take into account "what is at stake" (Kleinman and Benson 2006, e294) for people within these encounters.

In many ways, these encounters of physicians with patients labeled as "failure to thrive" represent the problem of witnessing and confronting a suffering other. In my case, I feel conflicted by shifting roles and obligations as a human being, as part of a community plagued by social inequalities in which some people lack or shirk adequate social and financial supports, and as a physician with a specific professional obligation to individual patients. What am I to do if I cannot prescribe you the community supports you need? Can I write you a prescription for love, for a friend? Can I write your children a work note every day for a month so that they can spend more time with you, check on you every day, and help you bathe and shower and toilet and take your medications? Can I get you a 24-hour home health aide if you and your family don't have the resources to do so?

This genealogy of failure to thrive is perhaps ironically considered within the realm of my medical internship and residency training, where I work approximately eighty hours a week in the hospital as part of ongoing medical training. What does it mean to be well within this context? What does it mean, generally speaking, to cultivate the conditions of wellness, prosperity, happiness, or self-care of the caregivers? U.S. doctors know our colleagues in Europe work about half the number of hours (approximately 37 to 48 hours per week) and emerge with similar competencies as part of more effective health care and public health systems with overall better health outcomes (Temple 2014).

In the United States, "intern year," the first year of medical residency training, is often discussed as one of the hardest years of a physician's life. Sometimes it is chalked up to "hazing." Intern year is largely defined by the impossibility of addressing higher-order complex social and cognitive processes in the absence of meeting biological and physiological needs such as adequate sleep and food. As young physicians training in the United States, we are asked to think critically and analytically about the everyday dilemmas faced by our patients and respond to them empathetically, but this analysis is not applied to ourselves as caregivers.

On the face of it, the task of caring for FTT patients that falls onto medical trainees seems impossible. And physicians don't like dealing with the spaces in-between. "Failure to thrive" is precisely that messy in-between that both patients and their caregivers want to avoid. Yet it is a diagnostic category that reflects ongoing temporality and a dynamic, uncertain process. It is increasingly becoming a part of aging in America, reflecting social isolation and the thin threads of community and unpaid hours spent by family members grappling with the very same dilemmas. As Michael Jackson (2011, xiii) reflects on his work with the Kuranko people in Sierra Leone:

> Just as human existence is never simply an unfolding from within but rather an outcome of a situation, of a relationship with others, so human understanding is never born of contemplating the world from afar; it is an emergent and perpetually renegotiated outcome of social interaction, dialogue and engagement. And though something of one's own experience—of hope or despair, affinity or estrangement, well-being or illness—is always one's point of departure, this experience continually undergoes a sea change in the course of one's encounters and conversations with others. Life transpires in the subjective in-between, in a space that remains indeterminate despite our attempts to fix our position within it.

While anthropologists have tried to understand upstream sources of suffering—what is here called "failure to thrive" in Emma's case—Kleinman and Wilkinson (2016) argue that the social sciences, anthropology included, have largely failed to enact the reparative visions of society laid out by eighteenth- and nineteenth-century thinkers like Adam Smith, John Stuart Mill, John Locke, and Voltaire. So both anthropology and medicine have, in their own ways, done inadequate jobs of addressing the root causes of inequality and their consequent social suffering. The denotation of "failure to thrive" should beget the question of why only some fail to thrive. In many ways, failure to thrive is the result of the unequal distribution of political and socioeconomic power and capital.

When I think about the cases of patients like Emma, I am positioned between often-conflicting worldviews and stances toward individual and social suffering. Yet in my role as a doctor, I am compelled to take action every day. These are decisions that can and do have a long-lasting impact on others' lives, an impact that I may never entirely know the consequences of. I often wonder how we can maintain our humanity in the face of all of this, including the pressures from hospital systems to move patients quickly out of the hospital, toward an ultimate "disposition." How can we attend to these patients with care, acknowledging the specificities of their individual situations and the very real constraints in their social milieus that cannot be solved with a three-day hospital admission?

As essayist Leslie Jamison (2014, 23) writes in her book *The Empathy Exams*, we should not necessarily lose hope in our abilities to care for others: "Empathy isn't just something that happens to us—a meteor shower of synapses firing across the brain—it's also a choice we make: to pay attention, to extend ourselves . . . the labor, the motions, the dance—of getting inside another person's state of heart or mind." This we can do confidently. We can attend patiently the particulars of individual situations. We can listen. But we must remember to do this while also addressing the overall structures of power and vulnerability, whereby those at the social margins are most affected. And we cannot forget that how these structures are assembled and interact influences our ability to attend to one another as we envision alternate ways of living, caring, and dying.

REFERENCES

Altemeier, William, Susan O'Connor, Kathryn Sherrod, and Peter Vietze. 1985. "Prospective Study of Antecedents of Nonorganic Failure to Thrive." *Journal of Pediatrics* 106: 360–365.

Barbero, Giulio, and Eleanor Shaheen. 1967. "Environmental Failure to Thrive: A Clinical View." *Journal of Pediatrics* 71: 639–644.

Bullard, Dexter, Helen Glaser, Margaret Heagarty, and Elizabeth Pivchik. 1967. "Failure to Thrive in the 'Neglected' Child." *American Journal of Orthopsychiatry* 37: 680–690.

Elmer, Elizabeth. 1960. "Failure to Thrive: Role of the Mother." *Pediatrics* 25: 717–725.

Frank, D., and S. Zeisel. 1988. "Failure to Thrive." *Pediatric Clinics of North America* 35: 1187–1206.

Jackson, Michael. 2011. *Life within Limits*. Durham, NC: Duke University Press.

Jamison, Leslie. 2014. *The Empathy Exams*. Minneapolis, MN: Graywolf Press.

Kaufman, Sharon. 2005. *And a Time to Die*. Chicago: University of Chicago Press.

Kleinfeld, N.R. 2015. "The Lonely Death of George Bell." *New York Times*, 18 October, A1.

Kleinman, Arthur. 1998. "Experience and Its Moral Modes: Culture, Human Conditions, and Disorder. The Tanner Lecture on Human Values." Presentation at Stanford University, Palo Alto, CA, 13–16 April.

Kleinman, Arthur, and Peter Benson. "Anthropology in the Clinic: The Problem of Cultural Competency and How to Fix It." *PLoS Medicine* 3, no. 10: e294. https://doi.org/10.1371/journal.pmed.0030294.

Kleinman, Arthur, and Iain Wilkinson. 2016. *A Passion for Society: How We Think about Human Suffering.* Berkeley: University of California Press.

Klinenberg, Eric. 2001. "Dying Alone: The Social Production of Urban Isolation." *Ethnography* 2: 501–531.

Klinenberg, Eric. 2012. *Going Solo: The Extraordinary Rise and Surprising Appeal of Living Alone.* New York: Penguin.

Marcovitch, Harvey. 1994. "Failure to Thrive." *British Medical Journal* 308: 35–38.

Markowitz, Robert, John Watkins, and Christopher Duggan. 2008. "Failure to Thrive: Malnutrition in the Pediatric Outpatient Setting." *Nutrition in Pediatrics.* 4th ed., 479–89. Hamilton, Ontario: BC Decker Inc.

Robertson, Russell, and Marcos Montagnini. 2004. "Geriatric Failure to Thrive." *American Family Physician* 70: 343–350.

Temple, John. 2014. "Resident Duty Hours around the Globe: Where Are We Now?" *BMC Medical Education* 14: S1–S8.

World Health Organization. 2016. "International Statistical Classification of Diseases and Related Health Problems," 10th Revision. http://apps.who.int/classifications/icd10/browse/2014/en.

The Dead Donor Rule and Organ Transplantation

Robert D. Truog and Franklin G. Miller

Since its inception, organ transplantation has been guided by the overarching ethical requirement known as the dead donor rule, which simply states that patients must be declared dead before the removal of any vital organs for transplantation. Before the development of modern critical care, the diagnosis of death was relatively straightforward: patients were dead when they were cold, blue, and stiff. Unfortunately, organs from these traditional cadavers cannot be used for transplantation. Forty years ago, an ad hoc committee at Harvard Medical School, chaired by Henry Beecher, suggested revising the definition of death in a way that would make some patients with devastating neurologic injury suitable for organ transplantation under the dead donor rule.[1]

The concept of brain death has served us well and has been the ethical and legal justification for thousands of lifesaving donations and transplantations. Even so, there have been persistent questions about whether patients with massive brain injury, apnea, and loss of brain-stem reflexes are really dead. After all, when the injury is entirely intracranial, these patients look very much alive: they are warm and pink; they digest and metabolize food, excrete waste, undergo sexual maturation, and can even reproduce. To a casual observer, they look just like patients who are receiving long-term artificial ventilation and are asleep.

The arguments about why these patients should be considered dead have never been fully convincing. The definition of brain death requires the complete absence of all functions of the entire brain, yet many of these patients retain essential neurologic function, such as the regulated

Robert D. Truog and Franklin G. Miller, "The Dead Donor Rule and Organ Transplantation," from *New England Journal of Medicine* 359 (2008): 674–675. © 2008 by Massachusetts Medical Society. Reprinted by permission of Massachusetts Medical Society.

secretion of hypothalamic hormones.[2] Some have argued that these patients are dead because they are permanently unconscious (which is true), but if this is the justification, then patients in a permanent vegetative state, who breathe spontaneously, should also be diagnosed as dead, a characterization that most regard as implausible. Others have claimed that "brain-dead" patients are dead because their brain damage has led to the "permanent cessation of functioning of the organism as a whole."[3] Yet evidence shows that if these patients are supported beyond the acute phase of their illness (which is rarely done), they can survive for many years.[4] The uncomfortable conclusion to be drawn from this literature is that although it may be perfectly ethical to remove vital organs for transplantation from patients who satisfy the diagnostic criteria of brain death, the reason it is ethical cannot be that we are convinced they are really dead.

Over the past few years, our reliance on the dead donor rule has again been challenged, this time by the emergence of donation after cardiac death as a pathway for organ donation. Under protocols for this type of donation, patients who are not brain-dead but who are undergoing an orchestrated withdrawal of life support are monitored for the onset of cardiac arrest. In typical protocols, patients are pronounced dead 2 to 5 minutes after the onset of asystole (on the basis of cardiac criteria), and their organs are expeditiously removed for transplantation. Although everyone agrees that many patients could be resuscitated after an interval of 2 to 5 minutes, advocates of this approach to donation say that these patients can be regarded as dead because a decision has been made not to attempt resuscitation.

This understanding of death is problematic at several levels. The cardiac definition of death requires the irreversible cessation of cardiac function. Whereas the common understanding of "irreversible" is "impossible to reverse," in this context irreversibility is interpreted as the result of a choice not to reverse. This interpretation creates the paradox that the hearts of patients who have been declared dead on the basis of the irreversible loss of cardiac function have in fact been transplanted and have successfully functioned in the chest of another. Again, although it may be ethical to remove vital organs from these patients, we believe that the reason it is ethical cannot convincingly be that the donors are dead.

At the dawn of organ transplantation, the dead donor rule was accepted as an ethical premise that did not require reflection or justification, presumably because it appeared to be necessary as a safeguard against the unethical removal of vital organs from vulnerable patients. In retrospect, however, it appears that reliance on the dead donor rule has greater potential to undermine trust in the transplantation enterprise than to preserve it. At worst, this ongoing reliance suggests that the medical profession has been gerrymandering the definition of death to carefully conform with conditions that are most favorable for transplantation. At best, the rule has provided misleading ethical cover that cannot withstand careful scrutiny. A better approach to procuring vital organs while protecting vulnerable patients against abuse would be to emphasize the importance of obtaining valid informed consent for organ donation from patients or surrogates before the withdrawal of life-sustaining treatment in situations of devastating and irreversible neurologic injury.[5]

What has been the cost of our continued dependence on the dead donor rule? In addition to fostering conceptual confusion about the ethical requirements of organ donation, it has compromised the goals of transplantation for donors and recipients alike. By requiring organ donors to meet flawed definitions of death before organ procurement, we deny patients and their families the opportunity to donate organs if the patients have devastating, irreversible neurologic injuries that do not meet the technical requirements of brain death. In the case of donation after cardiac death, the ischemia time inherent in the donation process necessarily diminishes the value of the transplants by reducing both the quantity and the quality of the organs that can be procured.

Many will object that transplantation surgeons cannot legally or ethically remove vital organs from patients before death, since doing so will cause their death. However, if the critiques of the current methods of diagnosing death are correct, then such actions are already taking place on a routine basis. Moreover, in modern intensive care units, ethically justified decisions and actions of physicians are already the proximate cause of death for many patients—for instance, when mechanical ventilation is withdrawn. Whether death occurs as the result of ventilator withdrawal or organ procurement, the ethically relevant precondition is valid consent by the patient or surrogate. With such consent, there is no harm or wrong done in retrieving vital organs before death, provided that anesthesia is administered. With proper safeguards, no patient will die from vital organ donation who would not otherwise die as a result of the withdrawal of life support. Finally, surveys suggest that issues related to respect for valid consent and the degree of neurologic injury may be more important to the public than concerns about whether the patient is already dead at the time the organs are removed.

In sum, as an ethical requirement for organ donation, the dead donor rule has required unnecessary and unsupportable revisions of the definition of death. Characterizing the ethical requirements of organ donation in terms of valid informed consent under the limited conditions of devastating neurologic injury is ethically sound, optimally respects the desires of those who wish to donate organs, and has the potential to maximize the number and quality of organs available to those in need.

NOTES

1 A definition of irreversible coma: report of the ad hoc committee of the Harvard Medical School to examine the definition of brain death. *JAMA*. 1968;205:337–440.

2 Truog RD. Is it time to abandon brain death? *Hastings Cent Rep*. 1997;27:29–37.

3 Bernat JL, Culver CM, Gert B. On the definition and criterion of death. *Ann Intern Med*. 1981;94:389–394.

4 Shewmon DA. Chronic "brain death": meta-analysis and conceptual consequences. *Neurology*. 1998;51:1538–1545.

5 Miller FG, Truog RD. Rethinking the ethics of vital organ donation. *Hastings Cent Rep*. 2008;38:38–46.

The Darkening Veil of "Do Everything"

Chris Feudtner and Wynne Morrison

The hour is late and the situation dire. Huddled by the patient's bedside, a nurse and respiratory therapist stand just behind the physician who speaks to the family members. Sometimes the patient is a child—perhaps an infant, just born, with severe congenital anomalies, or maybe a toddler who fell into a pool and nearly drowned. Other times, the patient is far older and may have had a sudden massive heart attack or may have been living with progressive cancer for months or years. The family members could be young parents or a spouse married half a century. The conversation focuses on the patient's history and diagnosis, the gravity of the predicament, and the possible treatment options, outlining the possible benefits and harms.

Then someone says: "Do everything." The physician may offer this up as a pledge: "We are going to do everything." Or asks the question: "Do you want us to do everything?" Alternatively, a family member may utter the phrase as a request or demand: "We want you to do everything." Heads nod in silent agreement. We will do everything.

Problem is, no one can really be clear about what has been said. What do the words "do everything" mean? The phrase is vague at best and vacuous at worst, permitting an increasingly harmful vacillation in the face of critical illness, which can eventually result in medical care that is harmful to the patient.[1,2]

First, we simply cannot do everything. There are so many—almost too many—possibilities. Medical care can go in many different directions, but not all at the same time. One cannot simultaneously cradle a grievously ill infant in one's arms and at the same time insert vascular cannulas for extracorporeal membrane oxygenation; nor can one hold a loved one's hand while they are dying at the same moment that the code team yells "clear" and attempts to defibrillate the patient's heart. One must choose. Whether acknowledged or not, choices are woven throughout the fabric of medical care. The phrase "do everything," though, seems to say otherwise: let's avoid any choice for now and do this and do that. Behind the veil of "do everything," the choices we inevitably are making—and the responsibility for those choices—are obfuscated.

Equally muddled is the mirror image phrase that "there is nothing more we can do"—full stop. Just as we cannot do everything, we can always do something. Intensive care is composed of both invasive care and intensive caring, and even if the former is failing, the latter can continue unabated. Our commitment to do the-best-something-that-we-can-do may make a world of difference. When operating within the confines of the increasingly tight constraints that progressive disease can cause, clinicians need to be more precise, complete, and empathetic:[3]

> I wish there was more that we could do that would halt the progress of this disease, but none of the treatments we have are able to do this. We are still devoted to taking care of your child and will do everything in our power to keep pain and discomfort away.

Second, the veil of "do everything" leaves a disturbing amount of room for misunderstanding what will actually be done. Families and physicians approach the patient's illness crisis from different frames of reference and thus infuse the "do everything" phrase with different meanings. Rather than assuming (often mistakenly) that the family understands the vast array of possible interventions and the detailed physical implications of what "doing everything" might mean, clinicians can respond to "do everything" statements by responding that "yes, we will do everything that we can do that can possibly help your loved one."

Third, when confronting the ominous circumstances that envelop the patient, the dark veil of "do everything" prevents families and clinicians from making genuine connections. The etiology of this vague and unattainable verbal imperative originates, in many instances, in an anguished outcry against how the critical illness threatens the patient in the bed and an urgent need to establish and affirm a basis of trust. For the family, "do everything" can be a way of asking that the clinicians stay committed and engaged with their loved one: "Don't give up." "Don't abandon us." In this sense, "everything" is not an object; rather, "everything" is an adverb, describing a "doing" that is vigorous and trustworthy.

Fourth, the "do everything" stance may stifle discussion by fostering an adversarial air in conversations. If a patient or family has framed the choices (or had them framed by others) as "do everything" versus not doing so, they may be more likely to fear that care is being rationed for some reason other than the patient's best interests. They may then become unwilling to consider alternatives to what they see as the one path that proves their loved one is not being shortchanged. Once a family mentions the phrase "do everything," clinicians may use it as an excuse to escape from or shorten a difficult conversation, thinking, "well, we know what they want." But to shy away from engaging in this discussion does not build a collaborative partnership between family and clinicians, nor does it serve the patient well.[4]

Ours is not an argument for confronting daunting choices bluntly—or, worse, brusquely—relying chiefly on medical facts and clinical logic to grapple with frightfully difficult situations. Rather, we argue for taking the time in these conversations to explore the choices that could be made. When confronted with requests or demands to "do everything," we view this as a starting point for a discussion, not an ending point.[5] The discussion should not so much debate the pros and cons of particular interventions but rather focus on and elaborate specific commitments. Our response might be:[6]

> I respect how deeply committed you are, and we are also absolutely committed to figuring out what the best thing to do is. Let's talk for a few minutes about what the different options might look like.

In the crisis that families confront when a loved one is critically ill, increased clarity of speech is not a cure-all. Still, being clear and forthright helps. When a family member talks about "doing everything," clinicians might pause to insert a reflective comment:[7]

> We always ask ourselves what we can do to help the patient. To answer this question, we have to be clear about what we are hoping for—recovery, comfort, dignity—and do all that we can that has a reasonable chance of getting us there.

Finally, with each passing year, this veil of "do everything" grows darker. A mere 60 years ago, "do everything" would have at most meant lying in a hospital bed on a regular ward, receiving oxygen by mask and antibiotic injections, and perhaps undergoing surgery. There were no intensive care units, no telemetry monitors, no mechanical ventilators, no dialysis, no transplantation, no extracorporeal membrane oxygenation, and no left ventricular assist devices. Over time, the medical and surgical interventions that we can do are increasingly invasive and effective, all of which is nothing short of marvelous; yet, these miraculous technologies are also effective at merely forestalling death even in those cases where recovery never happens, and most likely never could have, while nonetheless creating in their wake the pain and suffering associated with invasive care, bereft of any benefits.[8]

The bottom line is simple: saying that we are going to "do everything" is dangerous nonsense. If we really don't mean it, then we really must not say it. A moratorium is warranted, halting all medical personnel from further casual utterances of "do everything."

NOTES

1 Tulsky JA. Beyond advance directives: importance of communication skills at the end of life. *JAMA*. 2005;294(3):359–365.

2 Levetown M; American Academy of Pediatrics Committee on Bioethics. Communicating with children and families: from everyday interactions to skill in conveying distressing information. *Pediatrics*. 2008;121(5):e1441–e1460.

3 Selph RB, Shiang J, Engelberg R, Curtis JR, White DB. Empathy and life support decisions in intensive care units. *J Gen Intern Med*. 2008;23(9):1311–1317.

4 Feudtner C. Collaborative communication in pediatric palliative care: a foundation for problem-solving and decision-making. *Pediatr Clin North Am*. 2007;54(5):583–607.

5 Quill TE, Arnold R, Back AL. Discussing treatment preferences with patients who want "everything." *Ann Intern Med*. 2009;151(5):345–349.

6 Back AL, Arnold RM, Baile WF, Edwards KA, Tulsky JA. When praise is worth considering in a difficult conversation. *Lancet*. 2010;376(9744):866–867.

7 Feudtner C. The breadth of hopes. *N Engl J Med*. 2009;361(24):2306–2307.

8 Rosenberg CE. *Our Present Complaint: American Medicine, Then and Now*. Baltimore: Johns Hopkins University Press; 2007.

Death and Dignity

A Case of Individualized Decision Making

Timothy E. Quill

Diane was feeling tired and had a rash. A common scenario, though there was something subliminally worrisome that prompted me to check her blood count. Her hematocrit was 22, and the white-cell count was 4.3 with some metamyelocytes and unusual white cells. I wanted it to be viral, trying to deny what was staring me in the face. Perhaps in a repeated count it would disappear. I called Diane and told her it might be more serious than I had initially thought—that the test needed to be repeated and that if she felt worse, we might have to move quickly. When she pressed for the possibilities, I reluctantly opened the door to leukemia. Hearing the word seemed to make it exist. "Oh, shit!" she said. "Don't tell me that." Oh, shit! I thought, I wish I didn't have to.

Diane was no ordinary person (although no one I have ever come to know has been really ordinary). She was raised in an alcoholic family and had felt alone for much of her life. She had vaginal cancer as a young woman. Through much of her adult life, she had struggled with depression and her own alcoholism. I had come to know, respect, and admire her over the previous eight years as she confronted these problems and gradually overcame them. She was an incredibly clear, at times brutally honest, thinker and communicator. As she took control of her life, she developed a strong sense of independence and confidence. In the previous 3½ years, her hard work had paid off. She was completely abstinent from alcohol, she had established much deeper connections with her husband, college-age son, and several friends, and her business and her artistic work were blossoming. She felt she was really living fully for the first time.

Timothy E. Quill, "Death and Dignity: A Case of Individualized Decision Making," from *New England Journal of Medicine* 324 (1991): 691–694. © 1991 by Massachusetts Medical Society. Reprinted by permission of Massachusetts Medical Society.

Not surprisingly, the repeated blood count was abnormal, and detailed examination of the peripheral-blood smear showed myelocytes. I advised her to come into the hospital, explaining that we needed to do a bone marrow biopsy and make some decisions relatively rapidly. She came to the hospital knowing what we would find. She was terrified, angry, and sad. Although we knew the odds, we both clung to the thread of possibility that it might be something else.

The bone marrow confirmed the worst: acute myelomonocytic leukemia. In the face of this tragedy, we looked for signs of hope. This is an area of medicine in which technological intervention has been successful, with cures 25 percent of the time—long-term cures. As I probed the costs of these cures, I heard about induction chemotherapy (three weeks in the hospital, prolonged neutropenia, probable infectious complications, and hair loss; 75 percent of patients respond, 25 percent do not). For the survivors, this is followed by consolidation chemotherapy (with similar side effects; another 25 percent die, for a net survival of 50 percent). Those still alive, to have a reasonable chance of long-term survival, then need bone marrow transplantation (hospitalization for two months and whole-body irradiation, with complete killing of the bone marrow, infectious complications, and the possibility for graft-versus-host disease—with a survival of approximately 50 percent, or 25 percent of the original group). Though hematologists may argue over the exact percentages, they don't argue about the outcome of no treatment—certain death in days, weeks, or at most a few months.

Believing that delay was dangerous, our oncologist broke the news to Diane and began making plans to insert a Hickman catheter and begin induction chemotherapy that afternoon. When I saw her shortly thereafter, she was enraged at his presumption that she would want treatment, and devastated by the finality of the diagnosis. All she wanted to do was go home and be with her family. She had no further questions about treatment and in fact had decided that she wanted none. Together we lamented her tragedy and the unfairness of life. Before she left, I felt the need to be sure that she and her husband understood that there was some risk in delay, that the problem was not going to go away, and that we needed to keep considering the options over the next several days. We agreed to meet in two days.

She returned in two days with her husband and son. They had talked extensively about the problem and the options. She remained very clear about her wish not to undergo chemotherapy and to live whatever time she had left outside the hospital. As we explored her thinking further, it became clear that she was convinced she would die during the period of treatment and would suffer unspeakably in the process (from hospitalization, from lack of control over her body, from the side effects of chemotherapy, and from pain and anguish). Although I could offer support and my best effort to minimize her suffering if she chose treatment, there was no way I could say any of this would not occur. In fact, the last four patients with acute leukemia at our hospital had died very painful deaths in the hospital during various stages of treatment (a fact I did not share with her). Her family wished she would choose treatment but sadly accepted her decision. She articulated very clearly that it was she who would be experiencing all the side effects of treatment and that odds of 25 percent were not good enough for her to undergo so toxic a course of therapy, given her expectations of chemotherapy and hospitalization and the absence of a closely matched bone marrow donor. I had her repeat her understanding of the treatment, the odds, and what to expect if there were no treatment. I clarified a few misunderstandings, but she had a remarkable grasp of the options and implications.

I have been a longtime advocate of active, informed patient choice of treatment or nontreatment, and of a patient's right to die with as much control and dignity as possible. Yet there was something about her giving up a 25 percent chance of long-term survival in favor of almost certain death that disturbed me. I had seen Diane fight and use her considerable inner resources to overcome alcoholism and depression, and I half expected her to change her mind over the next week. Since the window of time in which effective treatment can be initiated is rather narrow, we met several times that week. We obtained a second hematology consultation and talked at length about the meaning and implications of treatment and nontreatment. She talked to a psychologist she had seen in the past. I gradually understood the decision from her perspective and became convinced that it was the right decision for her. We arranged for home hospice care (although at that time Diane felt reasonably well, was active, and looked healthy), left the door open for her to change her mind, and tried to anticipate how to keep her comfortable in the time she had left.

Just as I was adjusting to her decision, she opened up another area that would stretch me profoundly. It was extraordinarily important to Diane to maintain control of herself and her own dignity during the time remaining to her. When this was no longer possible, she clearly wanted to die. As a former director of a hospice program, I know how to use pain medicines to keep patients comfortable and lessen suffering. I explained the philosophy of comfort care, which I strongly believe in. Although Diane understood and appreciated this, she had known of people lingering in what was called relative comfort, and she wanted no part of it. When the time came, she wanted to take her life in the least painful way possible. Knowing of her desire for independence and her decision to stay in control, I thought this request made perfect sense. I acknowledged and explored this wish but also thought that it was out of the realm of currently accepted medical practice and that it was more than I could offer or promise. In our discussion, it became clear that preoccupation with her fear of a lingering death would interfere with Diane's getting the most out of the time she had left until she found a safe way to ensure her death. I feared the effects of a violent death on her family, the consequences of an ineffective suicide that would leave her lingering in precisely the state she dreaded so much, and the possibility that a family member would be forced to assist her, with all the legal and personal repercussions that would follow. She discussed this at length with her family. They believed that they should respect her choice. With this in mind, I told Diane that information was available from the Hemlock Society that might be helpful to her.

A week later she phoned me with a request for barbiturates for sleep. Since I knew that this was an essential ingredient in a Hemlock Society sui- cide, I asked her to come to the office to talk things over. She was more than willing to protect me by participating in a superficial conversation about her insomnia, but it was important to me to know how she planned to use the drugs and to be sure that she was not in despair or overwhelmed in a way that might color her judgment. In our discussion, it was apparent that she was having trouble sleeping, but it was also evident that the security of having enough barbiturates available to commit suicide when and if the time came would leave her secure enough to live fully and concentrate on the present. It was clear that she was not despondent and that in fact she was making deep, personal connections with her family and close friends. I made sure that she knew how to use the barbiturates for sleep, and also that she knew the amount needed to commit suicide. We agreed to meet regularly, and she promised to meet with me before taking her life to ensure that all other avenues had been exhausted. I wrote the prescription with an uneasy feeling about the boundaries I was exploring—spiritual, legal, pro- fessional, and personal. Yet I also felt strongly that I was setting her free to get the most out of the time she had left and to maintain dignity and control on her own terms until her death.

The next several months were very intense and important for Diane. Her son stayed home from college, and they were able to be with one another and say much that had not been said earlier. Her husband did his work at home so that he and Diane could spend more time together. She spent time with her closest friends. I had her come into the hospital for a conference with our residents, at which she illustrated in a most profound and personal way the importance of informed decision making, the right to refuse treatment, and the extraordinarily personal effects of illness and interaction with the medical system. There were emotional and physical hardships as well. She had periods of intense sadness and anger. Several times she became very weak, but she received transfusions as an outpatient and responded with marked improvement of symptoms. She had two serious infections that responded surprisingly well to empirical courses of oral antibiotics. After three tumultuous months, there were two weeks of relative calm and well-being, and fantasies of a miracle began to surface.

Unfortunately, we had no miracle. Bone pain, weakness, fatigue, and fevers began to dominate her life. Although the hospice workers, family members, and I tried our best to minimize the suffering and promote comfort, it was clear that the end was approaching. Diane's immediate future held what she feared the most—increasing discomfort, dependence, and hard choices between pain and sedation. She called up her closest friends and asked them to come over to say goodbye, telling them that she would be leaving soon. As we had agreed, she let me know as well. When we met, it was clear that she knew what she was doing, that she was sad and frightened to be leaving, but that she would be even more terrified to stay and suffer. In our tearful goodbye, she promised a reunion in the future at her favorite spot on the edge of Lake Geneva, with dragons swimming in the sunset.

Two days later her husband called to say that Diane had died. She had said her final goodbyes to her husband and son that morning, and asked them to leave her alone for an hour. After an hour, which must have seemed an eternity, they found her on the couch, lying very still and covered by her favorite shawl. There was no sign of struggle. She seemed to be at peace. They called me for advice about how to proceed. When I arrived at their house, Diane indeed seemed peaceful. Her husband and son were quiet. We talked about what a remarkable person she had been. They seemed to have no doubts about the course she had chosen or about their cooperation, although the unfairness of her illness and the finality of her death were overwhelming to us all.

I called the medical examiner to inform him that a hospice patient had died. When asked about the cause of death, I said, "Acute leukemia." He said that was fine and that we should call a funeral director. Although acute leukemia was the truth, it was not the whole story. Yet any mention of suicide would have given rise to a police investigation and probably brought the arrival of an ambulance crew for resuscitation. Diane would have become a "coroner's case," and the decision to perform an autopsy would have been made at the discretion of the medical examiner. The family or I could have been subject to criminal prosecution, and I to professional review, for our roles in support of Diane's choices. Although I truly believe that the family and I gave her the best care possible, allowing her to define her limits and directions as much as possible, I am not sure the law, society, or the medical profession would agree. So I said "acute leukemia" to protect all of us, to protect Diane from an invasion into her past and her body, and to continue to shield society from the knowledge of the degree of suffering that people often undergo in the process of dying. Suffering can be lessened to some extent, but in no way eliminated or made benign, by the careful intervention of a competent, caring physician, given current social constraints.

Diane taught me about the range of help I can provide if I know people well and if I allow them to say what they really want. She taught me about life, death, and honesty and about taking charge and facing tragedy squarely when it strikes. She taught me that I can take small risks for people that I really know and care about. Although I did not assist in her suicide directly, I helped indirectly to make it possible, successful, and relatively painless. Although I know we have measures to help control pain and lessen suffering, to think that people do not suffer in the process of dying is an illusion. Prolonged dying can occasionally be peaceful, but more often the role of the physician and family is limited to lessening but not eliminating severe suffering.

I wonder how many families and physicians secretly help patients over the edge into death in the face of such severe suffering. I wonder how many severely ill or dying patients secretly take their lives, dying alone in despair. I wonder whether the image of Diane's final aloneness will persist in the minds of her family, or if they will remember more the intense, meaningful months they had together before she died. I wonder whether Diane struggled in that last hour, and whether the Hemlock Society's way of death by suicide is the most benign. I wonder why Diane, who gave so much to so many of us, had to be alone for the last hour of her life. I wonder whether I will see Diane again, on the shore of Lake Geneva at sunset, with dragons swimming on the horizon.

Active and Passive Euthanasia

James A. Rachels

The distinction between active and passive euthanasia is thought to be crucial for medical ethics. The idea is that it is permissible, at least in some cases, to withhold treatment and allow a patient to die, but it is never permissible to take any direct action designed to kill the patient. This doctrine seems to be accepted by most doctors, and it is endorsed in a statement adopted by the House of Delegates of the American Medical Association on December 4, 1973:

> The intentional termination of the life of one human being by another—mercy killing—is contrary to that for which the medical profession stands and is contrary to the policy of the American Medical Association.
>
> The cessation of the employment of extraordinary means to prolong the life of the body when there is irrefutable evidence that biological death is imminent is the decision of the patient and/or his immediate family. The advice and judgment of the physician should be freely available to the patient and/or his immediate family.

However, a strong case can be made against this doctrine. In what follows I will set out some of the relevant arguments and urge doctors to reconsider their views on this matter.

To begin with a familiar type of situation, a patient who is dying of incurable cancer of the throat is in terrible pain, which can no longer be satisfactorily alleviated. He is certain to die within a few days, even if present treatment is continued, but he does not want to go on living for those days since the pain is unbearable. So he asks the doctor for an end to it, and his family joins in the request.

James A. Rachels, "Active and Passive Euthanasia," *New England Journal of Medicine* 292 (1975): 78–80. © 1975 by Massachusetts Medical Society. Reprinted by permission of Massachusetts Medical Society.

Suppose the doctor agrees to withhold treatment, as the conventional doctrine says he may. The justification for his doing so is that the patient is in terrible agony, and since he is going to die anyway, it would be wrong to prolong his suffering needlessly. But now notice this. If one simply withholds treatment, it may take the patient longer to die, and so he may suffer more than he would if more direct action were taken and a lethal injection given. This fact provides strong reason for thinking that, once the initial decision not to prolong his agony has been made, active euthanasia is actually preferable to passive euthanasia, rather than the reverse. To say otherwise is to endorse the option that leads to more suffering rather than less and is contrary to the humanitarian impulse that prompts the decision not to prolong his life in the first place.

Part of my point is that the process of being "allowed to die" can be relatively slow and painful, whereas being given a lethal injection is relatively quick and painless. Let me give a different sort of example. In the United States about one in 600 babies is born with Down's syndrome. Most of these babies are otherwise healthy—that is, with only the usual pediatric care, they will proceed to an otherwise normal infancy. Some, however, are born with congenital defects such as intestinal obstructions that require operations if they are to live. Sometimes, the parents and the doctor will decide not to operate and let the infant die. Anthony Shaw describes what happens then:

> When surgery is denied [the doctor] must try to keep the infant from suffering while natural forces sap the baby's life away. As a surgeon whose natural inclination is to use the scalpel to fight off death, standing by and watching a salvageable baby die is the most emotionally exhausting experience I know. It is easy at a conference, in a theoretical discussion, to decide that such infants should be allowed to die. It is altogether different to stand by in the nursery and watch as dehydration and infection wither a tiny being over hours and days. This is a terrible ordeal for me and the hospital staff—much more so than for the parents who never set foot in the nursery.*

I can understand why some people are opposed to all euthanasia and insist that such infants must be allowed to live. I think I can also understand why other people favor destroying these babies quickly and painlessly. But why should anyone favor letting "dehydration and infection wither a tiny being over hours and days"? The doctrine that says that a baby may be allowed to dehydrate and wither but may not be given an injection that would end its life without suffering seems so patently cruel as to require no further refutation.

The strong language is not intended to offend, but only to put the point in the clearest possible way.

My second argument is that the conventional doctrine leads to decisions concerning life and death made on irrelevant grounds.

Consider again the case of the infants with Down's syndrome who need operations for congenital defects unrelated to the syndrome to live. Sometimes, there is no operation, and the baby dies, but when there is no such defect, the baby lives on. Now, an operation such as that to remove an intestinal obstruction is not prohibitively difficult. The reason why such operations are not performed in these cases is, clearly, that the child has Down's syndrome and the parents and doctor judge that because of that fact it is better for the child to die.

But notice that this situation is absurd, no matter what view one takes of the lives and potentials of such babies. If the life of such an infant is worth preserving, what does it matter if it needs a simple operation? Or, if one thinks it better that such a baby should not live on, what difference does it make that it happens to have an unobstructed intestinal tract? In either case, the matter of life and death is being decided on irrelevant grounds. It is the Down's syndrome, and not the intestines, that is the issue. The matter should be decided, if at all, on that basis, and not be allowed to depend on the essentially irrelevant question of whether the intestinal tract is blocked.

What makes this situation possible, of course, is the idea that when there is an intestinal blockage, one can "let the baby die," but when there is no such defect there is nothing that can be done, for one must not "kill" it. The fact that this idea leads to such results as deciding life or death on irrelevant grounds is another good reason why the doctrine should be rejected.

One reason why so many people think that there is an important moral difference between active and passive euthanasia is that they think killing someone is morally worse than letting someone die. But is it? Is killing, in itself, worse than letting die? To investigate this issue, two cases may be considered that are exactly alike except that one involves killing whereas the other involves letting someone die. Then, it can be asked whether this difference makes any difference to the moral assessments. It is important that the cases be exactly alike, except for this one difference, since otherwise one cannot be confident that it is this difference and not some other that accounts for any variation in the assessments of the two cases. So, let us consider this pair of cases:

In the first, Smith stands to gain a large inheritance if anything should happen to his 6-year-old cousin. One evening while the child is taking his bath, Smith sneaks into the bathroom and drowns the child, and then arranges things so that it will look like an accident.

In the second, Jones also stands to gain if anything should happen to his 6-year-old cousin. Like Smith, Jones sneaks in planning to drown the child in his bath. However, just as he enters the bathroom Jones sees the child slip and hit his head, and fall face down in the water. Jones is delighted; he stands by, ready to push the child's head back under if it is necessary, but it is not necessary. With only a little thrashing about, the child drowns all by himself, "accidentally," as Jones watches and does nothing.

Now Smith killed the child, whereas Jones "merely" let the child die. That is the only difference between them. Did either man behave better, from a moral point of view? If the difference between killing and letting die were in itself a morally important matter, one should say that Jones's behavior was less reprehensible than Smith's. But does one really want to say that? I think not. In the first place, both men acted from the same motive, personal gain, and both had exactly the same end in view when they acted. It may be inferred from Smith's conduct that he is a bad man, although that judgment may be withdrawn or modified if certain further facts are learned about him—for example, that he is mentally deranged. But would not the very same thing be inferred about Jones from his conduct? And would not the same further considerations also be relevant to any modification of this judgment? Moreover, suppose Jones pleaded, in his own defense, "After all, I didn't do anything except just stand there and watch the child drown. I didn't kill him; I only let him die." Again, if letting die were in itself less bad than killing, this defense should have at least some weight. But it does not. Such a "defense" can only be regarded as a grotesque perversion of moral reasoning. Morally speaking, it is no defense at all.

Now, it may be pointed out, quite properly, that the cases of euthanasia with which doctors are concerned are not like this at all. They do not involve personal gain or the destruction of normal healthy children. Doctors are concerned only with cases in which the patient's life is of no further use to him, or in which the patient's life has become or will soon become a terrible burden. However, the point is the same in these cases: the bare difference between killing and letting die does not, in itself, make a moral difference. If a doctor lets a patient die, for humane reasons, he is in the same moral position as if he had given the patient a lethal injection for humane reasons. If his decision was wrong—if, for example, the patient's illness was in fact curable—the decision would be equally regrettable no matter which method was used to carry it out. And if the doctor's decision was the right one, the method used is not in itself important.

The AMA policy statement isolates the crucial issue very well; the crucial issue is "the intentional termination of the life of one human being by another." But after identifying this issue, and forbidding "mercy killing," the statement goes on to deny that the cessation of treatment is the intentional termination of a life. This is where the mistake comes in, for what is the cessation of treatment, in these circumstances, if it is not "the intentional termination of the life of one human being by another"? Of course it is exactly that, and if it were not, there would be no point to it.

Many people will find this judgment hard to accept. One reason, I think, is that it is very easy to conflate the question of whether killing is, in itself, worse than letting die, with the very different question of whether most actual cases of killing are more reprehensible than most actual cases of letting die. Most actual cases of killing are clearly terrible (think, for example, of all the murders reported in the newspapers), and one hears of such cases every day. On the other hand, one hardly ever hears of a case of letting die, except for the actions of doctors who are motivated by humanitarian reasons. So one learns to think of killing in a much worse light than of letting die. But this does not mean that there is something about killing that makes it in itself worse than letting die, for it is not the bare difference between killing and letting die that makes the difference in these cases. Rather, the other factors—the murderer's motive of personal gain, for example, contrasted with the doctor's humanitarian motivation—account for different reactions to the different cases.

I have argued that killing is not in itself any worse than letting die; if my contention is right, it follows that active euthanasia is not any worse than passive euthanasia. What arguments can be given on the other side? The most common, I believe, is the following:

> The important difference between active and passive euthanasia is that, in passive euthanasia, the doctor does not do anything to bring about the patient's death. The doctor does nothing, and the patient dies of whatever ills already afflict him. In active euthanasia, however, the doctor does something to bring about the patient's death: he kills him. The doctor who gives the patient with cancer a lethal injection has himself caused his patient's death; whereas if he merely ceases treatment, the cancer is the cause of the death.

A number of points need to be made here. The first is that it is not exactly correct to say that in passive euthanasia the doctor does nothing, for he does do one thing that is very important: he lets the patient die. "Letting someone die" is certainly different, in some respects, from other types of action—mainly in that it is a kind of action that one may perform by way of not performing certain other actions. For example, one may let a patient die by way of not giving medication, just as one may insult someone by way of not shaking his hand. But for any purpose of moral assessment, it is a type of action nonetheless. The decision to let a patient die is subject to moral appraisal in the same way that a decision to kill him would be subject to moral appraisal: it may be assessed as wise or unwise, compassionate or sadistic, right or wrong. If a doctor deliberately let a patient die who was suffering from a routinely curable illness, the doctor would certainly be to blame for what he had done, just as he would be to blame if he had needlessly killed the patient. Charges against him would then be appropriate. If so, it would be no defense at all for him to insist that he didn't "do anything." He would have done something very serious indeed, for he let his patient die.

Fixing the cause of death may be very important from a legal point of view, for it may determine whether criminal charges are brought against the doctor. But I do not think that this notion can be used to show a moral difference between active and passive euthanasia. The reason why it is considered bad to be the cause of someone's death is that death is regarded as a great evil—and so it is. However, if it has been decided that euthanasia—even passive euthanasia—is desirable in a given case, it has also been decided that in this instance death is no greater an evil than the patient's continued existence. And if this is true, the usual reason for not wanting to be the cause of someone's death simply does not apply.

Finally, doctors may think that all of this is only of academic interest—the sort of thing that philosophers may worry about but that has no practical bearing on their own work. After all, doctors must be concerned about the legal consequences of what they do, and active euthanasia is clearly forbidden by the law. But even so, doctors should also be concerned with the fact that the law is forcing upon them a moral doctrine that may well be indefensible, and has a considerable effect on their practices. Of course, most doctors are not now in the position of being coerced in this matter, for they do not regard themselves as merely going along with what the law requires. Rather, in statements such as the AMA policy statement that I have quoted, they are endorsing this doctrine as a central point of medical ethics. In that statement, active euthanasia is condemned not merely as illegal but as "con-

trary to that for which the medical profession stands," whereas passive euthanasia is approved. However, the preceding considerations suggest that there
is really no moral difference between the two, considered in themselves (there
may be important moral differences in some cases in their *consequences*, but,
as I pointed out, these differences may make active euthanasia, and not passive euthanasia, the morally preferable option). So, whereas doctors may
have to discriminate between active and passive euthanasia to satisfy the
law, they should not do any more than that. In particular, they should not
give the distinction any added authority and weight by writing it into official
statements of medical ethics.

NOTE

*Anthony Shaw, "Doctor, Do We Have a Choice?," *New York Times Magazine*, January 30,
1972, 54.

Clinician-Patient Interactions about Requests for Physician-Assisted Suicide

A Patient and Family View

Anthony L. Back, Helene Starks, Clarissa Hsu,
Judith R. Gordon, Ashok Bharucha, and Robert A. Pearlman

For physicians and other clinicians who care for patients with life-threatening illnesses, responding to a patient's request for physician-assisted suicide (PAS) is an important clinical skill. Although Oregon is the only state to have legalized PAS, patients in every state report that they think about PAS, and physicians in every state discuss PAS.[1] In a national survey involving 988 terminally ill patients, 60 percent of patients supported PAS in a hypothetical situation, and 10 percent had seriously considered PAS for themselves.[2] In physician surveys, 18 to 24 percent of primary care physicians and 46 to 57 percent of oncologists stated that they have received a request for PAS.[3-5]

When a patient asks for PAS, how should a clinician respond? Experts agree that an initial clinical response should include the following: the clinician should ask why the patient is interested in PAS, explore the meanings underlying the request, assess whether palliative care is adequate (especially in addressing depression), and revise the care plan to respond to the patient's concerns.[6-11] Since PAS requests may not persist, these initial clinical responses are extremely important. Beyond the initial response, however, there is controversy about whether clinicians should disclose their own

Anthony L. Back, Helene Starks, Clarissa Hsu, Judith R. Gordon, Ashok Bharucha, and Robert A. Pearlman, "Clinician-Patient Interactions about Requests for Physician-Assisted Suicide: A Patient and Family View," from *Archives of Internal Medicine* 162, no. 11 (2002): 1257–1265.

moral beliefs about PAS, offer sedation for refractory symptoms or intolerable suffering, or provide a prescription for PAS in a state where it is illegal.[12–15]

Although expert recommendations for responding to PAS requests presume that clinicians possess communication skills and palliative care expertise, little empirical research has been conducted to identify exactly what skills and expertise are required.[7–9,11] Previous surveys of physicians suggest that the most prominent concerns for patients considering PAS are nonphysical concerns about dying, such as loss of control and loss of dignity.[3,16] Yet a qualitative study of physicians who dealt with PAS requests indicated that physicians felt least competent in addressing existential suffering.[17] Judging by these studies in the medical literature and anecdotes in the lay press,[18–20] it appears that the nonphysical concerns about dying that prompt patients to consider PAS are issues that many physicians feel poorly equipped to address.

We conducted an intensive qualitative interview study with patients who seriously pursued PAS and with their family members. The primary study objectives were to describe the reasons that the patient was pursuing PAS, the narrative of events leading to death, and interactions with physicians and other clinicians. This article reports our findings about interactions with clinicians. We asked our participants to describe their conversations with their physicians and other medical clinicians about PAS. From these data, we identified themes that describe qualities of clinician-patient interactions about PAS that patients and family members valued. In describing what patients and family members valued when discussing PAS, we hope to provide guidance for clinicians faced with these difficult conversations, regardless of their willingness to provide PAS or its legal status.

A qualitative design was chosen for this study because of the lack of empirical data describing how clinicians respond to requests for PAS. We used semistructured interviews to yield data that we analyzed and developed into a description of important qualities of clinician-patient communication about PAS from the perspectives of patients and their family members.

The sampling frame for this study included patients and family members who were actively seeking information and access to PAS because we wanted to describe the process of planning and implementing PAS. This sample includes a self-selected group of patients and family members who sought out advocacy organizations that specifically help patients organize a PAS. Therefore, the sample is limited to those patients and their families who were engaged in assessing PAS as a concrete option for determining the timing and circumstances of their death.

We focused on two groups of participants: (1) a prospective cohort of patients who were currently pursuing PAS (and their family members); and (2) a retrospective cohort of family members who had been involved with a patient pursuing PAS. Based on other qualitative studies, we estimated that about 30 families would provide enough data such that additional data would fail to contribute further to explaining the phenomena being studied, a condition called *theoretical saturation*. Our sample size of 35 families was not intended to be a comprehensive view of all patients seeking PAS, but it was adequate to describe this particular group of patients and family members. Thirty of the 35 cases occurred in a state where PAS is illegal. (For more on the study participants and methods, see the appendix at the end of this chapter.)

Results

Participant Characteristics

We studied 35 cases of patients who pursued PAS and their family members. Table 1 and table 2 give the characteristics of the participants. Table 1 also lists the manner of death and where the patients obtained their lethal prescription. For the prospective cohort, the mean time between the first interview with patients and death was 10.6 months (range, 0.1–30.6 months). For the retrospective cohort, the mean time between the patient's death and the first interview with a family member was 20.2 months (range, 2.4–49.5 months).

Themes

Most patients and family members could recall the PAS discussions with their clinicians in substantial detail. Their first-hand accounts of clinician interactions regarding a PAS request provide important data about their perceptions of clinical care related to PAS. The themes summarize what patient and family members valued in communicating with clinicians about PAS.

Openness to Discussion about PAS

Patients and family members highly valued clinicians who were willing and open to discussing PAS. When they encountered a clinician who was willing to discuss PAS, they felt able to disclose many concerns about dying. They also felt lucky because they knew PAS was controversial. As one family member put it, what she wanted was "another sane adult" who could "talk in terms . . . that remove the taboo from the process" by giving "a real, clear picture of possible

TABLE 1 Patient Characteristics

Characteristic	Prospective Cases (n = 12)	Retrospective Cases (n = 23)	Total Patients (N = 35)
Age, mean (SD) [range], y	72 (10) [60–89]	66 (19) [33–99]	68 (16) [33–99]
Female	6	11	17
White	12	23	35
Marital status			
Married or living with partner	4	14	18
Divorced or separated	1	4	5
Widowed	5	4	9
Never married	2	1	3
Education			
High school or less	1	3	4
Some college	6	5	11
Bachelor's degree	4	3	7
Graduate degree	1	5	6
Unknown	0	7	7
Underlying illness			
Cancer	8	14	22
AIDS	1	4	5
Neurologic	1	4	5
Other†	2	1	3
Received hospice and/or home health care	7	18	25
Manner of death			
Physician-assisted suicide‡	5	13	18
Euthanasia§	2	5	7
Underlying illness	4	4	8
Self-inflicted gunshot wound	0	1	1
Still alive at the end of the study	1	0	1

TABLE 1 continued

Characteristic	Prospective Cases (*n*=12)	Retrospective Cases (*n*=23)	Total Patients (*N*=35)
Source of lethal prescription			
Primary or specialty care provider	6	13	19
Friends or acquaintances	3	6	9
Did not obtain medications	2	4	6
Declined to report	0	1	1
Health insurance			
HMO (includes Veterans Affairs)	2	9	11
Fee for service	3	8	11
Medicaid only	0	3	3
Medicare + supplemental	5	2	7
Medicare + Medicaid	2	1	3

*Data are given as number of patients, except for age. Data for prospective cases are reported from 12 patients and 20 of their family members; data for retrospective cases are reported about 23 patients by 28 of their family members. AIDS indicates acquired immunodeficiency syndrome; HMO, health maintenance organization.

†Other includes the following diagnoses: autoimmune disease, bronchiolitis obliterans, and debilitating unexplained pain syndrome.

‡Death by physician-assisted suicide included patients who had medications that they voluntarily ingested with the primary intention of ending their lives.

§Death by euthanasia included patients who asked clinicans or family members to administer a lethal dose of medication with the primary intent of causing death. Patients who died by euthanasia either were competent at the time of death but not able to self-administer medications, or were decisionally incapacitated but had specifically requested that medications be administered if they lost decisional capacity.

TABLE 2 Family Member Characteristics

Characteristic	Family Members of Prospective Cases (*n*=20)	Family Members of Retrospective Cases (*n*=28)	Total Family Members (*N*=48)
Family members interviewed per case, mean (range)	1.7 (1–4)	1.2 (1–3)	1.4 (1–4)
Relationship to patient			
Spouse or partner	5	10	15
Daughter	5	10	15
Son	6	2	8
Other in-law	1	3	4
Friend	3	3	6
Age, mean (range), y	51 (31–82)	52 (29–74)	51 (29–82)
Female sex	11	17	28
White race	20	27	47
Education			
High school or less	3	0	3
Some college	5	3	8
Bachelor's degree	5	4	9
Graduate degree	6	15	21
Unknown	1	6	7

Note: Data are given as number of members, except for age.

approaches without advocating [PAS]." The following counterexample underscores the importance of clinician openness to discussion about PAS.

> I know the physician that we had—the conversations were a struggle with him because we couldn't talk about hastening the death. So there was, like, a part of us that we could not talk about, which made our questions limited. So it was like we didn't have access to information that would have allowed our conversations to be more full and more fully informed.

Patients and family members attributed clinician unwillingness to discuss PAS to a variety of reasons. Some clinicians were unwilling to discuss PAS because it was illegal. These clinicians behaved as if discussions of PAS in and of themselves were illegal and dangerous. One patient observed that "all [my physicians] talk about is the legality of it," and another concluded that clinicians "have to hide their feelings about [PAS], so as not to jeopardize their careers." In other cases, patients and family members reported that the topic of PAS provoked a strong emotional response from clinicians that made further conversation awkward. For example, one family member described a neurologist who was "so adamant that PAS was a terrible thing and the wrong thing to do . . . it was kind of awful." Another subject described a physician's reaction to a PAS request as "protective [of himself] . . . not at all sympathetic or comforting." One patient described how she could detect that her oncologist became "really uncomfortable" talking about PAS or "anything" about dying, and she changed the subject for him. She said, "I learned that he's a baseball fan and much more comfortable if I change the topic to baseball. . . . It's awful when you have to try to make them feel comfortable, but that's the way it is." Other clinicians seemed to want to maintain a biomedical focus. One family member said, "They won't talk to you about [PAS] even as a possibility. It's like, 'I know that happens, but—what about let's do the chemotherapy.'"

The value of clinician openness to discussing PAS went beyond this topic alone. Patients felt that a clinician willing to talk about PAS might also be willing to discuss other worries, fears, and vulnerabilities about illness and dying. As one patient said, "Everything was laid out on the table. Oh, you bet, yeah. Because he can't help you—nobody can help you if they don't know what's going on in your life." In a different case, a family member described how her father's relationship with the caseworker from an advocacy organization provided a different dimension of care than he received from his oncologist. The family member said, "It provided a place where he could talk about his illness. He didn't talk about hastening his death [because he was prepared and did not think it was time]. He's just describing to them what's going on with him and so on. But it's good to have a place like that." Thus, patients may use talking about PAS as a gateway to talk about dying.

> It's not that she [my friend, the patient] doesn't want to [talk about dying]; that's the sad thing. She's sitting here holding all of this stuff in, and to me the most important events in your life are your transitions, your birth and your death . . . the beginning and the end of this physical existence. But you can't talk to your doctor about it without them getting all weird, [thinking] that you're suicidal or something.

This patient, during her own interview, wept as she described her frustration trying to talk to one of her doctors. She said, "You're trying to get a doctor to sit down and listen to you . . . but they never, ever get the overall picture." Her clinicians' unwillingness to discuss PAS resulted in missed opportunities to connect with this patient's deepest concerns, which included her quality of life, her prognosis, and her suffering.

Another value of clinician openness is that it facilitated a complete evaluation of a PAS request. Participants described clinicians who were willing to assist patients and families but who avoided discussing PAS openly or explicitly. In these cases, the clinicians fulfilled PAS requests with little evaluation. One patient's wife said, "My husband, with the advice of a doctor friend that lives in [another state], went to his cardiologist . . . And he told the doctor that he needed Seconal. And this doctor has known my husband for a long time, and all he said was, I trust you have a good reason, and gave it to him, a prescription for it." In this case, a family member obtained a prescription for PAS from a physician who had never met the patient. This is an extreme case in our sample but it is not unique. Two other patients in our study obtained prescriptions without any medical evaluation. In one of these cases, a family member found that after a visit with the patient's oncologist, the necessary prescriptions had been tucked into her purse without her knowledge. Clinicians who deal obliquely with PAS requests may miss opportunities to fully evaluate and understand the issues underlying the request.

Expertise in Dealing with the Dying Process

One important type of clinician expertise was the ability to describe the natural history of illness and care options in the last days of life. Patients and families were extremely sensitive to the ways in which clinicians talked— or avoided talking—about these issues. A woman with metastatic ovarian cancer found that she could not get information from her oncologist about how she would die, so she went to a medical library and read a textbook on gynecologic cancer. What she learned was that dying of ovarian cancer was "long, protracted, not very happy . . . organ failures or blockages or blood poisoning or pneumonia, and it takes a whole combination of things to finally just be fatal." Although she confronted her oncologist with this information, she left without reassurance that she could avoid a long, agonizing death. She concluded that PAS was probably the least worst way for her to die. In a different case, another patient was told by his physician that in "all the AIDS cases in the city, it was the worst thrush they'd ever seen." His partner reported:

Our doctor was like, you do not want to die of thrush, and then kind of described how it would happen. Basically, he said the thrush would grow and shut off your esophagus, so that you'd not be able to swallow ... [my partner] would drool constantly and end up starving to death, because he wouldn't be able to pass any food down. The doctor said, "You don't want to die like that." And that's when [my partner] decided to do a hastened death.

The patient and his partner interpreted the physician's statements, which did not include a medical response to fears of drooling and starving to death, as a tacit endorsement of PAS as the best option in their circumstances. Before this conversation, the patient was already considering PAS, but this conversation marked a turning point in his interest.

Another valued type of clinical expertise was defining reasonable expectations about dying and then delivering the care necessary to fulfill those expectations. One woman with lung cancer was very suspicious of doctors and hospitals, believing that "cancer is big business." She declined anticancer therapies but was willing to explore palliative care options. Her physician referred her to hospice, and her experience there made her rethink her commitment to PAS:

Before Thanksgiving, I went over to the hospice [an inpatient unit] for respite care. It's a wonderful place. It's absolutely wonderful. Unlike a hospital, you don't see any uniforms; you are not No. 14 or No. 12; you are a person. The only thing that resembles a hospital is the bed and the tray table. Outside of that, there is absolutely nothing that resembles a hospital. There is no noise of anyone being in pain. It's wonderful; it really is. [My] main concern is to be pain free, and they do take care of that.

She ultimately died of progressive cancer at home with hospice care.

Another case of a patient with advanced acquired immunodeficiency syndrome exemplifies what can happen when clinicians overpromise a "pain-free" death:

The physician encouraged [stopping total parenteral nutrition] as a nice way to go and said that that would be probably a 3-week process, maybe 4 at the most, but probably 3. "That's a very pleasant way to die. It's pain free." ... We went in and out of the emergency room 3 times over pain in the last 2 weeks of his life ... and he had great, agonizing, lower abdominal pain through it all. So I felt real cheated about that. It wasn't this quiet, pain-free existence. ... If you're going to make a guarantee that a person is really not going to be in pain, you need to make sure that they're not. And if you don't think that you can make sure, you shouldn't promise.

When dying proved to be neither quiet nor pain free, the patient and his partner began to plan a PAS.

A third type of expertise was individualizing pain control to meet patient goals. In one case, the absence of this expertise led to a death by a self-inflicted gunshot wound. The patient had painful bony metastases to his spine and was "on 800 milligrams of morphine a day. Besides all the Roxicet he could manage to keep down." His oncologist referred him to hospice for better pain management. However, the patient and his wife found that their hospice providers had an agenda about pain control that did not allow for the fact that his top priority was to maintain a sense of control over his situation.

> They put him on a morphine pump. It took him a couple of days to adjust it, and they were extremely caring. They hovered. They just about drove him up the wall. [They said,] "We're going to kill your pain." Well, they killed his pain. He was unconscious for almost 24 hours. Flat on his back. He had not been able to lay on his back. He was totally out of it. He got up the next day and he said, "I feel like Ray Milland's 'Lost Weekend.'" [That movie was about] an alcoholic who just went through all sorts of, just, DTs and, you know, it just—really hell on wheels. And that's exactly how my husband felt. He said, "I can't think; I can't do this."

The next morning, the patient fired the hospice and discontinued the pain regimen. "Once the hospice people had knocked him for 1 loop, he wasn't going to let it happen again," explained his wife. The following day, the patient warned his wife not to follow him outside, where he positioned himself out of sight and shot himself in the head. The hospice nurse wrote in her bereavement card, "At least he got one good night's sleep," to which his wife responded, "I almost went through the ceiling."

A final type of expertise involved clinician knowledge about the lethal potential of medications. In cases in which clinicians had this knowledge and were willing to provide a prescription for PAS, patients and families were reassured that if they ultimately decided to implement a PAS, it would be successful. As one family member said:

> The psychiatrist that [my husband] saw said that he didn't understand why my husband needed to be in hell anymore, or myself, and that he was seeing that a lot had been tried, and he thought that [my husband]

should be able to end his life if he wanted. So he began describing the correct pills, and so there—and so then when he had it, I remember there was just a huge relief on both of our parts and deep gratefulness to that person.

In other cases, however, patients or family members received instructions from clinicians to increase doses of morphine and diazepam to hasten death that proved to be incorrect. One family member recalled how a hospice nurse, with explicit instructions from the physician, taught him how to unlock an intravenous patient-controlled analgesia device and how to administer a lethal dose of morphine. "They told us that within 3 to 4 hours his heart would stop and it would be over. . . . Very specific. And we were never told any alternative. We were never told it might not work. . . . And of course, it didn't work." After 12 hours, the patient woke up, and his partner spent days frantically searching for information and support. The patient finally came up with the idea of dissolving secobarbital tablets in saline and injecting them intravenously. The family member called the physician and hospice nurse for help, but "when I asked what went wrong, they had no idea." Despite these frustrations with clinician expertise, patients and family members remained genuinely appreciative of clinicians' efforts on their behalf.

Maintenance of a Therapeutic Patient-Clinician Relationship, Even When Patient and Clinician Disagree about PAS

Every patient and family member in this study recognized that asking for PAS was a special request that went beyond the usual boundaries of a clinician-patient relationship. Maintaining the clinician-patient relationship was made possible by clinician openness to discussion and clinician expertise. Also, it involved explicit negotiation about the roles of each party in the relationship as well as clinician self-awareness of emotional vulnerabilities. Patients and family members were relieved and reassured when clinicians made an explicit commitment to assist with PAS in some way. However, when clinicians declined to participate and were able to set clear boundaries about their role, as in the example below, they could still maintain an important relationship with a patient and family member.

My internist simply will not do [PAS], not just because of fear of the law, [but] because his approach is he will not end life. . . . I adore my internist who, when he had more time, used to make house visits to see [my late husband when he was dying] and pep him up. Wonderful. So I love this guy; I really do, even though I disagree with him on this issue. I love him, and I respect him as a doctor.

When patients had had meaningful relationships with their clinicians, family members often wanted some closure with them. In our study, this occurred both when clinicians assisted PAS in some way and when clinicians evaluated and discussed PAS but did not assist in any way. For example, members of one family went to the physician's office the day after their mother's death: "We took some living flowers and a card and a sweater . . . [my mother] sent him her favorite sweater; it was a men's sweater anyway. So we saw him, and that was our closure with him." In another example, one patient's physician was sympathetic to her situation, said she would help as much as she could with maximizing comfort, but also said that she could not provide a prescription for PAS for legal reasons. The family obtained a prescription elsewhere, and made plans for PAS, all the while maintaining close contact with the physician. The family called this physician the day after the patient died of PAS, in part to reassure the physician that she had done a good job. "[We] told her it went well and that she hadn't failed. She had cried. I mean she wanted to totally help us and just felt her hands were tied." Thus, the therapeutic aspect of a clinician-patient relationship does not rest on a clinician's willingness to provide a lethal prescription.

One case illustrates the importance of clinician self-awareness of emotional needs and vulnerabilities in maintaining a therapeutic relationship. As the family member put it, their physician "lacked boundaries." This physician had an intense relationship with the patient that included daily telephone calls and home visits, and on the night the patient attempted PAS, the physician implemented a backup plan after oral medications failed. After the patient's death, the family member reported that "[the physician] would go over to the hospital to see a patient, and she'd call me at 10 o'clock P.M. and say she wanted to come over [to our house] and sit in the room where he died and 'hang out.' And I'd say no, and she'd come over anyway." After a couple of these incidents, the family member wrote the physician requesting that they have no further contact because he felt burdened by these requests. Regardless of their own beliefs about PAS, clinicians can maintain therapeutic relationships with their patients when open communication, expertise, and appropriate boundaries are present.

Comment

This report describes clinician-patient interactions from a unique set of data involving 35 patients (and their family members) who seriously pursued PAS. The qualitative methodology we used provides an in-depth, behind-the-scenes look from the patient and family perspective on how clinicians dealt with requests for PAS. From more than 3,600 pages of transcribed interviews, we identified three themes describing qualities of clinician-patient interactions that patients and family members valued highly. These themes raise important considerations for physicians and other clinicians about the skills, attitudes, and knowledge needed to handle requests for PAS.

The controversy over the morality of PAS, including surveys of the general public,[22] extensive media coverage of Jack Kevorkian,[23] the 1997 U.S. Supreme Court decision,[13,24] and medical journals,[6,25] has created a context for discussing PAS that highlights potential conflict between patients and clinicians. Discussions about death and dying—even without PAS—engender intense emotions in patients, family members, and clinicians.[26,27] It comes as no surprise that many clinicians would rather avoid the topic altogether. Our finding that clinicians had varying degrees of openness to discussion about PAS (theme 1), and broader discussions of dying as well, leads us to wonder whether published surveys of physicians actually underestimate the degree to which patients wish to talk about PAS. When physicians say that their patients never ask about PAS, it may be because they block the discussion. Maguire[28] has described how clinicians block and avoid the concerns that patients with cancer have about dying. Our data suggest that PAS is another patient concern that is frequently blocked.

The medical literature on responding to PAS requests acknowledges that these discussions can be uncomfortable and awkward, characteristics that can be barriers for physicians. But what has not been described in the literature is the way that patients in our study used discussions about PAS as a starting point for discussions about dying that ranged far beyond PAS. In a medical culture that views death as a failure, dying patients may feel as if they have failed.[29] Physician-assisted suicide provides a different kind of end-of-life story for patients, one that emphasizes individual values and personal choice,[30] and data from patients in Oregon underscore the importance of autonomy for patients who choose PAS.[1] Our data indicate that PAS can serve as the entry point for discussions that go beyond the right to die to explore concerns about dying. Recognizing this can enable clinicians to probe beyond the issue of PAS. In addition to asking, "Why are you considering PAS?" it might be useful to ask, "How do you want your death to go?" or, "How do you want it to look?"

A lack of openness to discussing PAS may result in a "don't ask, don't tell" policy for both patient and clinician. Clinician openness may be crucial for patients to feel comfortable in extending a PAS discussion beyond technical medical issues, such as a lethal prescription, and toward difficult topics such as dying and suffering, which can constitute an unacknowledged "elephant in the room."[31,32] The lack of communication that we observed about PAS suggests that a kind of collusion may occur that enables both patient and clinician to avoid difficult subjects, as has been described in other situations.[28,33] Collusion may allow a clinician to avoid a PAS discussion that is awkward and difficult, but at the cost of missing an opportunity to reassure patients that their concerns will be addressed and that they will not be abandoned.[34,35] Our data suggest that the presence of collusion may be a marker for inadequate clinician communication skills or clinician discomfort with dying, and may lead to the provision of a lethal prescription for PAS without patient evaluation.

Patients and family members also valued expertise in dealing with the dying process (theme 2). The specific aspects of expertise that our subjects mentioned included communication skills, setting reasonable expectations, individualizing pain control, and knowledge about the lethal potential of commonly used medications. The combination of cognitive and affective skills encompassed in these observations resonates with other work describing curricular needs for clinicians in end-of-life care.[36] Our work also underscores the need for clinicians to have both specific content knowledge in discussing and managing dying and patient-centered communications skills in order to respond to requests for PAS.[37,38]

The combination of openness to discussions about PAS and expertise in dealing with the dying process are what make a continued clinician-patient relationship possible when a patient pursues a hastened death. Our data suggest that even for this highly selected group, a therapeutic clinician-patient relationship may be as or more important to patients and family members interested in PAS than a lethal prescription. When the patients in this study approached their clinicians about PAS, they were usually looking for more than just a prescription. They were looking for someone with whom they could build a therapeutic alliance—a person who could act as a sounding board or guide them through the dying process. Although some existing guidelines for responding to PAS requests address the request as a single event, our data emphasize the importance of the process of responding to a request over time in the context of a clinician-patient relationship.

Patients and family members were mindful of the importance of boundaries in therapeutic relationships. Our data show how underinvolvement or overinvolvement by a clinician can be problematic in dealing with patients requesting PAS. These behaviors may reflect the clinician's personal emotions. Block and Billings[9] and Miles[39] have outlined, based on clinical experience and a careful reading of psychological and psychiatric literature, how the personal emotions of clinicians might influence their behavior in dealing with a patient considering PAS. For clinicians, these issues of personal emotion, which may include self-awareness, boundaries, transference, or countertransference, require attention because they can facilitate or complicate the clinical relationship.[40–42] Our findings reinforce other work stressing the importance for clinicians to monitor their own feelings and to establish boundaries in their relationships with patients.

While the strengths of this study are in its detailed, "thick" description of a small group of patients and family members, it also has corresponding limitations. The study participants were a self-selected sample of patients and their family members who were highly motivated to pursue PAS, interested in telling their stories, and physically able to search for and find people willing to help facilitate PAS. Nearly all our participants obtained access to lethal prescriptions despite the illegality. These participants may not be directly comparable to those of other PAS studies in which the patients were enrolled from inpatient palliative care units[43] or had a uniform medical diagnosis.[44,45] In addition, our participants not only exhibited a desire for PAS, as has been studied in other outpatients,[46] but also actively made plans and tried to implement them in order to have a hastened death.

Another study limitation is that we were not able to interview the clinicians involved with our study participants. It is possible that patients and families themselves contributed to the communication issues described here. For example, patients who were secretive about their intention to pursue PAS may not have alerted their clinician to their need to explore a desire for PAS, or they may have colluded with their clinician to avoid discussing PAS.[33]

TABLE 3 Guidelines for Responding to a Patient Requesting Physician-Assisted Suicide (PAS) Suggested by These Data

1. Address the PAS request explicitly and openly.
2. Ask about what kind of death the patient would like to have.
3. After understanding patient wishes and expectations, offer to discuss how dying could be managed.
4. Check patient perception by asking, "What are you taking away from our talk today?"
5. Remember that the process of building a therapeutic relationship is more important than providing a lethal prescription.
6. Monitor yourself for underinvolvement or overinvolvement in the clinician-patient relationship.

Finally, the themes we report are based on patient and family member reports of their perceptions of communication rather than on transcripts or videotapes of actual conversations. However, patient and family perceptions are extremely important, and the three themes that we describe articulate patient and family member concerns that were present in the majority of interviews we conducted.

Based on this study, we suggest a set of guidelines that clinicians might use when responding to patient requests for PAS (Table 3). These guidelines may also be useful for educators who are teaching communication skills that are relevant to end-of-life care.

Conclusions

Responding to a patient request for PAS is an important and complex clinical skill. These clinical discussions occur amid profound moral controversy, the emotions engendered by death and dying, and the technical complexities of contemporary medical care. Our patient and family accounts reveal many missed opportunities for clinicians to engage in therapeutic relationships involving discussions about PAS, dying, and end-of-life care. Clinicians responding to patients requesting PAS need communication skills that will enable them to discuss PAS and dying openly, an ability to talk about dying in a patient-centered way, and palliative care expertise. They also need expertise in setting reasonable expectations, individualizing pain control, and providing accurate information about the lethal potential of medications.

APPENDIX: PARTICIPANTS AND METHODS

Participant Recruitment and Informed Consent

We asked intermediate sources such as patient advocacy organizations that counsel persons interested in PAS, hospices, and grief counselors to introduce our study to potential participants. Our intermediate sources gave detailed written information statements describing the study to prospective patients with life-threatening illnesses (and their family members) who expressed a serious interest in PAS and were attempting to obtain medications for PAS. Our definition of *family member* included unmarried partners and close friends. We also asked our sources to mail information statements to family members who had been involved in PAS. These information statements asked potential participants to call our office if they wished to participate or ask questions about the study. One investigator (H.S.) spoke with each potential participant to explain study procedures, answer questions, obtain verbal informed consent, enroll participants, and collect demographic data.

To protect the confidentiality of our participants, no written consent forms or any other forms with identifying data were maintained by the investigators. The detailed information statements described the purpose of the study, interview procedures, and participants' right to refuse to answer questions or to withdraw from the study at any time. Prospective patients had to have an ongoing relationship with a case manager and medical care providers to be eligible for the study. Subjects in the prospective cohort were informed verbally and in the written information statement that if interviewers identified a serious medical or psychiatric issue that was not being addressed, or if a psychiatric issue was causing decisional incapacity, investigators would inform the patient's case manager and we would discontinue interviews with the patient and his or her family. These issues were discussed with participants in detail, and informed consent was obtained verbally before each interview. Also, the interview guide for prospective patients contained a statement assuring patients that we were interested in their concerns and decision-making processes and would continue to follow them regardless of whether or not they ultimately decided to pursue PAS. Study procedures were reviewed and approved by the Institutional Review Board of the University of Washington, Seattle.

Data Collection

We conducted multiple qualitative, semistructured interviews with patients and family members. Five investigators conducted interviews, and the same investigator interviewed all participating members of a family. The prospective cases included interviews with 12 patients and 20 family members. The retrospective cases included interviews with 28 family members concerning 23 patients. In total, we conducted 159 interviews with 60 participants from about 35 families (12 prospective and 23 retrospective), resulting in 3,613 pages of transcripts. The interview guide included questions about (1) patient and family interactions with health care providers regarding PAS requests, (2) how these requests were evaluated, and (3) the provider's involvement with PAS implementation. We asked participants to provide details about the manner of death and any complications of a PAS attempt. We also asked family members to describe their personal reactions to the PAS request and subsequent events. Other topics were covered but are not included in this analysis.

Coding and Analytic Methods

All interviews were audiotaped and transcribed, with identifying data deleted. Each case was discussed at weekly meetings by the multidisciplinary research team representing medical oncology, palliative care, health services, psychology, anthropology, psychiatry, geriatrics, and bioethics. The analytic approach was based on grounded theory, which involves open coding (a process of examining, comparing, conceptualizing, and categorizing data), followed by axial coding (a process of reassembling data into groupings based on relationships discovered in the data) and, finally, selective coding (a process of identifying and describing central phenomena in the data).

We coded patients' and family members' firsthand accounts of interactions with clinicians, and did not code hearsay accounts. Examples of primary codes include "reasons for pursuing PAS," "interactions with health care providers," and "planning for death." The interviewer and another investigator independently coded all transcripts, compared coding, and resolved disagreements in coding. Significant coding discrepancies were discussed at the weekly team meeting.

Axial coding involved all sections of transcripts assigned the primary code "interactions with health care providers" for the analysis presented here. Two investigators (A.L.B. and H.S.) developed secondary codes that classified clinician-patient interactions. The intent of the secondary coding was to characterize clinician-patient communication about PAS, non-PAS end-of-life issues, and palliative care. Secondary codes were used to classify subject perceptions of PAS conversations; clinician knowledge, attitudes, and skills; and clinician-patient relationship issues. Examples of secondary codes include "explicit PAS discussion," "clinician willingness to discuss dying," and "clinician empathy." The secondary codes were refined through review with the multidisciplinary research team. At this stage, participants' statements about what they valued in their clinician's response to a PAS request, or what they wanted but did not get in their clinician's response to a PAS request, emerged as central issues.

Finally, in selective coding, the key phenomena that related to the issue of how patients and family members wanted clinicians to respond to PAS requests were identified. Our analysis at this step differs from some other grounded-theory studies in that we did not attempt to build a completely new theory of clinician-patient communication. Rather, we focused on patient and family perceptions of clinician-patient communication in order to describe key attributes of communication about PAS. The three major themes we report are the products of this analysis. These themes were shared among patients and family members and did not differ between prospective and retrospective subjects.

To enhance trustworthiness, each step of the analysis was reviewed in weekly investigator meetings to ensure that the analysis was anchored to specific identifiable data from transcripts. ATLAS.ti software was used to facilitate data management and analysis.[21] The themes from this analysis were presented at a meeting of our patient advocacy intermediate sources (a group that includes clinicians, advocates, and family members), and we received verbal and written feedback confirming the validity of our analysis. No major changes were made as a result of this presentation.

NOTES

1 Chin AE, Hedberg K, Higginson GK, Fleming DW. Legalized physician-assisted suicide in Oregon—the first year's experience. *N Engl J Med.* 1999;340:577–583.

2 Emanuel EJ, Fairclough DL, Emanuel LL. Attitudes and desires related to euthanasia and physician-assisted suicide among terminally ill patients and their caregivers. *JAMA.* 2000;284:2460–2468.

3 Back AL, Wallace JI, Starks HE, Pearlman RA. Physician-assisted suicide and euthanasia in Washington State: patient requests and physician responses. *JAMA.* 1996;275:919–925.

4 Meier DE, Emmons CA, Wallenstein S, Quill T, Morrison RS, Cassel CK. A national survey of physician-assisted suicide and euthanasia in the United States. *N Engl J Med.* 1998;338:1193–1201.

5 Emanuel EJ, Fairclough DL, Daniels ER, Clarridge BR. Euthanasia and physician-assisted suicide: attitudes and experiences of oncology patients, oncologists, and the public. *Lancet.* 1996;347:1805–1810.

6 Foley KM. Competent care for the dying instead of physician-assisted suicide. *N Engl J Med.* 1997;336:54–58.

7 Emanuel LL. Facing requests for physician-assisted suicide: toward a practical and principled clinical skill set. *JAMA.* 1998;280:643–647.

8 Quill TE, Cassel CK, Meier DE. Care of the hopelessly ill: proposed clinical criteria for physician-assisted suicide. *N Engl J Med.* 1992;327:1380–1384.

9 Block SD, Billings JA. Patient requests to hasten death: evaluation and management in terminal care. *Arch Intern Med.* 1994;154:2039–2047.

10 Block SD, Billings JA. Patient requests for euthanasia and assisted suicide in terminal illness: the role of the psychiatrist. *Psychosomatics.* 1995;36:445–457.

11 Emanuel LL, von Gunten CF, Ferris FD, Portenoy RK. *Education for Physicians in End-of-Life Care (EPEC) Trainer's Guide.* Chicago, IL: American Medical Association; 1999.

12 Quill TE, Byock IR. Responding to intractable terminal suffering: the role of terminal sedation and voluntary refusal of food and fluids: ACP-ASIM End-of-Life Care Consensus Panel: American College of Physicians–American Society of Internal Medicine. *Ann Intern Med.* 2000;132:408–414.

13 Orentlicher D. The Supreme Court and physician-assisted suicide—rejecting assisted suicide but embracing euthanasia. *N Engl J Med.* 1997;337:1236–1239.

14 Sulmasy DP, Ury WA, Ahronheim JC, et al. Publication of papers on assisted suicide and terminal sedation. *Ann Intern Med.* 2000;133:564–566.

15 Quill TE. Death and dignity: a case of individualized decision making. *N Engl J Med.* 1991;324:691–694.

16 Van der Wal G, van Eijk JT, Leenen HJ, Spreeuwenberg C. Euthanasia and assisted suicide, II: do Dutch family doctors act prudently? *Fam Pract.* 1992;9:135–140.

17 Kohlwes RJ, Koepsell TD, Rhodes LA, Pearlman RA. Physicians' responses to patients' requests for assisted suicide. *Arch Intern Med.* 2000;161:657–663.

18 Duin S, Barnett E. Brian's journey. *Oregonian.* November 25, 1998:A1.

19 Rollin B. *Last Wish.* New York: Simon & Schuster; 1985.

20 Jamison S. *Final Acts of Love: Family, Friends, and Assisted Dying.* New York: GP Putnam's Sons; 1995.

21 Muhr T. *ATLAS.ti* [computer program]. Version 4.0. Berlin, Germany: Scientific Software; 1999.

22 Blendon RJ, Szalay US, Knox RA. Should physicians aid their patients in dying? the public perspective. *JAMA.* 1992;267:2658–2662.

23 Brody H. Kevorkian and assisted death in the United States. *BMJ.* 1999;318:953–954.

24 Burt RA. The Supreme Court speaks—not assisted suicide but a constitutional right to palliative care. *N Engl J Med.* 1997;337:1234–1236.

25 Angell M. The Supreme Court and physician-assisted suicide—the ultimate right. *N Engl J Med.* 1997;336:50–53.

26 Siegel B. Crying in stairwells: how should we grieve for dying patients? *JAMA.* 1994;272:659.

27 Parkes CM. The dying adult. *BMJ.* 1998;316:1313–1315.

28 Maguire P. Improving communication with cancer patients. *Eur J Cancer.* 1999;35: 1415–1422.

29 Field MJ, Cassel CK. *Approaching Death: Improving Care at the End of Life.* Washington, DC: National Academy Press; 1997.

30 Humphry D. *Final Exit.* Eugene, OR: Hemlock Society; 1991.

31 Quill TE. Initiating end-of-life discussions with seriously ill patients: addressing the "elephant in the room." *JAMA.* 2000;284:2502–2507.

32 Lo B, Quill T, Tulsky J. Discussing palliative care with patients: ACP-ASIM End-of-Life Care Consensus Panel: American College of Physicians-American Society of Internal Medicine. *Ann Intern Med.* 1999;130:744–749.

33 The AM, Hak T, Koeter G, van der Wal G. Collusion in doctor-patient communication about imminent death: an ethnographic study. *West J Med.* 2001;174:247–253.

34 Quill TE, Cassell CK. Nonabandonment: a central obligation for physicians. *Ann Intern Med.* 1995;5:368–374.

35 Epstein RM, Morse DS, Frankel RM, Frarey L, Anderson K, Beckman HB. Awkward moments in patient-physician communication about HIV risk. *Ann Intern Med.* 1998;128:435–442.

36 Curtis JR, Wenrich MD, Carline JD, Shannon SE, Ambrozy DM, Ramsey PG. Understanding physicians' skills at providing end-of-life care perspectives of patients, families, and health care workers. *J Gen Intern Med.* 2001;16:41–49.

37 Roter DL, Larson S, Fischer GS, Arnold RM, Tulsky JA. Experts practice what they preach: a descriptive study of best and normative practices in end-of-life discussions. *Arch Intern Med.* 2000;160:3477–3485.

38 Emanuel EJ, Fairclough D, Clarridge BC, et al. Attitudes and practices of U.S. oncologists regarding euthanasia and physician-assisted suicide. *Ann Intern Med.* 2000;133:527–532.

39 Miles SH. Physicians and their patients' suicides. *JAMA.* 1994;271:1786–1788.

40 Novack DH, Suchman AL, Clark W, Epstein RM, Najberg E, Kaplan C. Calibrating the physician: personal awareness and effective patient care: Working Group on Promoting Physician Personal Awareness, American Academy on Physician and Patient. *JAMA.* 1997;278:502–509.

41 Farber NJ, Novack DH, O'Brien MK. Love, boundaries, and the patient-physician relationship. *Arch Intern Med.* 1997;157:2291–2294.

42 Balint M. *The Doctor, His Patient, and the Illness.* New York: International Universities Press Inc; 1957.

43 Breitbart W, Rosenfeld B, Pessin H, et al. Depression, hopelessness, and desire for hastened death in terminally ill patients with cancer. *JAMA.* 2000;284:2907–2911.

44 Ganzini L, Johnston WS, McFarland BH, Tolle SW, Lee MA. Attitudes of patients with amyotrophic lateral sclerosis and their care givers toward assisted suicide. *N Engl J Med.* 1998;339:967–973.

45 Chochinov HM, Wilson KG, Enns M, et al. Desire for death in the terminally ill. *Am J Psychiatry.* 1995;152:1185–1191.

46 Lavery JV, Boyle J, Dickens BM, Maclean H, Singer PA. Origins of the desire for euthanasia and assisted suicide in people with HIV-1 or AIDS: a qualitative study. *Lancet.* 2001;358:362–367.

My Father's Death

Susan M. Wolf

Duty: An act . . . required of one by position, social custom, law, or
religion. . . . Moral obligation.
—*American Heritage Dictionary of the English Language*, 4TH ED.

My father's death forced me to rethink all I had written over two decades
opposing legalization of physician-assisted suicide and euthanasia.[1] That
should not have surprised me. Years ago, when I started working on end-of-
life care, he challenged my views on advance directives by insisting that he
would want "everything," even in a persistent vegetative state. "I made the
money, so I can spend it." More deeply, he argued that the Holocaust was
incompatible with the existence of God. There is no afterlife, he claimed.
This is it, and he wanted every last bit of "it" on any terms.

My father was a smart, savvy lawyer, the family patriarch. He was force-
ful, even intimidating at times. We had fought over the years, especially as I
neared college. That was probably necessary—my separating and our disen-
gaging. When I was a child, it was a family joke how often he and I said the
same thing at the same time. We were alike in many ways.

My father was diagnosed with a metastatic head and neck cancer in 2002.
His predictable view was "spare no effort." A top head and neck surgeon
worked through conflicting pathology reports to locate the primary tumor
in the thyroid and excise the gland. Metastases would crop up from time to
time, but radiation and then CyberKnife radiosurgery kept them in check.
For five years he did well.

Things changed in June of 2007. The last CyberKnife treatment was billed
as the worst, with significant pain likely to follow. Sure enough, ten days later,
my father's pain on swallowing became severe. He began losing weight—a

Susan M. Wolf, "Confronting Physician-Assisted Suicide and Euthanasia: My Father's Death,"
from *Hastings Center Report* 38, no. 5 (2008): 23–26. Reprinted by permission of John Wiley
and Sons.

lot of it. He weakened. He fell twice in his apartment. His regular internist was out of town, so he went to the emergency room of a local hospital. Doctors did little for this 79-year-old man with a 5-year history of metastatic thyroid cancer plus emphysema and chronic obstructive pulmonary disease.

He was briefly discharged to home but finally made it to the head and neck surgeon who had found the primary tumor in 2002. One look at my father and the surgeon admitted him, ordering a gastrostomy tube to deliver nutrition. Now my father was in an excellent hospital, with the head and neck, pulmonology, and gastroenterology services working him up. The mood brightened and the family gathered around him. I spent days in his sunny hospital room reminiscing, plowing through the *New York Times* with him, singing the college fight songs he offered as lullabies when I was little.

With multiple services focusing on my father's condition, I hoped the picture would soon come clear. I waited for a single physician to put the pieces together. And the medical picture was becoming worse. A surgical procedure revealed cancer in the liver. Pulmonology added pneumonia to the roster of lung ailments. Meanwhile, dipping oxygen saturation numbers drove a trip to the intensive care unit. Attempted endoscopy revealed a tumor between the esophagus and trachea, narrowing the esophagus. But no physician was putting the whole picture together. What treatment and palliative options remained, if any? What pathways should he—and we—be considering at this point?

He Said He Wanted to Stop

My father was becoming increasingly weak. He was finding it difficult to "focus," as he put it. He could not read, do the *New York Times* crossword puzzles he used to knock off in an hour, or even watch TV. Fortunately, he could talk, and we spent hours on trips he had taken around the world, family history, his adventures as a litigator. But he was confined to bed and did little when he was alone.

Then one morning he said he wanted to stop. No more tube feeding. No one was prepared for this switch from a lifetime of "spare no effort." He told me he feared he was now a terrible burden. I protested, knowing that I would willingly bear the "burden" of his illness. I suspect that what others said was more powerful, though. I was later told that the doctor urged him not to stop, warning that he would suffer a painful death, that morphine would be required to control the discomfort, and that my father would lose consciousness before the day was out. Instead of assuring my father that health professionals know how to maintain comfort after termination of artificial nutrition and hydration, my father was scared away from this option. Weeks later, my father would wish aloud that he had carried through with this decision.

Convinced now that he had no choice, my father soldiered on. But hospital personnel announced that it was time for him to leave the hospital. We were incredulous. He could not stand, walk, or eat. He had bedsores. Even transferring him from bed to a chair was difficult. And the rigors of transporting him in the early August heat were worrisome. But they urged transfer to a rehabilitation facility. My father was assured that with continued tube feeding and rehab, he could be walking into the surgeon's office in October.

It seemed to me my father was being abandoned. His prognosis was clearly bad and he himself had now raised the prospect of stopping tube feeding and dying, but it shocked me to see the hospital try to get rid of him. Yes, the hospital said he could return (somehow) in late September to see the ENT oncologist. But as far as I knew, that physician had never even met my father. And I doubted my father would make it to September. Still, no one was integrating the big picture. There seemed to be little choice. My father was successfully transported by ambulance to another hospital with a well-regarded rehabilitation unit.

The transfer provided brief respite. My father was delighted that he was now only blocks from his apartment, and the enticing possibility of actually going home beckoned. But the rehab unit demanded hours per day of rigorous work from each patient. My father was too weak. And his pneumonia was an issue. He was moved off rehab to the medical floor. A compassionate and attentive hospitalist appeared, trying to put together the big picture. She set about collecting the reports from the prior two hospitals and integrating them. Again, many teams were on board, including rheumatology now for flaring gout.

I requested the palliative care team. Even though my father could be lucid and "himself," I listened painfully as he faltered through the questions on their mini–mental exam. It was hard to accept that this paragon of analytic and verbal precision was failing. I alerted a member of the palliative care team that my father had evidently been misinformed at the prior hospital about the consequences of stopping artificial nutrition and hydration. I urged her to find a time to reassure him that he indeed had choices, could refuse treatments if he wanted to, and could be confident that his comfort would be maintained. I made clear to her that I hoped he would choose to stay the course for now and remain with us, but that he deserved to know that he had the choice. My father had designated his two proxy decision makers (one of them me), but could still participate in the medical decision making. His values and his subjective experience—whether he wanted more interventions or had reached his limit—were key.

Still unresolved, though, was the question of where we were headed. Could tube feeding and rehab bring him home and even walking into the surgeon's office in October? Was there treatment that could slow the growth of the newly discovered cancer in his lung? Should we instead pursue hospice care? At times, my father's illness seemed like *Rashomon*, a story with conflicting versions and possible trajectories. But soon my father was back in the ICU, with oxygen saturation percentages dipping into the seventies. Tube feeding was so uncomfortable that it was administered slowly through the night. Pain medication was a constant. Despite this, he held court in his room, enjoying the banter, and offering his own with that wry smile and cocked eyebrow.

He was briefly transferred to the pulmonary care unit, as the most pressing issues at this point were actually not cancer but lung mucus and secretions, as well as pneumonia. I arrived one morning to find him upset. His nurse was not answering his calls, and his immobility left him at her mercy. I summoned the highly experienced and empathetic supervisor, but even behind closed doors with her he was afraid to speak plainly. I saw this tough-as-nails litigator reduced to fearful dependence.

"Can We Accelerate?"

By morning there was a new problem. My father had developed a massive bleed. Nursing had found him in a pool of his own blood, lying among the clots. The gastroenterologists took him in for a procedure, spending hours trying to find the source of the bleed. They never found it. My father required transfusion of most of his blood volume. The bleeding abated, but we knew it could resume any time.

That was it—the final blow. My father was back in the ICU now, but the bleed and the hours spent searching for its source were too much. He waited until we gathered at his bedside. His speech was halting now, but his determination obvious. "Tell me my choices." We went through each option—you can keep going like this, or you can go back to the floor if the ICU is bothering you, or you can halt the tube feeding and IV hydration. You also can wait, rather than deciding right now.

For close to an hour we stayed in a tight circle around his bed, straining to hear his every word, crying, responding to each question. At one point, I thought he wanted to wait, but he called us back. "It could happen again. At 2 A.M.," he said. He wanted a decision now. "That's what I want. To terminate." He made it clear he wanted to stop tube feeding and IV hydration. But that wasn't enough. He wanted consensus.

With the decision made, we set about communicating it to the caregivers and getting new orders written. It was then that he uttered three words that shook me. "Can we accelerate?" It seemed he was asking for more—a fast death, by assisted suicide or euthanasia. Reflexively, I said no, but with a promise—we can make absolutely certain they keep you comfortable. Even if you can't talk, even if you appear comatose, if you merely furrow your brow, we'll know you need more pain medication.

I knew right away that I needed to think through my "no." In reality, we were in the ICU of a major hospital in a jurisdiction that allowed neither assisted suicide nor euthanasia. Indeed, no jurisdiction in the United States allows euthanasia, and my father was beyond assisted suicide by swallowing prescribed lethal medication, as he couldn't swallow anything. But I still needed to think this through.

I knew that in some ways, my father presented what proponents of assisted suicide and euthanasia would regard as a strong case. He was clearly dying of physical causes, unlike the controversial 1991 *Chabot* case in the Netherlands involving a patient who was merely depressed. He certainly had less than six months to live. He was probably depressed by his illness, but in a way that was appropriate to his situation. His decisional capacity had surely declined, but he was able to express definite treatment preferences.

Moreover, he wasn't asking for a change in policy or law. Statewide or national changes in policy require considering a huge range of patients, anticipating the predictable errors and abuses. The Dutch have bravely documented all of this through empirical study of their practice of legalized euthanasia—violations of the requirement for a contemporaneous request by a competent patient, doctors failing to report the practice as required, and practice falling down the slippery slope to euthanasia of newborns.[2] Oregon has documented its experience with legalized assisted suicide, too, but only the cases reported as required, leaving great uncertainty about cases not reported.[3] My father wasn't asking for societal change, though, only whether he himself could "accelerate." I faced the highly individual question of how to do right by my own father.

In truth, it was life that answered the question, not logic. In some ways, it would have been psychologically easier, or at least faster, to bring the ordeal we all were experiencing to a quick end. I was in a city far from my husband and children, doing shifts at my father's bedside at all hours, fearful of more looming medical disasters increasing his discomfort. But instead of ending all of this and fleeing, we stayed, redoubling our attention to him. I stroked his thick white hair. He and I reminisced. He was always a great raconteur. We talked and talked over the next days. The decision to stop tube feeding actually seemed to lighten his load. A decision. In a way, it was a relief.

And executing the decision took work, itself a devotion. It was around 6 P.M. when the decision was made. The ICU doctor came to the bedside to confirm the new plan and assure my father that he would be kept comfortable. But the palliative care professional, about to go off-duty, insisted that my father would need to leave the hospital. I was astonished. Was she saying he could not terminate treatment here? That the hospital had no in-patient hospice care? That you could accept invasive treatment at this hospital, but not refuse it? After years of working on end-of-life issues, I knew better. I confronted her: "You know that my father has a constitutional and common law right to refuse invasive treatment, including in this hospital." She acceded, but insisted that he would no longer meet the criteria for hospitalization; he would need to leave, to a hospice facility or home. The hospital evidently had no hospice to offer. Fine, we would set about arranging admission to hospice.

There was more—concerns over whether the fluid flowing through a remaining line would wrongly prolong his life and whether giving morphine by pump rather than through his line would do the same. I reached out by cell phone and email to colleagues who were expert in maintaining comfort when artificial nutrition and hydration are stopped. We signed the papers requesting transfer to hospice. At one point, my father asked, "Will I see the end coming or fade away?" No one in the hospital was counseling my father. I worked my cell phone for answers and carried them to my father's bedside. To a man who could hold no faith after the Holocaust, I even brought the words and experience of my rabbi.

We kept vigil, around the clock. He was out of the ICU now, in a hospital room awaiting transfer to hospice. As he began to doze more and talk less, we watched carefully for the slightest sign of discomfort. We had promised we would assure his comfort. That meant constant vigilance.

The last time I saw my father, he was motionless. His eyes were closed. He had stopped speaking. He appeared unresponsive. His breathing was quieter, rasps gone with dehydration. I took his hand. I told him I loved him. I stroked his hair, still full and silvered. I spoke to him from the heart, words that remain between him and me. Then I heard myself say, "If I am a good mother, it's because you were a great father." And to my surprise, he moved his jaw. Not his lips or his mouth. But he opened his jaw three times. It was our signal, the one we'd worked out in the ICU. Three means "I-love-you." Tears streamed down my face. I struggled, remembering the rabbi's caution that the ones we love most may need permission to leave us, to die. "I know you may have to leave before I get back. That's okay." It felt nearly impossible to let him go. My chest was bursting. The pain was crushing.

When I finally left, I was working to breathe. Taking one step then another. Breaking down, collecting myself, breaking down again. He died not long after.

In the End

I will not pretend—there was a price to be paid for going the longer way, not the shorter. My father died slowly. He had to trust that we would keep a ferocious vigil, demanding whatever palliative care he needed. It was he who traveled that road, not me. I paid my own price, though. I felt the heavy weight of his trust and the obligation to fight for him. I was scared I might fail. I felt very close to the jaws of death.

But with every memory we shared while he could speak, every lilt of his eyebrow and wry smile, we basked together in life, reveled in a bit more of 54 years together and his nearly 80 on this earth. Family and caregivers did manage to keep him comfortable. He died loved and loving.

I grieve still. I reread the letters he wrote home from Oxford in his 20s, I pore over the genealogy charts he painstakingly constructed over decades, I finger the abacus he kept in his law office. I go to email him, then remember. I would not want to bear the burden of having "accelerated," of causing his death by euthanasia or assisted suicide; this is hard enough. My father's death made me rethink my objections to legalizing assisted suicide and euthanasia, but in the end it left me at ease with what I've written. Staying, keeping vigil, fighting to secure a comfortable death, stroking his hair, standing guard as death approached was my duty. It was the final ripening of my love. We both changed, even closer at the end.

NOTES

1 In the mid-1980s, I had led the Hastings Center project that developed *Guidelines on the Termination of Life-Sustaining Treatment and the Care of the Dying* (Indianapolis: Indiana University Press, 1987). For a sample of my subsequent work on physician-assisted suicide, see "Gender, Feminism, and Death: Physician-Assisted Suicide and Euthanasia," in *Feminism and Bioethics: Beyond Reproduction*, ed. S. M. Wolf (New York: Oxford University Press, 1996), 282–317; "Physician-Assisted Suicide in the Context of Managed Care," *Duquesne Law Review* 35 (1996): 455–479; "Physician-Assisted Suicide, Abortion, and Treatment Refusal: Using Gender to Analyze the Difference," in *Physician-Assisted Suicide*, ed. R. Weir (Indianapolis: Indiana University Press, 1997), 167–201; "Facing Assisted Suicide and Euthanasia in Children and Adolescents," in *Regulating How We Die: The Ethical, Medical, and Legal Issues Surrounding Physician-Assisted Suicide*, ed. L. L. Emanuel (Cambridge, MA.: Harvard University Press, 1998), 92–119, 274–294; "Pragmatism in the Face of Death: The Role of Facts in the Assisted Suicide Debate," *Minnesota Law Review* 82 (1998): 1063–1101; and "Assessing Physician Compliance with the Rules for Euthanasia and Assisted Suicide," *Archives of Internal Medicine* 165 (2005): 1677–1679.

2 I discuss all of this in my work cited above. See also P. J. van der Maas et al., "Euthanasia and Other Medical Decisions Concerning the End of Life," *Lancet* 338 (1991): 669–674; L. Pijnenborg et al., "Life-Terminating Acts without Explicit Request of Patient," *Lancet* 341 (1993): 1196–1199; P. J. van der Maas et al., "Euthanasia, Physician-Assisted Suicide, and Other Medical Practices Involving the End of Life in the Netherlands, 1990–1995," *New England Journal of Medicine* 335 (1996): 1699–1705; G. van der Wal et al., "Evaluation of the Notification Procedure for Physician-Assisted Death in the Netherlands," *New England Journal of Medicine* 335 (1996): 1706–1711; A. van der Heide and P. J. van der Maas, "Medical End-of-Life Decisions Made for Neonates and Infants in the Netherlands," *Lancet* 350 (1997): 251–255; B. D. Onwuteaka-Philipsen et al., "Euthanasia and Other End-of-Life Decisions in the Netherlands in 1990, 1995, and 2001," *Lancet* 362 (2003): 395–399; T. Sheldon, "Only Half of Dutch Doctors Report Euthanasia, Report Says," *British Medical Journal* 326 (2003): 1164; T. Sheldon, "Dutch Reporting of Euthanasia Cases Falls—Despite Legal Reporting Requirements," *British Medical Journal* 328 (2004): 1336; B. D. Onwuteaka-Philipsen et al., "Dutch Experience of Monitoring Euthanasia," *British Medical Journal* 331 (2005): 691–693; E. Verhagen and P. J. J. Sauer, "The Groningen Protocol: Euthanasia in Severely Ill Newborns," *New England Journal of Medicine* 352 (2005): 959–962; A. van der Heide et al., "End-of-Life Practices in the Netherlands under the Euthanasia Act," *New England Journal of Medicine* 356 (2007): 1957–1965.

3 See K. Foley and H. Hendin, "The Oregon Report: Don't Ask, Don't Tell," *Hastings Center Report* 29, no. 3 (1999): 37–42; E. J. Emanuel, "Oregon's Physician-Assisted Suicide Law: Provisions and Problems," *Archives of Internal Medicine* 156 (1996): 825–829.

ALLOCATION AND JUSTICE

V

Glossary

Justice and the Allocation of Health Resources

Rebecca L. Walker and Larry R. Churchill

Health-related resources are allocated in a vast array of different ways and by multiple agents. Among the many allocating agents are individual clinicians, institutions such as hospitals, insurers, and communities, as well as legal and government bodies. The levels of allocation also range from micro to macro. For example, resources can be allocated between and among individual patients, groups of patients, and communities, and by using criteria such as insurance type, residency, and institutional affiliation, among many others. Health-related resources are much broader than medical interventions, drugs, and devices. Other, perhaps more significant, resources include *health care access* (including adequate insurance and available and attentive providers), *public health resources* (including clean water, immunizations, and health behavior programs), and the *social determinants* that help shape health outcomes (including wealth, education, and social status). How we allocate health-related resources has much to do with the type of resource, the agents doing the allocation, and the level at which the resource is being distributed.

For example, allocation of solid organs from deceased donors is managed within the United States by a single body—the United Network for Organ Sharing—a private network that the federal government has contracted with since 1986 to run the nation's Organ Procurement and Transplantation Network. The network uses multiple criteria for different organ systems to allocate, by region, among individuals on a national wait list. Allocation of health insurance, on the other hand, depends on multiple factors including individual ability to pay, government allocation of funds and policies determining enrollment (for example, for Medicaid), job status (for insurance through employers), and immigration status.

No matter the level at which health-related resources are allocated, however, ethical considerations of justice come into play. Larger-scale philosophical theories regarding *distributive justice* have included *egalitarian* theories, which track the moral equality of persons by aiming for some kind of equality in the distribution of social goods; *utilitarian* theories, which aim to maximize the collective welfare outcomes for all those affected by a particular allocation; and *libertarian* theories, which emphasize freedom by envisioning that *whatever* distribution arises from the free exchange of goods and services between politically equal individuals is just. Such broad-scale theories, however, must be interpreted through the lens of particular allocation principles and methods that further the underlying values that the theories promote. Below we list a number of principles and methods of allocation that have been proposed as relevant to the allocation of health resources. It is important to note that most real-world allocation methods appeal to or include multiple allocation principles.

WILLINGNESS TO PAY · According to this method, people's willingness to pay for health resources (or health insurance) mirrors the value they place on these resources as opposed to other goods they also value. Distributing according to willingness to pay by using markets thus allows maximum freedom of choice between different kinds of goods. This method is in keeping with philosophical libertarian theories of distributive justice that place a premium on both individual freedom of choice and responsibility for choices. It does not attend to social determinants of choices or to equality of outcomes.

MERIT JUSTICE · is "backward looking" in that it considers a person's past actions in deciding how to allocate health resources. With respect to health care, this principle takes into account the role of individual responsibility for health outcomes. Those who appear to be the most blameless with regard to their health care needs receive resources and services first and/or those seen as negligently responsible for their health might receive lesser priority. Merit justice might also take a broader view of individual "merit" and allocate fewer resources to those persons who have committed crimes or have otherwise "earned" less support from society. This principle may be in keeping with a libertarian theory of distributive justice in so far as it emphasizes personal choice and responsibility.

JUSTICE AS SOCIAL WORTH · is "forward looking" because it takes into consideration future societal contributions when allocating health care. This is not merely preference for those with greater social status (such as the president or famous people), but rather promotes those who contribute in various ways to other people in society (those caring for dependents, those with jobs supporting social infrastructure, those whose ideas may lead to great future health care breakthroughs, or even those who can entertain others). In general, more effort is expended on those who can recover and be productive. A utilitarian theory of distributive justice, according to which we allocate so as to achieve the greatest happiness for the greatest number, will take such considerations into account (as long as taking such considerations into account doesn't itself unduly undermine utility).

———

COST-BENEFIT ANALYSIS (CBA) · is closely related to social worth considerations but focuses on social contributions in dollar amounts and future financial drain as well as on costs of the health interventions. The aim is to allocate health resources in ways that give the most overall financial gain and the least overall financial expenditure for the greatest health benefit. This method takes into account such nonhealth outcomes as ability to return to work and the overall cost of a person's continued ill health on social resources. CBA is compatible with a limited-scope utilitarian analysis (e.g., one focused not on broader welfare, but on social contribution as measured economically).

———

COST-EFFECTIVENESS ANALYSIS (CEA) · is closely related to cost-benefit analysis, but does not take into account nonhealth outcomes or future costs. CEA aims to achieve the most healthy life years overall for the population served at the least financial cost for the intervention at issue. This method is often seen as synonymous with choosing the most "efficient" health resource distribution. Like CBA, CEA is compatible with a limited-scope utilitarian analysis (focused on health-related quality of life measures).

———

RESOURCE EGALITARIANISM · aims to give each person an equal share of social resources. Social resources are those resources that everyone has some claim on because they are gained through social cooperation. For example, those resources that the government legitimately gains through taxation may be called "social resources." With respect to health care, this type of theory might support equal health insurance for all. Other health-related egalitarian principles, in addition to those listed below, strive for equality in health outcomes or in health satisfaction.

CAPACITY EGALITARIANISM · aims for all to have equal capacities to choose between various visions of "the good life." On this theory, distributing resources equally is not really equitable since people have different views of what they want to do and who they want to be, and also start off with very different capacities. What we really want is to distribute equally the *capacity* or *freedom* to achieve those ends.

PRIORITARIAN PRINCIPLE · According to this principle, we should distribute resources in a way that maximizes the position of the least well-off person. With respect to health resources, this will mean that we have to assist the *most ill first*. In an emergency situation, for example, this principle prioritizes rescue for those nearest to death. In a different context, like providing insurance, this principle would prioritize insuring those most in need of health care and with the least ability to self-pay. This principle is often seen as following from an egalitarian theory of justice.

PRINCIPLE OF RESTORATIVE JUSTICE · Using this principle, resources are prioritized for those whose maladies are caused or exacerbated by previous social or economic injustices. For example, the current concentration of some racial or ethnic minority populations in neighborhoods with high rates of environmental hazards (leading to higher rates of childhood asthma, lead poisoning, and other illness) may be linked to past social and economic injustices, including discriminatory lending policies. Restorative justice is compatible with both egalitarian and libertarian theories. Most clearly, restorative justice is compatible with egalitarian theories that are interested in rectifying persistent inequalities. However, because libertarian theories take political equality as a normative starting place, those individuals who are not politically equally situated because of past injustice should be compensated.

HONOR LONG-STANDING OBLIGATIONS · Here a moral criterion for distributing resources is loyalty to those who have been previously treated, or to whom fidelity is owed because of prior obligations—such as the elderly and persons already dependent on existing programs, services, and technologies. It is not clear which theories of justice this principle is compatible with, though it seems to play a role in medical ethics norms by appealing to moral principles like fidelity and the duty not to abandon patients.

———————

DRAW THE WINNERS FROM A HAT · This lottery approach might be used when all services or recipients are thought to be equally meritorious, or when their relative worth cannot be (or should not be) judged. Proponents of a lottery method say it gives everyone an equal chance. Opponents call it gambling and consider it a choice by default. This method could be appealing to different theories of justice under the right circumstances. For example, an egalitarian theory could support this allocation method if all participants truly are otherwise equal. A utilitarian theory could support the method if introduction of randomness in the distributive mechanism makes people happier overall with the allocation.

Dead Man Walking

Michael Stillman and Monalisa Tailor

"Shocked" wouldn't be accurate, since we were accustomed to our uninsured patients receiving inadequate medical care. "Saddened" wasn't right, either, only pecking at the edge of our response. And "disheartened" just smacked of victimhood. After hearing this story, we were neither shocked nor saddened nor disheartened. We were simply appalled.

We met Tommy Davis in our hospital's clinic for indigent persons in March 2013 (the name and date have been changed to protect the patient's privacy). He and his wife had been chronically uninsured despite working full-time jobs and were now facing disastrous consequences.

The week before this appointment, Mr. Davis had come to our emergency department with abdominal pain and obstipation. His examination, laboratory tests, and CT scan had cost him $10,000 (his entire life savings), and at evening's end he'd been sent home with a diagnosis of metastatic colon cancer.

The year before, he'd had similar symptoms and visited a primary care physician, who had taken a cursory history, told Mr. Davis he'd need insurance to be adequately evaluated, and billed him $200 for the appointment. Since Mr. Davis was poor and ineligible for Kentucky Medicaid, however, he'd simply used enemas until he was unable to defecate. By the time of his emergency department evaluation, he had a fully obstructed colon and widespread disease and chose to forgo treatment.

Mr. Davis had had an inkling that something was awry, but he'd been unable to pay for an evaluation. As his wife sobbed next to him in our examination room, he recounted his months of weight loss, the unbearable pain of his bowel movements, and his gnawing suspicion that he had cancer. "If we'd found it sooner," he contended, "it would have made a difference. But now I'm just a dead man walking."

For many of our patients, poverty alone limits access to care. We recently saw a man with AIDS and a full-body rash who couldn't afford bus fare to a dermatology appointment. We sometimes pay for our patients' medications because they are unable to cover even a $4 copayment. But a fair number of our patients—the medical "have-nots"—are denied basic services simply because they lack insurance, and our country's response to this problem has, at times, seemed toothless.

In our clinic, uninsured patients frequently find necessary care unobtainable. An obese 60-year-old woman with symptoms and signs of congestive heart failure was recently evaluated in the clinic. She couldn't afford the echocardiogram and evaluation for ischemic heart disease that most internists would have ordered, so furosemide treatment was initiated and adjusted to relieve her symptoms. This past spring, our colleagues saw a woman with a newly discovered lung nodule that was highly suspicious for cancer. She was referred to a thoracic surgeon, but he insisted that she first have a PET scan—a test for which she couldn't possibly pay.

However unconscionable we may find the story of Mr. Davis, a U.S. citizen who will die because he was uninsured, the literature suggests that it's a common tale. A 2009 study revealed a direct correlation between lack of insurance and increased mortality and suggested that nearly 45,000 American adults die each year because they have no medical coverage.[1] And although we can't confidently argue that Mr. Davis would have survived had he been insured, research suggests that possibility; formerly uninsured adults given access to Oregon Medicaid were more likely than those who remained uninsured to have a usual place of care and a personal physician, to attend outpatient medical visits, and to receive recommended preventive care.[2] Had Mr. Davis been insured, he might well have been offered timely and appropriate screening for colorectal cancer, and his abdominal pain and obstipation would surely have been urgently evaluated.

Elected officials bear a great deal of blame for the appalling vulnerability of the 22 percent of American adults who currently lack insurance. The Affordable Care Act (ACA)—the only legitimate legislative attempt to provide near-universal health coverage—remains under attack from some members of Congress, and our own two senators argue that enhancing marketplace competition and enacting tort reform will provide security enough for our nation's poor.

In discussing (and grieving over) what has happened to Mr. Davis and our many clinic patients whose health suffers for lack of insurance, we have considered our own obligations. As some congresspeople attempt to defund

Obamacare, and as some states' governors and attorneys general deliberate over whether to implement health insurance exchanges and expand Medicaid eligibility, how can we as physicians ensure that the needs of patients like Mr. Davis are met?

First, we can honor our fundamental professional duty to help. Some have argued that the onus for providing access to health care rests on society at large rather than on individual physicians,[3] yet the Hippocratic Oath compels us to treat the sick according to our ability and judgment and to keep them from harm and injustice. Even as we continue to hope for and work toward a future in which all Americans have health insurance, we believe it's our individual professional responsibility to treat people in need.

Second, we can familiarize ourselves with legislative details and educate our patients about proposed health care reforms. During our appointment with Mr. Davis, he worried aloud that under the ACA, "the government would tax him for not having insurance." He was unaware (as many of our poor and uninsured patients may be) that under that law's final rule, he and his family would meet the eligibility criteria for Medicaid and hence have access to comprehensive and affordable care.

Finally, we can pressure our professional organizations to demand health care for all. The American College of Physicians, the American Medical Association, and the Society of General Internal Medicine have endorsed the principle of universal health care coverage yet have generally remained silent during years of political debate. Lack of insurance can be lethal, and we believe our professional community should treat inaccessible coverage as a public health catastrophe and stand behind people who are at risk.

Seventy percent of our clinic patients have no health insurance, and they are all frighteningly vulnerable; their care is erratic, they are disqualified from receiving certain preventive and screening measures, and their lack of resources prevents them from participating in the medical system. And this is not a community- or state-specific problem. A recent study showed that underinsured patients have higher mortality rates after myocardial infarction,[4] and it is well documented that our country's uninsured present with later-stage cancers and more poorly controlled chronic diseases than do patients with insurance.[5] We find it terribly and tragically inhumane that Mr. Davis and tens of thousands of other citizens of this wealthy country will die this year for lack of insurance.

1   Wilper AP, Woolhandler S, Lasser KE, McCormick D, Bor DH, Himmelstein DU. Health insurance and mortality in US adults. *Am J Public Health*. 2009;99:2289–2295.

2   Finkelstein A, Taubman S, Wright B, et al. The Oregon health insurance experiment: evidence from the first year. *Q J Econ*. 2012;127:1057–1106.

3   Huddle TS, Centor RM. Retainer medicine: an ethically legitimate form of practice that can improve primary care. *Ann Intern Med*. 2011;155:633–635.

4   Ng DK, Brotman DJ, Lau B, Young JH. Insurance status, not race, is associated with mortality after an acute cardiovascular event in Maryland. *J Gen Intern Med*. 2012;27:1368–1376.

5   Institute of Medicine. *America's Uninsured Crisis: Consequences for Health and Health Care*. Washington, DC: National Academies Press; February 23, 2009. http://www.nationalacademies.org/hmd/Reports/2009/Americas-Uninsured-Crisis-Consequences-for-Health-and-Health-Care.aspx.

Full Disclosure

Out-of-Pocket Costs as Side Effects

Peter A. Ubel, Amy P. Abernethy, and S. Yousuf Zafar

Few physicians would prescribe treatments to their patients without first discussing important side effects. When a chemotherapy regimen prolongs survival, for example, but also causes serious side effects such as immuno-suppression or hair loss, physicians are typically thorough about informing patients about those effects, allowing them to decide whether the benefits outweigh the risks. Nevertheless, many patients in the United States experience substantial harm from medical interventions whose risks have not been fully discussed. The undisclosed toxicity? High cost, which can cause considerable financial strain.

Since health care providers don't often discuss potential costs before ordering diagnostic tests or making treatment decisions, patients may unknowingly face daunting and potentially avoidable health care bills. Because treatments can be "financially toxic,"[1] imposing out-of-pocket costs that may impair patients' well-being, we contend that physicians need to disclose the financial consequences of treatment alternatives just as they inform patients about treatments' side effects. Health care costs have risen faster than the Consumer Price Index for most of the past 40 years. This growth in expenditures has increasingly placed a direct burden on patients, either because they are uninsured and must pay out of pocket for all their care or because insurance plans shift a portion of the costs back to patients through deductibles, copayments, and coinsurance. The current reality is that it is very difficult, and often impossible, for the clinician to know the actual out-of-pocket costs for each patient, since costs vary by intervention, insurer, location of care, choice of pharmacy or radiology service, and so on; nonetheless, some general information is known, and solutions that provide patient-level details are in development.

Consider a Medicare patient with metastatic colorectal cancer. Commonly, a component of first-line therapy for this disease is bevacizumab. The addition of bevacizumab to chemotherapy extends life by an average of approximately 5 months over chemotherapy alone. The drug is fairly well tolerated, but among other risks, patients receiving bevacizumab have a 2 percent increase in the risk of severe cardiovascular toxic effects. Over the course of a median of 10 months of therapy, bevacizumab costs $44,000.[1] A patient with Medicare coverage alone would be responsible for paying 20 percent of that cost, or $8,800, out of pocket, and that price tag doesn't include payments for other chemotherapy, doctor's fees, supportive medications, or diagnostic tests. Most physicians insist on discussing the 2 percent risk of adverse cardiovascular effects associated with bevacizumab, but few would mention the drug's potential financial toxicity.

This example is not isolated, and the consequences for patients are grim. The problem is perhaps starkest in cancer care, but it applies to all complex illness. The Center for American Progress has estimated that in Massachusetts, out-of-pocket costs for breast-cancer treatment are as high as $55,250 for women with high-deductible insurance plans; the out-of-pocket costs of managing uncomplicated diabetes amount to more than $4,000 per year; and out-of-pocket costs can approach $40,000 per year for a patient with a myocardial infarction requiring hospitalization.[2] The Centers for Disease Control and Prevention estimates that, owing in part to such high out-of-pocket costs, in 2011 about a third of U.S. families were either struggling to pay medical bills or defaulting on their payments (see figure 1).[3]

This health care–related financial burden can cause substantial distress, forcing people to cut corners in ways that may affect their health and well-being. In our research, we discovered that many insured patients burdened by high out-of-pocket costs from cancer treatment reduce their spending on food and clothing to make ends meet, or they reduce the frequency with which they take prescribed medications.[4]

Whether because of insufficient training or time, many physicians don't include information about the cost of care in the decision-making process.[5] But discussing costs is a crucial component of clinical decision making. First, discussing out-of-pocket costs enables patients to choose lower-cost treatments when there are viable alternatives. Patients experience unnecessary financial distress when physicians do not inform them of alternative treatments that are less expensive but equally or nearly as effective. We

A Americans <65 Yr of Age

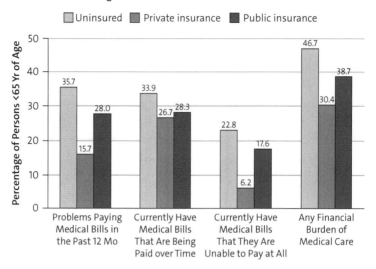

B Americans ≥65 Yr of Age

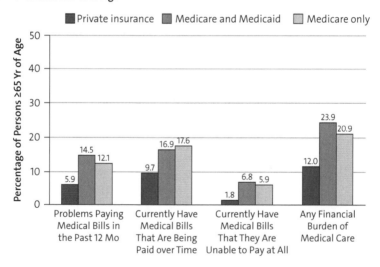

FIGURE 1 Financial burden of medical care. Source: Data are from the National Center for Health Statistics, Centers for Disease Control and Prevention.

discovered this phenomenon when interviewing a convenience sample of breast-cancer survivors who had participated in a national study of financial burden. Many women reported discussing treatment-related costs with their physicians only after they had begun to experience financial distress. One woman reported that only after she told her clinician "I am not taking this if it is going to be $500 a month" did the clinician inform her that "We can put you on something [less expensive] which is just as effective."

Second, such discussions could assist patients who are willing to trade off some chance of medical benefit for less financial distress. Admittedly, the trade-off between cost and potential benefit is complex and ethically charged. Yet when costs are not included in decision making, patients are deprived of the option, and patient engagement is harmed. Presenting this trade-off to patients makes clinical sense if we think of financial costs as treatment side effects.

Third, discussing out-of-pocket costs could benefit patients by enabling them to seek financial assistance early enough in their care to avoid financial distress. One of the patients we interviewed explained, "My husband died and we were in debt. I was sick, he was sick. I lost my house. . . . And I told [my doctor] that I could not afford to take the Femara. She said, 'Well, you can apply for help' . . . and I got help!" One has to wonder whether an earlier discussion of out-of-pocket costs might have prevented the patient from losing her home.

Fourth, a growing body of evidence suggests that including consideration of costs in clinical decision making might reduce costs for patients and society in the long term.

Although we believe that physicians should discuss out-of-pocket costs with their patients, we recognize that such discussions will not always be easy. As previously acknowledged, it is often difficult to determine a patient's out-of-pocket costs for any given intervention. Efforts are under way to address this informational barrier: insurance companies are developing technologies to better estimate patients' costs, and several states have passed price-transparency legislation. But these efforts are imperfect and incomplete, so for now, physicians and patients will often have a difficult time estimating cost differentials between viable treatment options. In addition, patients and physicians face social barriers to discussing costs of care. No doubt, many doctors and patients find discussions of money uncomfortable; they have not been coached in ways of having the conversation. Patients worry that asking about costs will put them at odds with their doctors or result in subpar treatment. And some physicians believe that their duty is to provide the best medical care regardless of cost.

We believe that given the distress created by out-of-pocket costs, it is well within physicians' traditional duties to discuss such matters with our patients. Admittedly, out-of-pocket costs are difficult to predict, but so are many medical outcomes that are nevertheless included in clinical discussions. Policymakers need to continue the push for greater transparency in medical costs, especially those borne by patients. Health care stakeholders should advocate for high-value care that reduces cost while improving outcomes. But that change will not occur overnight, and in the meantime, patients will continue to suffer from treatment-related financial burden. Physicians should discuss what is known about these costs with our patients, so that the personal financial impact of medical care is incorporated into the selection of the best care for any given patient, in the same way that any other potential toxic effect is considered. We can no longer afford to divorce costs from our discussion of patients' treatment alternatives.

NOTES

1 Centers for Medicare and Medicaid Services. 2013 ASP drug pricing files. 2013. http:// www.cms.gov/Medicare/Medicare-Fee-for-Service-Part-B-Drugs/McrPartBDrugAvg-SalesPrice/2013ASPFiles.html.

2 Center for American Progress Action Fund. Coverage when it counts: how much protection does health insurance offer and how can consumers know? May 2009. http://www.americanprogressaction.org/wp-content/uploads/issues/2009/05/pdf /CoverageWhenItCounts.pdf.

3 National Center for Health Statistics. Financial burden of medical care: early release of estimates from the National Health Interview Survey, January–June 2011. 2012. http:// www.cdc.gov/nchs/data/nhis/earlyrelease/financial_burden_of_medical_care_032012 .pdf.

4 Zafar SY, Peppercorn JM, Schrag D, et al. The financial toxicity of cancer treatment: a pilot study assessing out-of-pocket expenses and the insured cancer patient's experience. *Oncologist.* 2013;18:381–390.

5 Alexander GC, Casalino LP, Meltzer DO. Patient-physician communication about out-of-pocket costs. *JAMA.* 2003;290:953–958.

Seven Sins of Humanitarian Medicine

David R. Welling, James M. Ryan, David G. Burris,
and Norman M. Rich

The Catholic Church during the Middle Ages had a list of seven cardinal sins.[1] Commission of any of these sins was considered to be a severe act. The list addressed many of our human foibles and included extravagance, gluttony, greed, sloth, wrath, envy, and pride. These "deadly" sins were more serious than the "venial" sins that we all commit more regularly. Forgiveness from the seven sins required confession, penitence, and extraordinary efforts. When considering the topic of humanitarian medicine, it has occurred to us that we could craft a list of seven areas of concern, seven mistakes that are common and continue to challenge those who go forth on humanitarian missions (box 1). With each area mentioned, we provide examples. Finally, we propose the ideal humanitarian mission, with its features.

The Seven Sins of Humanitarian Medicine

Sin #1: Leaving a mess behind

Sin #2: Failing to match technology to local needs and abilities

Sin #3: Failing of NGOs to cooperate and help each other, and to cooperate and accept help from military organizations

Sin #4: Failing to have a follow-up plan

Sin #5: Allowing politics, training, or other distracting goals to trump service, while representing the mission as "service"

David R. Welling, James M. Ryan, David G. Burris, and Norman M. Rich, "Seven Sins of Humanitarian Medicine," from *World Journal of Surgery* 34 (2010): 466–470. © 2010 by Société Internationale de Chirurgie. Reprinted by permission of Springer.

Sin #6: Going where we are not wanted or needed and/or being poor guests

Sin #7: Doing the right thing for the wrong reason

Almost invariably, applicants for medical school when asked why they have decided to become a physician, give as an answer: "the desire to help others." Humanitarian medicine provides the almost perfect opportunity to do just that. To go to an area where good care is not available, to provide services that can make a huge difference in the health and welfare of a fellow human being, to provide this service freely and without personal gain—surely these sorts of activities can be life-altering for both provider and recipient of care. And yet we do not always successfully accomplish our goals of providing safe, modern, successful, appropriate care.

This article is in no way meant to denigrate the good works of those who participate in humanitarian missions. We salute all those in these sorts of activities, realizing that there often is real sacrifice made, including the sacrifice of time, money, and equipment. Occasionally, humanitarian missions can even expose us to serious disease, accidents, or assaults. We have great respect for all who go forth to serve. Surely those who aspire to help others almost always do so with honorable intent, and almost never set out to satisfy selfish desires. However, despite our good intentions, mistakes continue to be made, which we attempt to demonstrate in this paper. In our view, there are (at least) seven major opportunities for improvement in the art and science of humanitarian medicine.

The following are major reasons for failures in humanitarian medicine:

SIN #1 · Leaving a mess behind. Complications can ruin everything. The death of a child can quickly erase the memories of a thousand successful operations. A good example of this principle is found in reviewing the story of Operation Smile. Operation Smile had been described as a "model charity." It was founded in 1982 to increase vastly the ability to treat cleft palate and cleft lip cases throughout the developing world. This humanitarian effort quickly gained popularity and traction. Supporters of this organization have even included Mother Theresa, Goldie Hawn, and Bill Gates. It became a well-funded charity. The problems with Operation Smile began in 1998 with the death of a child in China. It was alleged that "It was the direct result of a poorly run mission with far too much attention being paid to publicity and not enough to patient safety and standard operating techniques." Medical professionals at the Beijing hospital where Operation Smile conducted the mission also were severely critical, saying, "There was a high number of serious complications where children suffered from excessive bleeding or had to have emergency surgery because their palates had collapsed." Besides the criticism of the Chinese mission, there was a child who died because the oxygen supply had run out in Kenya, and another child died in Viet Nam of unrecognized asthma. This sort of adverse publicity has had a predictable, negative effect upon the organization, which continues to operate missions throughout the world. Major contributors withdrew offers of support, and the organization has undergone some serious restructuring and introspection as a result of these accusations. "After Operation Smile came to Bolivia, several children needed extensive follow-up care at San Gabriel Hospital," according to Dr. Roberto Rosa, a pediatric surgeon there who was sharply critical of Operation Smile and other charities. "This is a form of neo-colonialism," argued Dr. Rosa, saying that Operation Smile had committed "surgical safaris against our children," who are from poor families who are unlikely to complain.[2]

Perhaps some of the difficulty encountered by Operation Smile revolved around the complexity of the cases they attempted. As a rule, the more difficult cases should not be routinely done by humanitarian medicine transient teams, in our view. Sometimes "No" is the best answer when pressed. Surely it is wise to always review the capabilities of the team and never allow providers to do more than they should be doing, given limitations of equipment, time, etc. Numbers of cases performed should not be allowed to trump patient safety and proper monitoring. Large and complex cases should be reviewed and only performed when the team is convinced that the case can be done safely, and that the patient will receive good care when the humanitarian team is no longer on the scene. This implies a great degree of trust and cooperation with local health care providers, which Operation Smile apparently did not always have. We also believe that, ideally, visiting surgeons should be teaching local surgeons how to do the operations and have them fully onboard in the decision-making and care, especially if the visitors plan to leave patients with unresolved issues. If local surgeons feel that they lack expertise in a particular operation and ask for training by the visiting surgeons, then certainly that sort of training is sensible and more likely will have a positive outcome.

One good rule is to offer the types of procedures that are minimally invasive, to relieve immediate discomfort, and that require little follow-up care, especially for missions that are short-term. Thus, removal of abscessed teeth, removal of ingrown toenails, fitting of eyeglasses—simple acts of this sort will create good will and a positive memory of the care given, with little risk of leaving a mess behind.[3]

SIN #2 · Failing to match technology to local needs and abilities. Despite what we may think, a vast part of our world does not have high-speed Internet access, or even electricity, or potable water. As we prepare to go off on a mission to a disadvantaged country, we ought to be asking ourselves how we might best go about helping. Generally, bringing the latest and the greatest new technology into a society that is impoverished can be more a cruel joke than a boon for the people. Yet, as we prepare to go, we generally like to surround ourselves with equipment that we normally use, and so this error is very easily understood. Here is a telling quote from a Belgian plastic surgeon, Dr. Christian Dupuis, who has volunteered to go to Southeast Asia for several months each year since the 1970s: "I have seen professors from fancy American universities teaching endoscopy skills in Laos to internists who don't have access to an endoscope. . . ."[4] Perhaps this foible is somewhat tied into the desire to do a "first," as in doing the first laparoscopic adrenalectomy in the Amazon basin. It is more about bragging rights than about solid, needed care that will be sustainable after we leave.

SIN #3 · Failing of NGOs to cooperate and help each other and to cooperate and accept help from military organizations. Nongovernmental organizations (NGOs) are in a constant battle with each other as they compete for funding for their particular cause. If they can somehow show that their particular organization is doing more operations, or pulling more teeth, or treating more patients, this degree of activity can translate into getting more funds from the donors. It is well known that these organizations get into contests with each other and spend a good deal of energy and resources trying to look better than the competition. To quote Dr. Anthony Redmond, a British Professor of Accident and Emergency Medicine: "Teams must cooperate with each other. Competitive humanitarianism is destructive and very wasteful of resources, both human and material. There can be pressure, either real or imagined, to be seen to be doing something in the eyes of those who have sponsored the team. This must be resisted. Much useful work can be done away from the glare of publicity in support of the work of others."[5]

One area that certainly could be improved is the attitude of NGOs toward the military. Both U.S. and non-U.S. military capabilities for transportation of supplies and personnel, for setting up tent hospitals, for bringing in operating room capabilities and blood banks—this sort of amazing capability is available and has been proven effective throughout the world. And yet at times the NGOs would appear to rather go without than to be seen working with someone in a military uniform. Ultimately, that attitude hurts the mission. We believe that both sides, military and nonmilitary, could do more to foster cooperation in this regard. Perhaps some progress is being made. Very recently, Navy Captain Miguel Cubano, who is presently serving as the U.S. Southern Command Surgeon, reported that NGOs have been offered operating room time on board the USNS *Comfort*, and a number of NGOs were onboard as the ship was to sail into the Caribbean on its next mission, which began in April 2009 (Dr. Miguel Cubano, personal communication). This sort of planning, which is innovative and unusual, should be congratulated and encouraged in the future.

SIN #4 · Failing to have a follow-up plan. A good example of this foible has been the activity of the U.S. military in Africa during the past several decades. We have had a yearly mission to a given area, a humanitarian effort, which is a wonderful and unforgettable opportunity for those lucky enough to be chosen to go along. The problem with these missions is that they have generally never gone back to the same place twice; thus, perversely, instead of helping people, perhaps these efforts actually cause the good people of Africa to resent our well-intentioned efforts. One of us (David Welling) was involved in a humanitarian mission, called Operation Red Flag, to northern Cameroon in March 2000. This mission lasted almost a month. It involved several hundred medical and support military personnel, mainly stationed in Germany, who were transported via C-17 and B-747 aircraft to Garoua, Cameroon. Tons of supplies were brought in, as well as vehicles and other ancillary equipment. We presented the hospital with a vast array of new equipment, including autoclaves and operating room tables. Our teams built an X-ray suite at the military hospital. Teams went to villages, where wells were drilled, vaccinations were given, teeth pulled, and eyeglasses distributed. We were very kindly hosted by the local populace, and when we finally left, dinners were held in our honor, toasts were made, and we said goodbye to our new friends. But what must the good people of Garoua think of those Americans now? Surely the supplies are long gone, and the equipment needs maintenance or replacement. Those who had our care no doubt need follow-up. It was almost a cruel joke, tantamount to taking a little child to Disneyland for 15 minutes, and then getting back into the car and leaving forever. We had given the citizens of Garoua just a taste of modern medicine, just a brief look at what might be. And then we left. Surely we should never have one-time-only missions. We should have an ongoing, regular visit schedule. We should see our patients again and again. We should know and have ongoing dialogue with our medical colleagues in these countries. None of this was done after the Cameroon mission. It is much better to pick one country and continue to serve it well, than to hopscotch all over Africa, going everywhere and truly getting nowhere.

SIN #5 · Allowing politics, training, or other distracting goals to trump service, while representing the mission as "service." The U.S. Navy has two large hospital ships, the USNS *Comfort* and the USNS *Mercy*. The *Comfort* is berthed in Baltimore, Maryland, and the *Mercy* in California. Our Navy has fairly frequently used these ships to go on "humanitarian" cruises, as well as for response to natural and manmade disasters. For humanitarian missions, the *Comfort* usually goes to the Caribbean, while the *Mercy* goes to the South Pacific. Typically, at the end of a cruise, the Navy will announce the results of these missions, with invariably positive publicity. For example, a 2007 Caribbean tour by the *Comfort* involved more than 500 personnel and lasted several months; 98,000 patients were seen, 1,170 surgeries were performed, 32,322 shots were given, 122,245 prescriptions were filled, 24,242 eyeglasses were fitted, 3,968 teeth were pulled, and 17,772 animals were treated. Schools were built, and even the U.S. Navy Show Band participated.[6] On another mission, the *Mercy* left in May 2008, on a Southeast Pacific voyage, and after several months, reported that their providers had examined more than 90,000 patients and had performed almost 1,400 operations.[7] Obviously, for those aboard for these missions, this was a remarkable experience. But truly it was more about photo opportunities, training, diplomacy, and "showing the flag" than about service. These huge ships (894 feet long) are not well-suited to these missions. At times in the Caribbean, the *Comfort* was required to anchor a dozen miles offshore, relying on helicopters and smaller boats to ferry patients back and forth. Each port in the Caribbean was visited for about a week, and the visits were not always well-coordinated with local organizations, which at times were not even consulted. Thus, resources were not maximized. Even Fidel Castro weighed in on this mission and was quoted as saying this about our efforts, and he has a good point: "You can't carry out medical programs in episodes."[8] Interestingly, President Barack Obama, while attending a summit of the hemisphere's leaders in Trinidad and Tobago in April 2009, seemed to validate what Castro had previously inferred. President Obama felt that the United States could learn a lesson from Cuba, which for decades has sent doctors to other countries throughout Latin America to care for the poor. The policy has won Cuban leaders Fidel and Raul Castro deep goodwill in the region.[9] Apparently, the Cuban doctors have correctly realized that by staying in one place for a prolonged period of time, they can have maximum impact with the local populace. For a small and poor country, Cuba has made remarkable contributions to reducing infant mortality and helping disaster victims throughout the world. During the past four decades, some 52,000 doctors and nurses have been sent to 95 needy countries. Recently large numbers of doctors and nurses have been sent to Venezuela, with some subsequent discontent voiced by Cuban citizens, who now are noticing increased waiting times, and difficulty gaining access to routine care.[10] Cuba also has helped to establish medical schools in a number of third-world countries.[11]

These U.S. Navy missions must be great for training and for projecting power and showing the flag, but probably could be modified by using smaller ships and more frequent missions to the same places. The *Comfort* and the *Mercy* have never been proven able to reach a disaster site in a timely manner, and their attempts at humanitarian medicine have not always been convincing in the aggregate. The last USNS *Comfort* mission to the Caribbean began on April 1, 2009.[12]

SIN #6 · Going where we are not wanted or needed and/or being poor guests. Dr. Anthony Redmond teaches us that we need an official request to go into an area in need, asking for our specific help. He states this: "The pressure to do something immediately can be considerable. Emotive television and press reports galvanize public opinion into demands for immediate action. However, without recognized terms of reference and a clear mandate to enter and work in another country, foreign teams will at best be stranded at airports and at worst add considerably to the problems of an already beleaguered nation. Time spent in securing a safe passage through and identifying a task to be completed will result in a shorter journey to the scene."[5] Dr. Redmond also talks about the necessity of doing what the local officials want, instead of what we think they may need. "If assistance is to be most effective it has to be organized. Local officials are in charge and must be allowed to develop and execute their plans with foreign teams there as a resource and not a threat. When a team has gained local confidence and developed good local relationships they will have a better knowledge of local requirements. This process of 'bedding in' to the local network can be completed within 24 hours."[5] Mr. Jim Ryan, a surgeon from the United Kingdom and someone well-experienced in humanitarian medicine, relates seeing a whole team from Scandinavia, which had, with the very best of intentions, responded to the tsunami disaster in Sri Lanka without first getting permission from the government. Despite their great expertise and extensive equipment, they were sequestered and were not allowed to leave their compound, let alone go out and help the victims. As to how one should conduct oneself when on a humanitarian mission, a dose of humility might get us off on the right foot as we begin. Anything that looks like boorish behavior, or condescension, or a patronizing attitude—any such behavior is detrimental to our efforts and will leave an unpleasant memory of us for those who would be our patients and our colleagues. We need to be very careful with local customs and mores. How we dress, how we act, what we drink—all of these activities will define us to our hosts. We can learn much from third-world providers, as they maximize what they have in supplies, and innovate to give their patients the very best care possible. We should go with the desire to see a different way to render care, instead of insisting that our way is the only correct way possible.

SIN #7 · Doing the right thing for the wrong reason. In *Murder in the Cathedral*, T.S. Eliot wrote about the various temptations that Thomas the Archbishop suffered through, and the very last was the most difficult. As Thomas proclaimed: "The last temptation is the greatest treason: To do the right deed for the wrong reason."[13] The list of wrong reasons to go off on a humanitarian mission is potentially a long list, and no doubt would vary somewhat from person to person. To name a few reasons not to go, one might include the desire to go on an unusual vacation, bragging rights for having done a "first," the desire to perform a large number of complex cases quickly (without the niceties of informed consent, proper monitoring, planned follow-up, and without training the local surgeons to do the procedures themselves), to gain fame, to have a free trip to an exotic land, or to somehow get an advantage in academia. The corollary to this last observation would be that we should go forth with pure motives, with a well-thought-out plan of action, including host nation physicians, avoiding the types of operations that lend themselves to long-term complications, and with a teachable, humble attitude.

Summary

We have listed some of the common mistakes and pitfalls that can beset those who would go on humanitarian missions, with thoughts about how we might improve in this regard. The importance of doing humanitarian medicine properly cannot be overemphasized. To maximize our effectiveness as humanitarian providers, more time should be spent thinking about the details of a given mission. Motives should be questioned. We ought to aggressively plan activities that will do the most good for our patients, and we ought to shun those activities that are more designed for our own personal aggrandizement. There is an inexhaustible demand for modern medicine throughout the world, and we face that demand with finite resources and human foibles. How we go about doing humanitarian medicine can define us, for better or for worse.

NOTES

1   Seven deadly sins. *Wikipedia.* http://en.wikipedia.org/wiki/Seven_deadly_sins. Accessed March 26, 2009.

2   R. Abelson, E. Rosenthal. Charges of shoddy practices taint gifts of plastic surgery. November 24, 1999. http://www.nytimes.com/1999/11/24/world/charges-of-shoddy -practices-taint-gifts-of-plastic-surgery.html?=health&spon=&pagewanted=l. Accessed March 26, 2009.

3   Minken SL, Colgan R, Barish RA, Doyle J, Brown PR, Welling DR. Waging peace: a medical military mission to Bosnia-Herzegovina. *Surg Rounds.* 2008;31:128–135.

4   Wolfberg AJ. Volunteering overseas: lessons from surgical brigades. *N Engl J Med.* 2006;354:443–445

5   Lumley JSP, Ryan JM, Baxter PJ, Kirby N. *Handbook of the Medical Care of Catastrophes.* London: Royal Society of Medicine Press Limited; 1996:37.

6   http://www.southcom.mil/AppsSC/factfiles.php?id=6. Accessed April 20, 2009.

7   Davis KD, Douglas T, Kuncir E. Pacific Partnership 2008: U.S. Navy Fellows provide humanitarian assistance in Southeast Asia. *Bull Am Coll Surg.* 2009;94:14–23.

8   http://www.flacso.org/hemisferio/al-eeuu/boletines/02/86/rel_07.pdf. Accessed April 20, 2009.

9   Wilson S. Obama closes summit, vows broader engagement with Latin America. *Washington Post.* April 20, 2009;A6.

10 Lakshmanan, I. A. R. As Cuba loans doctors abroad, some patients object at home. *Boston Globe.* August 25, 2005.http://archive.boston.com/news/world/latinamerica/articles/2005/08/25/as_cuba_loans_doctors_abroad_some_patients_object_at_home/.

11 http://www.medicc.org/ns/index.php?s=46&p=12. Accessed May 20, 2009.

12 http://www.southcom.mil/appssc/factfiles.php?id=103. Accessed April 20, 2009.

13 Eliot TS. Murder in the cathedral. In: Brooks C, Purser JT, Warren RF, eds., *An Approach to Literature.* 4th ed. New York: Appleton-Century-Crofts; 1964:816.

Who Should Receive Life Support during a Public Health Emergency?

Using Ethical Principles to Improve Allocation Decisions

Douglas B. White, Mitchell H. Katz, John M. Luce, and Bernard Lo

The threat of pandemic influenza has produced large-scale federal, state, and local efforts to prepare for a public health disaster. Modeling studies suggest that a public health disaster similar in magnitude to the 1918 influenza pandemic would require 400 percent of current U.S. intensive care unit beds and 200 percent of all mechanical ventilators.[1,2] Even a smaller epidemic could be grave, because U.S. intensive care units typically run at greater than 90 percent occupancy and have little surge capacity.[3]

The U.S. Department of Health and Human Services acknowledges the possibility of ventilator and critical care shortages during a public health emergency but has been silent on what principles should guide allocation decisions.[4,5] In response, several groups have recently published guidelines for allocating ventilators and other life support during a public health emergency.[6–9] Each guideline recommends categorically excluding large groups of patients from life support and allocating life-sustaining treatments on the basis of patients' chances of survival to hospital discharge. These efforts to achieve a transparent process of allocation are an important first step to minimize the chance of arbitrary or biased decisions during a crisis. However,

Douglas B. White, Mitchell H. Katz, John M. Luce, and Bernard Lo, "Who Should Receive Life Support during a Public Health Emergency? Using Ethical Principles to Improve Allocation Decisions," from *Annals of Internal Medicine* 150, no. 2 (2009): 128–132. Reprinted by permission of American College of Physicians.

we believe that these guidelines omit morally relevant considerations that should be incorporated into allocation strategies.

To date, there has not been broad engagement of professionals and the public on what ethical principles should guide these difficult allocation decisions. Such debate is needed because a successful public health response will require public trust and cooperation with restrictive measures, such as the use of police powers, social distancing, and quarantine.[10] Moreover, advance discussion is essential because in-depth deliberations will not be feasible during a public health crisis.

To foster debate, we place these issues in the context of a clinical scenario during a hypothetical influenza pandemic, analyze the ethical principles that could guide allocation, propose an allocation strategy that balances multiple morally relevant considerations, and provide recommendations for meaningful public engagement in priority setting. Although we focus our discussion on the example of scarcity of mechanical ventilators during an influenza pandemic, the ethical considerations are similar for other types of public health emergencies during which there may be a scarcity of resources, such as critical care beds, health care personnel, and renal replacement therapy.

Decision Making during a Public Health Emergency

In everyday clinical practice, patients who require life-sustaining treatments receive them, except if they or their surrogates decline the treatments or in the rare circumstance that they are deemed medically futile.[11] This reflects the primacy of respect for patient autonomy in U.S. health care ethics and law, as well as the general availability of life support.[12,13] Physicians do not unilaterally withdraw mechanical ventilation against a patient's wishes in order to provide it to someone else.

Public health ethics differs from clinical ethics by giving priority to promoting the common good over protecting individual autonomy. The physician's primary duty in clinical medicine is to promote the well-being of individual patients,[14] but a shortage of ventilators in a public health emergency may require physicians to withhold or withdraw mechanical ventilation against their own clinical intuitions and against the wishes of some patients who otherwise might survive. Public health policies, which focus primarily on population-level health outcomes, may subordinate the inter-

TABLE 1 When the Demand for Ventilators Overwhelms the Supply

An influenza pandemic has caused severe shortages of ventilators and other life-saving resources in the United States. All critical care beds in the hospital in question are occupied by patients receiving mechanical ventilation, many of whom have respiratory failure from influenza. Patients are receiving mechanical ventilation in step-down units, and all nonemergency surgical cases have been canceled. Despite these measures, all but one of the hospital's ventilators are being used by patients who would die without them. All hospitals in the region are experiencing the same shortages.

Which of the following three patients should be prioritized for the one available ventilator?

A 32-year-old woman with severe primary pulmonary hypertension (pulmonary artery pressure, 55 mm Hg) who was intubated after an accidental overdose of narcotics and benzodiazepines. Her SOFA score is 4, predicting a roughly 90 percent chance of survival to discharge.

A housebound 83-year-old man with severe peripheral vascular disease and severe, inoperable coronary artery disease that substantially limits his long-term prognosis. His SOFA score is 10, predicting a roughly 50 percent chance of survival to hospital discharge.

A previously healthy 44-year-old man with sepsis and multiorgan failure. His SOFA score is 12, predicting a roughly 30 percent chance of survival to discharge.

SOFA = Sequential Organ Failure Assessment.

ests and rights of individuals to the common good.[15,16] The clinical scenario presented in table 1 highlights the dilemmas that may arise during a public health emergency if there are not enough mechanical ventilators to treat the patients who need them.

Although several strategies are used for allocating scarce medical resources (table 2), the notion that public health measures could shape life-or-death choices for all critically ill patients is foreign to most clinicians and patients. During a public health emergency, allocation decisions will be the responsibility of state public health departments, with federal guidance and support. In most states, the governor has the authority to declare a public health emergency, which then triggers public health police powers, including rationing of vaccines and medicines.[10,20] Individual health care systems, hospitals, and clinicians cannot set public health policy but will need to implement allocation decisions under the authority of public health departments.

TABLE 2 Examples of Existing Allocation Strategies

Situation	Allocation Strategy
Distribution of ICU beds during routine clinical circumstances	First-come, first-served.
Treating the wounded on battlefields	Regardless of rank, first treat soldiers with life-threatening injuries who are most likely to survive.[17]
Distributing limited supplies of intravenous fluid during cholera epidemics in refugee camps	Give fluids to persons with moderate dehydration who will probably recover with small amounts of fluid (rather than to those with the most advanced dehydration, who may or may not survive).[18]
Allocation of lungs for transplantation	Balance the patients' medical needs, defined by how likely they are to die within 1 year without transplantation, with their likelihood of benefit, defined as how likely they are to be alive 1 year after transplantation.[19]*
Allocation of livers for transplantation	Prioritize persons most likely to die without transplantation (using the Model for End-Stage Liver Disease score).*

ICU = intensive care unit.

* Some patients are deemed ineligible to be listed for transplantation on the basis of medical factors (such as severe comorbid conditions) and social factors (such as ongoing substance abuse or an inadequate social support structure).

Several other groups have suggested strategies to promote collaboration between public health officials and front-line clinicians, including training individual clinicians to function as triage officers under the supervision of public health officials.[7–9]

Critique of Existing Guidelines

Historically, allocation decisions in public health have been driven by the utilitarian goal of accomplishing the "greatest good for the greatest number."[15] Although this broad principle can be interpreted many ways, several recent guidelines for allocating life support during a public health emergency have specified it narrowly as "maximize the number of people who survive to hospital discharge."[7-9] We believe that this allocation strategy does not adequately incorporate other morally relevant considerations.

In addition, these published guidelines deny access to life support to certain patient groups who could potentially benefit from treatment. For example, one group advocates denying access to ventilatory support to persons who are functionally dependent from neurologic impairment.[6] Another group recommends excluding persons older than 85 years and persons with New York Heart Association class III or IV heart failure.[7-9] These exclusions are not explicitly justified. Moreover, they are ethically flawed because the criteria for exclusion (age, long-term prognosis, and functional status) are selectively applied to some types of patients, rather than to all patients who require life-sustaining interventions. Such selective application violates the principle of justice because patients who are similar in ethically relevant ways are treated differently. Categorical exclusion may also have the unintended negative effect of implying that some groups are "not worth saving," leading to perceptions of unfairness. In a public health emergency, public trust will be essential to ensure compliance with restrictive measures. Thus, an allocation system should make clear that all individuals are "worth saving." One way to do this is to keep all patients who would receive mechanical ventilation during routine clinical circumstances eligible, but allow the availability of ventilators to determine how many eligible patients receive it.

What Principles Should Guide Allocation?

The utilitarian rule of maximizing the number of lives saved is widely accepted during a public health emergency.[21] The Ontario and New York state working groups both propose modifying a relatively simple mortality prediction model—the Sequential Organ Failure Assessment score[22]—to determine an individual's priority. No compelling evidence suggests that one mortality prediction model will be more accurate than another, but the Sequential Organ Failure Assessment score is the easiest to implement and requires the fewest laboratory tests. Although existing models are imperfect, they are as accurate as physicians' prognostic estimates[23] and have the added appeal of being objective and transparent. Prioritizing treatment of individuals according to their chances for short-term survival also avoids ethically irrelevant considerations, such as race or socioeconomic status. Finally, it is appealing because it balances utilitarian claims for efficiency with egalitarian claims that because all lives have equal value, the goal should be to save the most lives.[21]

However, using the probability of short-term survival as the sole alloca-tion principle is problematic. It is hazardous to extrapolate mortality predic-tion models beyond the conditions for which they have been validated.[23,24] Perhaps because of this concern, existing guidelines recommend using the Sequential Organ Failure Assessment score only to stratify people into four prognostic groups, rather than to make finer distinctions among patients. On the basis of current experience with avian influenza, many patients with respiratory failure probably will also develop multiorgan failure.[25] Thus, there probably will be large clusters of patients who are indistinguishable on the basis of their prognoses for short-term survival.

Ethically, using only chance of survival to hospital discharge is insuffi-cient because it rests on a thin conception of "accomplishing the greatest good." We discuss additional principles that have been used in other situations to allocate scarce medical resources. We argue that two of these principles should be combined with the principle of "saving the most lives" to create a multiprinciple strategy to allocate scarce life-saving resources during a pub-lic health emergency.

Broad Social Value

Broad social value refers to one's overall worth to society. It involves summary judgments about whether a person's past and future contributions to soci-ety's goals merit prioritization for scarce resources.[21] When dialysis was first introduced, social value was a key consideration in allocating scarce dialysis machines. Patients who were professionals, heads of families, and caregiv-ers received priority over "creative non-conformists who rub the bourgeoisie the wrong way."[26] The public firestorm in response to revelations that social worth was a key factor in the Seattle Dialysis Committee's deliberations partly led Congress to authorize universal coverage for hemodialysis.[27]

In our morally pluralistic society, it has not been possible to agree on a set of criteria to assert that one person is intrinsically more worthy of saving than another. Even if such consensus could be reached, some philosophers argue that it should not be a guiding principle for allocation decisions. These indi-viduals defend the egalitarian view that all individuals have an equal moral claim to treatment regardless of whether they can contribute measurably to broad social goals.[28] Childress[29] writes that one's "dignity as a person . . . cannot be reduced to his past or future contribution to society." Given the lack of an accepted specification of broad social value and the sharp disagreement about whether it is a relevant consideration, we do not recommend using this principle to guide allocation of life support during a public health emergency.

Instrumental Value: The "Multiplier Effect"

Instrumental value refers to a person's ability to carry out a specific function that is essential to prevent social disintegration or a great number of deaths during a time of crisis. It has also been described as "narrow social utility" and the "multiplier effect."[21,30] The National Vaccine Advisory Committee recommends this principle to allocate vaccines and antiviral medications during a pandemic.[31] It gives first priority to workers in vaccine manufacturing and to health care providers. The ethical justification is that prioritizing certain key individuals will achieve a "multiplier effect," through which many more lives are ultimately saved by their work.

Instrumental value must be distinguished from judgments about broad social worth. With instrumental value, persons are prioritized not because they are judged to hold more "intrinsic worth," but because of their ability to perform a specific task that is essential to society. In this sense, instrumental value is a derivative allocation principle; it is desirable because it ensures an adequate workforce to achieve public health goals. Even critics of allocation based on broad social value accept the use of instrumental value in certain circumstances.[28]

However, using instrumental value to allocate ventilators may be ethically problematic for some public health emergencies, such as an influenza pandemic, which probably will be short and leave individuals with illnesses that require a long recovery. In general, to justify a restrictive public health measure, good evidence must suggest that the measure is necessary and will be effective.[20] It seems unlikely that persons with respiratory failure from influenza would recover in time to reenter the workforce and fulfill their instrumental roles. Moreover, it is not clear which roles are truly indispensable to saving a large number of lives during a pandemic. Because of the uncertainty about which key personnel will be in short supply and whether they will recover in time to achieve their instrumental value, we do not recommend that this principle be incorporated at this stage of planning. However, this principle should be openly debated with the public and "held in reserve" if convincing evidence emerges that its use would minimize mortality in a particular public health emergency.

Several other allocation principles can be rejected without extensive discussion. The "first-come, first-served" and "sickest first" principles are inconsistent with the public health goal of achieving the greatest good for the greatest number of persons.[32,33] Maximizing quality-adjusted life-years or disability-adjusted life-years would not be feasible to implement during a public health crisis because of the complexity of measuring these attributes. We next turn to two principles that can and, we contend, should be combined with the principle of "saving the most lives" to allocate life-saving resources during a public health emergency.

Maximizing Life-Years

A broader conceptualization of accomplishing the "greatest good" is to consider the years of life saved in addition to the number of lives saved. Assuming equal chances of short-term survival, giving priority to a 60-year-old woman who is otherwise healthy over a 60-year-old woman with a limited life expectancy from severe comorbid conditions will result in more "life-years" gained. The justification for incorporating this utilitarian claim is simply that, all other things being equal, it is better to save more years of life than fewer.

The principle of maximizing life-years was recently incorporated into the strategy to allocate lungs for transplantation. Rather than simply aiming to save the most lives, the lung allocation system now balances patients' medical need (prognosis without transplantation) against their expected duration of survival after transplantation.[19] We contend that explicitly adding considerations of "maximizing life-years saved" to "saving the most lives" yields a more complete specification of accomplishing the greatest good for the greatest number. Although current guidelines use this principle to exclude certain subgroups of patients from access to treatment, we think that this principle is relevant to all patients, not just those with extremely limited life expectancies. Moreover, applying it to all patients rather than an unfortunate few promotes consistency and fairness.

The Life-Cycle Principle

Under the life-cycle principle, the goal is to give each individual an equal opportunity to live through the various phases of life.[34] This principle has been called the "fair innings" argument and "intergenerational equity."[35] In practical terms, the life-cycle principle gives relative priority to younger individuals over older individuals. There is a precedent for incorporating life-cycle considerations into pandemic planning. The U.S. Department of Health and Human Services' plan to allocate vaccines and antivirals during an influenza pandemic prioritizes infants and children over adults.[31] The ethical justification of the life-cycle principle is that it is a valuable goal to give individuals equal opportunity to pass through the stages of life—childhood, young adulthood, middle age, and old age.[34] The justification for this principle does not rely on considerations of one's intrinsic worth or social utility. Rather, younger individuals receive priority because they have had the least opportunity to live through life's stages.

Empirical data suggest that, when individuals are asked to consider situations of absolute scarcity of life-sustaining resources, most believe younger patients should be prioritized over older ones.[36] Harris[37] summarizes the moral argument in favor of life-cycle–based allocation as follows: "[I]t is always a misfortune to die . . . it is both a misfortune and a tragedy [for life] to be cut off prematurely."

Some critics contend that the life-cycle principle unjustly discriminates against older persons. However, this principle is inherently egalitarian because it seeks to give all individuals equal opportunity to live a normal life span. It applies the notion of equality to individuals' whole lifetime experiences rather than just to their current situation.[35] Unlike prioritization based on sex or race, everyone faces the prospect of aging and everyone hopes to move through all stages of life.[34]

Can Multiple Principles Be Incorporated into an Allocation Strategy?

Past success in developing multiprinciple allocation systems for organ transplantation suggests that this is a feasible endeavor.[19] However, during a public health crisis, there will be little time for complex algorithms. Undoubtedly, there will be a tension between creating an allocation strategy that reflects the moral complexity of the issue and one that can be feasibly implemented. We propose an alternative to the single-principle strategy proposed by previous working groups—one that strives to incorporate and balance saving the most lives, saving the most life-years, and giving individuals equal opportunity to live through life's stages.

Table 3 describes an example of a very basic approach to specifying and incorporating these three principles into an allocation strategy. It is meant

TABLE 3 Illustration of a Multiprinciple Strategy to Allocate Ventilators during a Public Health Emergency

Principle	Specification	Point System*			
		1	2	3	4
Save the most lives	Prognosis for short-term survival (SOFA score)	SOFA score <6	SOFA score, 6–9	SOFA score, 10–12	SOFA score >12
Save the most life-years	Prognosis for long-term survival (medical assessment of comorbid conditions)	No comorbid conditions that limit long-term survival	Minor comorbid conditions with small impact on long-term survival	Major comorbid conditions with substantial impact on long-term survival	Severe comorbid conditions; death likely within 1 year
Life-cycle principle†	Prioritize those who have had the least chance to live through life's stages (age in years)	Age 12–40 y	Age 41–60 y	Age 61–74 y	Age ≥75 y

SOFA = Sequential Organ Failure Assessment.

* Persons with the lowest cumulative score would be given the highest priority to receive mechanical ventilation and critical care services.

† Pediatric patients may need to be considered separately, because their small size may require the use of different mechanical ventilators and personnel.

to be illustrative rather than definitive. Each principle is assessed on a four-point scale. Individual patients are evaluated on the basis of their likelihood for short-term survival, presence of comorbid conditions that would limit the duration of benefit, and phase of life. Patients with the lowest cumulative score would receive the highest priority for scarce, life-sustaining technologies. We make no claim that this specific, unweighted point system is the optimal way to balance and translate these three allocation principles into practice. Another approach is to treat each principle as a continuous variable and weigh each one according to judgments about its relative importance. Complex value judgments underlie decisions to weigh principles differently or arrange them hierarchically. Although these value judgments ultimately must be made, the first step—which is the goal of our article—is to establish that there are several relevant allocation principles. Thereafter, we should engage key stakeholders to determine how to fairly balance these principles.

To illustrate how the proposed multiprinciple system leads to different allocation decisions compared with the "save the most lives" approach, consider the vignette presented in table 1. By using the "save the most lives" strategy proposed by New York state, Ontario, and the Critical Care Initiative, the 83-year-old man with a 50 percent chance of hospital survival but multiple life-limiting comorbid conditions (which are not on the proposed lists of categorically excluded diseases) would receive highest priority. Even though the previously healthy 44-year-old man has a much better long-term prognosis and has had the least opportunity to live through life's stages, he is ranked less favorably because of his slightly worse prognosis for survival to hospital discharge. The woman with primary pulmonary hypertension and an accidental overdose would categorically be denied ventilation because of the severity of her pulmonary disease, even though the basis for that disqualification is not clearly justified in any of the proposals. Her case highlights the mistaken assertion that patients with severe comorbid conditions should be categorically denied life support on the grounds that they will always have poor intensive care unit outcomes.

In contrast, the multiprinciple allocation strategy we propose would result in priority going to the 32-year-old patient with pulmonary hypertension with a 90 percent chance of short-term survival. She is prioritized above the other 2 patients because of the combination of her excellent chances for short-term survival and her young age (total allocation score, 5). The previously healthy 44-year-old patient with no comorbid conditions and a 30 percent chance of short-term survival (total allocation score, 6) is prioritized over the 83-year-old man with severe comorbid conditions and 50 percent chance of short-term survival (total allocation score, 11) even though the younger man has a worse prognosis for short-term survival. Although not relevant in these sample cases, patients with identical allocation scores should be viewed as having equal moral claims to receive life support. In such a circumstance, a lottery is a reasonable approach to determine which patient will receive priority.

Some may criticize the proposed multiprinciple system as overpenalizing older individuals, who are more likely to have more comorbid conditions and to have lived through life's stages. However, the multiprinciple system we propose draws an important distinction between healthy older adults and older adults with life-limiting comorbid conditions. This approach avoids using age as a "blunt" predictor of years of life remaining. Rather than overpenalizing older adults for the correlation between age and comorbid conditions, our system avoids "penalizing" healthy older adults. Others may criticize such a system for relying on probabilities of outcomes that may not accurately predict what will happen to any individual. We acknowledge that any probabilistic scoring system cannot perfectly predict outcomes for individual patients. This concern has limited the use of probabilistic scoring systems to make treatment decisions during routine clinical practice.[11] However, the rationale for their use is stronger during a public health emergency, when the goal is to maximize population-level outcomes. Such an objective approach may also be viewed by the public as fairer than decisions based on more subjective criteria.

Although more complex than the previously proposed single-principle allocation system, this multiprinciple allocation system better reflects the diverse moral considerations relevant to these difficult decisions. In addition, this approach avoids the need to categorically deny treatment to certain groups, a problem that one legal scholar calls a "political and legal minefield."[38]

The Need for Meaningful Public Engagement

In our pluralistic society, people will probably disagree over which principles should guide allocation of ventilators during a pandemic. Therefore, careful attention to procedural justice becomes very important. Daniels and Sabin[39,40] identified several aspects of procedural justice that should be followed when allocating scarce health care resources: public engagement, transparency in decision making, appeals to rationales and principles that all can accept as relevant, oversight by a legitimate institution, and procedures for appealing and revising individual decisions in light of challenges to them.

Public involvement is essential because deciding which principles will guide allocation of life-saving resources during a public health emergency is a value judgment rather than an expert scientific judgment. Citizens' values are crucial in this process because the public will bear the consequences of triage decisions.[15] Public input has been useful for developing allocation policies for influenza vaccines and organs for transplantation.[41] The public input for lung transplantation revealed fundamental differences in the attitudes of policymakers and the public, both of which ultimately shaped the allocation system.[19]

Striving for a fair process of decision making may also enhance public trust.[10,42] If citizens perceive the process of setting priorities as unfair, they may challenge the legitimacy of the public health response and not adhere to restrictive measures. Public engagement may be especially important during a public health emergency because another important aspect of procedural justice—an individual's right to a due process appeals mechanism—will be severely limited by the urgency of individual decisions.[39]

To date, public involvement in the debate over allocation of limited resources in a public health emergency has not occurred. The proposals from the Critical Care Initiative and the Ontario working group were developed without broad public input.[7] In New York state, only after clinicians and policymakers determined their recommendations did they post the 52-page document on a Web site for public comment.[8] Because most individuals have not considered the possibility of ventilator scarcity during a pandemic and may not understand the range of potential allocation strategies, simple elicitation of comments is insufficient to allow informed public participation. Moreover, involving the public after the bulk of work on the policy has been completed reduces the likely impact of public comments. These represent serious deficiencies in both how and when public engagement occurs.

We propose three modifications to the process of public engagement that are feasible and methodologically rigorous. First, public engagement should occur before writing a draft policy, as well as after a draft is proposed. Second, the public needs adequate background information in order to be informed. Policymakers and ethicists should first delineate the range of feasible, ethically defensible allocation strategies, then collaborate with communication experts and social scientists to explain them to the public, including those of limited English proficiency and health literacy. Third, policymakers should engage a representative sample of citizens, rather than those with the knowledge and resources to seek out the draft guidelines on the Internet. This can be accomplished with research techniques from clinical and market

TABLE 4 Summary of Recommendations

Principles to Guide Allocation of Scarce Resources in a Public Health Emergency
1. Principles guiding allocation decisions should include maximizing survival to hospital discharge, maximizing the number of life-years saved, and maximizing individuals' chances to live through each of life's stages.
2. If it seems likely that there will be a severe shortage of providers of a key service and that personnel will recover in time to be useful, it is ethically permissible to incorporate considerations of instrumental value into prioritization considerations.

Creating a Fair Process of Decision Making
3. The public should be engaged early in the process of choosing among ethically permissible allocation strategies, both to identify the most acceptable approach and to achieve to the greatest possible extent a fair process of decision making.

research, such as in-depth qualitative interviews and focus groups. Focusing on community members rather than political or religious leaders may minimize the likelihood that the public engagement process will be dominated or co-opted by special interest groups. Other countries, such as the United Kingdom and Canada, have established procedures for public consultation on controversial health policies.[43]

Conclusion

Unresolved ethical and practical dilemmas about allocating ventilators and critical care resources could threaten the success of the response to a public health emergency. We contend that the previously proposed "save the most lives" allocation strategy is insufficient because it fails to incorporate morally relevant considerations, such as the expected years of life saved and the importance of giving individuals equal opportunity to pass through life's stages. We propose an alternative, multiprinciple allocation strategy that better reflects the moral complexity of the issue and applies the same allocation criteria to all patients (table 4). We hope that our proposal will stimulate a broad debate about how to ethically allocate scarce life-sustaining resources during a public health emergency.

1 Toner E, Waldhorn R, Maldin B, Borio L, Nuzzo JB, Lam C, et al. Hospital preparedness for pandemic influenza. *Biosecur Bioterror.* 2006;4:207–217. [PMID: 16792490]

2 Hearings (Roundtable Format) before the U.S. Senate Subcommittee on Bioterrorism and Public Health Preparedness on All Hazards Medical Preparedness and Response. April 5, 2006 (comments from Thomas Inglesby, MD).

3 Rubinson L, Nuzzo JB, Talmor DS, O'Toole T, Kramer BR, Inglesby TV. Augmentation of hospital critical care capacity after bioterrorist attacks or epidemics: recommendations of the Working Group on Emergency Mass Critical Care. *Crit Care Med.* 2005;33:2393–2403. [PMID: 16215397]

4 Phillips SJ, Knebel A, eds. *Providing Mass Medical Care with Scarce Resources: A Community Planning Guide.* Prepared by Health Systems Research, Inc., under contract no. 290-04-0010. AHRQ publication no. 07-0001. Rockville, MD: Agency for Health Research and Quality; 2006.

5 *Altered Standards of Care in Mass Casualty Events.* Prepared by Health Systems Research, Inc., under contract no. 290-04-0010. AHRQ publication no. 05-0043. Rockville, MD: Agency for Healthcare Research and Quality; April 2005.

6 Hick JL, O'Laughlin DT. Concept of operations for triage of mechanical ventilation in an epidemic. *Acad Emerg Med.* 2006;13:223–229. [PMID: 16400088]

7 Christian MD, Hawryluck L, Wax RS, Cook T, Lazar NM, Herridge MS, et al. Development of a triage protocol for critical care during an influenza pandemic. *CMAJ.* 2006;175:1377–1381. [PMID: 17116904]

8 Powell T, Christ KC, Birkhead GS. Allocation of ventilators in a public health disaster. *Disaster Med Public Health Prep.* 2008;2:20–26. [PMID: 18388654]

9 Devereaux AV, Dichter JR, Christian MD, Dubler NN, Sandrock CE, Hick JL, et al. Task Force for Mass Critical Care. Definitive care for the critically ill during a disaster: a framework for allocation of scarce resources in mass critical care: from a Task Force for Mass Critical Care summit meeting, January 26–27, 2007, Chicago, IL. *Chest.* 2008;133:s51–s66. [PMID: 18460506]

10 Gostin LO. Medical countermeasures for pandemic influenza: ethics and the law. *JAMA.* 2006;295:554–556. [PMID: 16449621]

11 Consensus statement of the Society of Critical Care Medicine's Ethics Committee regarding futile and other possibly inadvisable treatments. *Crit Care Med.* 1997;25:887–891. [PMID: 9187612]

12 Levinsky NG. The doctor's master. *N Engl J Med.* 1984;311:1573–1575. [PMID: 6438510]

13 Veatch RM. Who should manage care? The case for patients. *Kennedy Inst Ethics J.* 1997;7:391–401. [PMID: 11655372]

14 Beauchamp TL, Childress JF. *Principles of Biomedical Ethics.* 5th ed. New York: Oxford University Press; 2001.

15 Childress JF, Faden RR, Gaare RD, Gostin LO, Kahn J, Bonnie RJ, et al. Public health ethics: mapping the terrain. *J Law Med Ethics.* 2002;30:170–178. [PMID: 12066595]

16 Gostin L. Public health strategies for pandemic influenza: ethics and the law. *JAMA.* 2006;295:1700–1704. [PMID: 16609092]

17 Repine TB, Lisagor P, Cohen DJ. The dynamics and ethics of triage: rationing care in hard times. *Mil Med.* 2005;170:505–509. [PMID: 16001601]

18 Burkle FM Jr. Mass casualty management of a large-scale bioterrorist event: an epidemiological approach that shapes triage decisions. *Emerg Med Clin North Am.* 2002;20:409–436. [PMID: 12132490]

19 Egan TM, Kotloff RM. Pro/Con debate: lung allocation should be based on medical urgency and transplant survival and not on waiting time. *Chest.* 2005;128:407–415. [PMID: 16002964]

20 Gostin LO, Sapsin JW, Teret SP, Burris S, Mair JS, Hodge JG Jr, et al. The Model State Emergency Health Powers Act: planning for and response to bioterrorism and naturally occurring infectious diseases. *JAMA.* 2002;288:622–628. [PMID: 12150674]

21 Childress JF, ed. *Triage in Response to a Bioterrorist Attack.* Cambridge, MA: MIT Press; 2003.

22 Ferreira FL, Bota DP, Bross A, Mélot C, Vincent JL. Serial evaluation of the SOFA score to predict outcome in critically ill patients. *JAMA.* 2001;286:1754–1758. [PMID: 11594901]

23 Barnato AE, Angus DC. Value and role of intensive care unit outcome prediction models in end-of-life decision making. *Crit Care Clin.* 2004;20:345–362, vii–viii. [PMID: 15183207]

24 Justice AC, Covinsky KE, Berlin JA. Assessing the generalizability of prognostic information. *Ann Intern Med.* 1999;130:515–524. [PMID: 10075620]

25 Beigel JH, Farrar J, Han AM, Hayden FG, Hyer R, de Jong MD, et al. Writing Committee of the World Health Organization (WHO) Consultation on Human Influenza A/H5. Avian influenza A (H5N1) infection in humans. *N Engl J Med.* 2005;353:1374–1385. [PMID: 16192482]

26 Sanders D, Dukeminier J. Medical advance and legal lag: hemodialysis and kidney transplantation. *UCLA Law Rev.* 1968;15:366–380.

27 Rescher N. The allocation of exotic medical lifesaving therapy. *Ethics.* 1967:79;173–186.

28 Ramsey PG. *Patient as Person.* New Haven, CT: Yale University Press; 1970.

29 Childress JF. Who shall live when not all can live? *Soundings.* 1970;53:339–355.

30 Pesik N, Keim ME, Iserson KV. Terrorism and the ethics of emergency medical care. *Ann Emerg Med.* 2001;37:642–646. [PMID: 11385335]

31 Department of Health and Human Services. Draft Guidance on Allocating and Targeting Pandemic Influenza Vaccine. Washington, DC: U.S. Department of Health and Human Services; October 17, 2007. http://www.pandemicflu.gov/vaccine /prioritization.pdf. Accessed November 12, 2008.

32 Daniels N. Fair process in patient selection for antiretroviral treatment in WHO's goal of 3 by 5. *Lancet.* 2005;366:169–171. [PMID: 16005341]

33 Shortt SE. Waiting for medical care: is it who you know that counts? [Editorial]. *CMAJ.* 1999;161:823–824. [PMID: 10530299]

34 Emanuel EJ, Wertheimer A. Public health. Who should get influenza vaccine when not all can? *Science.* 2006;312:854–855. [PMID: 16690847]

35 Williams A. Intergenerational equity: an exploration of the "fair innings" argument. *Health Econ.* 1997;6:117–132. [PMID: 9158965]

36 Neuberger J, Adams D, MacMaster P, Maidment A, Speed M. Assessing priorities for allocation of donor liver grafts: survey of public and clinicians. *BMJ*. 1998;317:172–175. [PMID: 9665895]

37 Harris J. *The Value of Life*. London: Routledge and Kegan Paul; 1985.

38 Tanner L. Who should MDs let die in a pandemic? Report offers answers. *Washington Post*. May 5, 2008.

39 Daniels N. Accountability for reasonableness [Editorial]. *BMJ*. 2000;321:1300–1301. [PMID: 11090498]

40 Daniels N, Sabin J. Limits to health care: fair procedures, democratic deliberation, and the legitimacy problem for insurers. *Philos Public Aff*. 1997;26:303–350. [PMID: 11660435]

41 *Public Engagement Pilot Project on Pandemic Influenza: Citizen Voices on Pandemic Flu Choices*. Washington, DC: National Academies Press; 2005.

42 van den Bos K, Lind EA, Vermunt R, Wilke HA. How do I judge my outcome when I do not know the outcome of others? The psychology of the fair process effect. *J Pers Soc Psychol*. 1997;72:1034–1046. [PMID: 9150583]

43 Should we allow the creation of human/animal embryos? [news release]. London: Human Fertilisation and Embryonic Authority. April 26, 2007. http://www.hfea.gov.uk/en/1518.html. Accessed November 12, 2008.

About the Editors

JONATHAN OBERLANDER is Professor and Chair of Social Medicine in the School of Medicine and Professor of Health Policy and Management in the Gillings School of Global Public Health at the University of North Carolina at Chapel Hill.

MARA BUCHBINDER is Associate Professor of Social Medicine, Adjunct Associate Professor of Anthropology, and Core Faculty in the Center for Bioethics at the University of North Carolina at Chapel Hill.

LARRY R. CHURCHILL is Professor of Medical Ethics Emeritus at Vanderbilt University.

SUE E. ESTROFF is Professor of Social Medicine and Adjunct Professor of Anthropology and Psychiatry at the University of North Carolina at Chapel Hill.

NANCY M. P. KING is Professor in the Department of Social Sciences and Health Policy and the Wake Forest Institute for Regenerative Medicine at the Wake Forest School of Medicine, and Co-Director of the Center for Bioethics, Health and Society and Graduate Program in Bioethics at Wake Forest University.

BARRY F. SAUNDERS is Associate Professor of Social Medicine and holds adjunct appointments in the Departments of Anthropology, Religious Studies, and Communication Studies at the University of North Carolina at Chapel Hill.

RONALD P. STRAUSS is Executive Vice Provost and Chief International Officer, Dental Friends Distinguished Professor of Dental Ecology, and Professor of Social Medicine at the University of North Carolina at Chapel Hill.

REBECCA L. WALKER is Professor of Social Medicine, Core Faculty in the Center for Bioethics, and holds an adjunct appointment in the Department of Philosophy at the University of North Carolina at Chapel Hill.

Index